FIRST AID AND EMERGENCY CARE

James E. Aaron Ed.D

A. Frank Bridges H.S.D.

Dale O. Ritzel Ph.D

Larry B. Lindauer Ph.D

SOUTHERN ILLINOIS UNIVERSITY at Carbondale

FIRST AID AND EMERGENCY CARE PREVENTION AND PROTECTION OF INJURIES

Second Edition

Macmillan Publishing Co., Inc.
NEW YORK
Collier Macmillan Publishers
LONDON

Copyright © 1979, Macmillan Publishing Co., Inc.

Printed in the United States of America

All rights reserved. No part of this book may be reproduced or transmitted in any form or by any means, electronic or mechanical, including photocopying, recording, or any information storage and retrieval system, without permission in writing from the Publisher.

Earlier edition
copyright © 1972, Macmillan Publishing Co., Inc.

Macmillan Publishing Co., Inc.
866 Third Avenue, New York, New York 10022

Collier Macmillan Canada, Ltd.

Library of Congress Cataloging in Publication Data
Main entry under title:

First aid and emergency care.

   First ed. by J. E. Aaron published in 1972.
   Includes bibliographies and index.
   1. First aid in illness and injury.
2. Medical emergencies. I. Aaron, James E. First aid emergency care. II. Aaron, James E.
RC86.7.F56 1979   614.8'8   78-6134
ISBN 0-02-300060-0

Printing: 5 6 7 8   Year: 4 5

ISBN 0-02-300060-0

PREFACE

Never in the history of the nation has there been a time when the need for first-aid and emergency care training was more evident. Accidents kill over 100,000 Americans each year, and many thousands more are injured and disabled. With accidents the major cause of death among the age range 1 to 38 years, it bears stressing that one person in every family should be trained in first aid. An urgent need exists for trained first-aiders on the highway, at school, work, play, and in the home.

This book was written to serve primarily as a college-level first-aid textbook. However, the emphasis is such that the text can be used in first-aid training courses for police, nurses, civil defense workers, industrial employees, recreational leaders, and others. The teaching profession is one of the major groups for whom the book was intended. Even the family could use the book to great advantage.

One of the goals of the authors was to emphasize the role of the first-aider in *protection* rather than in treatment. While there are first-aid textbooks written by medical doctors or nurses, this is the first written by educators.

The material in this text is organized so that there is a logical progression from Chapter 1 through Chapter 25. However, each chapter can be taught as an independent unit of instruction. Part I deals with the accident problem, philosophy and principles of the safety movement, administrative procedures, and individual responsibility. Part II deals with the cursory examination of the victim and general first-aid problems such as wounds, shock, respiratory and cardiopulmonary resuscitation, body conditions resulting from extreme temperatures, poisons, and injuries to bones, joints, and muscles. In Part III there is a detailed discussion of psychological first-aid, animal bites and stings, poisonous plants, and special problems. Part IV is given over to a discussion of the various types of accident victims. The presentation includes victims of traffic, home, recreational, industrial, and school accidents. The final section, Part V, is primarily devoted to the practical application of first aid. Part V considers essential first-aid techniques, transportation of the injured, first-aid supplies, and the organization of emergency care services.

By definition, an accident is the unplanned event that causes death, injury, disability, or property damage. If people are to stay alive and enjoy living to the fullest, we must have a better organized society and eliminate hazards or learn to live with them.

First-aid courses are included in many college and university curricula. The teacher-training institution especially should offer such courses. It is recommended that teachers in the areas of safety, health, physical education, recreation, industrial education, home economics, and the sciences avail themselves of such training. If such training is not a requirement, then it is a most helpful elective. The college-level course should be structured so that the college-trained person will be qualified to instruct others in the community. It is important that the college course meet and surpass the American National Red Cross standards. College courses should be courses of record with the American National Red Cross.

The Highway Safety Standard, "Emergency Medical Services," published by the Department of Transportation, places a greater emphasis upon the training of first-aid personnel in all the states. First-aid courses at the college and university level can assist in accomplishing the objectives of this standard.

The two purposes of this textbook are accident prevention and protection of the injured in the event of an accident. It is an accepted fact that first-aid training helps to prevent or reduce the number of accidents. Industry has found that the first-aid-trained employee has fewer accidents and that first-aid training tends to develop a safety consciousness in the individual.

It is the role of the first-aider to protect, and this textbook has been written with this role in mind. The authors are hopeful that those students who use and study this book will gain some assurance and confidence in the practical application of first aid.

J. E. A.
A. F. B.
D. O. R.
L. B. L.

CONTENTS

Preface   v

PART I
INTRODUCTION—PRINCIPLES AND PHILOSOPHY

1 The Accident Problem   3

   Types of accidents—Accident causes

2 Safety: Philosophy and Movement   22

   The philosophy—Concept of safety—Emergency care—Organized safety movement—Organizations in the safety movement—Defining basic terms

3 Principles and Procedures in the Administration of Emergency Care   35

   Concept of protection—General first-aid principles—Records and accident-reporting system—Availability of trained personnel

4 Individual Responsibility and Legal Implications in Emergency Care   49

   Trends in personal liability—Basic definitions—Basis for liability—Scope of legal responsibility—Good Samaritan laws—Emergency care procedure

PART II
GENERAL EMERGENCY CARE PROBLEMS

5 Cursory Examination: Physical Check of the Injured   61

The accident itself—Hurry cases—The cursory examination—Additional problems to observe—Rules to follow after cursory check

6 Wounds   71

Open wounds—Closed wounds: contusions or bruises—Special wounds—Hemorrhage and bleeding—Use of the tourniquet—Infections

7 Shock   90

Traumatic shock—Psychological shock—Anaphylactic shock—Electric shock—Insufficient or excessive insulin supply

8 Respiratory and Cardiopulmonary Resuscitation (CPR)   103

The breathing system—Cardiovascular system—Respiratory arrest—Cardiac arrest—Other respiratory and cardiac arrest problems—Cardiopulmonary resuscitation (CPR)—Procedure for CPR—Infant CPR—Foreign body airway obstruction—Gastric distention—Chest-pressure arm-lift artificial ventilation method

9 Temperature Problems   130

Burns—Chemical burns—Major heat problems—Body temperature

10 Poisons   149

Prevention—Poison control centers—Noncorrosive poisoning—Corrosive poisoning—Petroleum products and distillate poisoning—Other cases of drug and chemical poisoning—Poisonous gases—Food poisoning

11 Bone, Joint, and Muscle Injuries   168

Broken bones or fractures—Sprains—Strains—Dislocations

PART III
SPECIFIC EMERGENCY CARE PROBLEMS

12 Psychological First Aid   187

Principles—Reactions to emergencies—General guidelines for psychological trauma—Suicidal tendencies

13 Poisonous Bites and Stings   196

Mammals—Reptiles—Arachnids—Insects

14 Poisonous Plants   214

Skin irritation plants—Oral poisoning plants

15 Special Problems   237

Unconsciousness—Apoplexy—Concussion—Convulsions—Epilepsy—Appendicitis—Fainting—Intoxication—Hernia—Hives—Emergency childbirth

16 Disaster Preparedness   254

The disaster shelter—The disaster volunteer—Emergency care training—Radiological monitors—Disaster supplies—Disaster warning signals

PART IV
TYPES OF EMERGENCY CARE VICTIMS

17 Traffic Accident Victims   265

Types of traffic collisions—Age of drivers—Causes of traffic collisions—Body part injured

18 Home Accident Victims   278

Types of home accidents—Causes of home accidents—Accidents among children—Accidents among adults—Farm home accidents

[x] Contents

19 Public Accident Victims 284

Types of public-recreational accidents—A special problem: epilepsy —Causes of public accidents

20 Industrial Accident Victims 294

Where accidents occur—Falls—Office accidents—Lifting—Cost of work accidents—Causes of industrial accidents—Part of body injured —Off-the-job injuries—Farm accidents

21 School Accident Victims 306

The elementary school—The secondary school—College and university accidents—Types of accidents—Accident reporting

PART V
PRACTICAL APPLICATIONS

22 Essential Techniques to Master: Bandaging and Splinting 319

Bandaging material—Bandaging techniques—Triangular bandage— Splinting—Splinting material—Types of splinting

23 Transportation for Protection 355

General precautions and directions—Methods of transportation— Transportation by vehicle—Transportation by air

24 First-Aid Supplies 374

Location and care of supplies—Home and farm—School—Motor vehicle—Recreation—Work or industry—Disaster shelter

25 Organizing Emergency Care Services 389

Need for organization—Highway Safety Program standards—The school—The police—Emergency crews—Disaster preparedness— Funeral directors—Industry—Evaluating emergency care needs— Medic alert—Ambulance design and equipment

Appendix—State-by-State EMS Survey 403

INDEX 413

PART I
INTRODUCTION: PRINCIPLES AND PHILOSOPHY

This first part contains four chapters which present the nature and scope of the accident and emergency care problems that need first-aid protection, the philosophy of the accident prevention movement, the principles of emergency care, and the legal implications.

Included in Part I are the following Chapters:

1. The Accident Problem
2. Safety: Philosophy and Movement
3. Principles and Procedures in the Administration of Emergency Care
4. Individual Responsibility and Legal Implications in Emergency Care

1. THE ACCIDENT PROBLEM

Accidents occur wherever there is human activity. They are as old as mankind. Throughout the world accidents cause millions of deaths each year. But because of inadequate worldwide reporting methods, the exact number of critical injuries and deaths is unknown.

Within the United States information regarding the nation's accident problem is more complete. In a recent year the National Safety Council [1] reported approximately 100,000 accidental deaths and 10.3 million accidental disabling injuries. Thus about one out of every 1,000 persons was killed as a result of an accident that year. Of the deaths, motor-vehicle crashes accounted for 46,700, home accidents 24,000, public accidents 21,500, and work accidents 12,500.[2] A current National Health Survey suggests that over 63 million persons are injured annually. This number includes the disabling injuries just mentioned. Over 40 million of the 63 million injured receive medical attention.[3]

An analysis of accident data reveals that accidents are the major cause of death of persons age 1 to 38 and the fourth leading cause of death for persons of all ages. Figure 1.1 compares accidental deaths with all other causes of death among the American populace.

Accidents cost the nation approximately $52.8 billion per annum. This figure encompasses wage losses, medical fees, insurance claims, property

---

[1] National Safety Council, *Accident Facts*. Chicago: The Council, 1977, pp. 1–96.

[2] Because some deaths are included in more than one accident classification, the four separate classifications total more than the national accident death figure of 100,000.

[3] U.S. Public Health Service, *Accidental Death and Injury Statistics*. Washington: U.S. Government Printing Office, Publ. No. 1111, 1963.

[3]

FIGURE 1.1 LEADING CAUSES OF ALL DEATHS IN THE UNITED STATES

	No. of Deaths	Death Rate*
ALL AGES	1,892,879	889
Heart disease	716,215	336
Cancer	365,693	172
Stroke	194,038	91
Accidents	**103,030**	**48**
Motor-vehicle	45,853	21
Falls	14,896	7
Drowning	8,000	4
Fires, burns	6,071	3
Other	28,210	13
UNDER 1 YEAR	50,525	1,641
Anoxia	12,577	408
Congenital anomalies	8,582	279
Complications of pregnancy and childbirth	6,344	206
Immaturity	4,398	143
Pneumonia	2,171	71
Accidents	**1,337**	**43**
Ingestion of food, object	360	12
Mech. suffocation	268	9
Motor-vehicle	255	8
Fires, burns	135	4
Falls	68	2
Other	251	8
1 TO 4 YEARS	9,060	71
Accidents	**3,611**	**28**
Motor-vehicle	1,321	10
Drowning	760	6
Fires, burns	617	5
Ingestion of food, object	144	1
Falls	129	1
Other	640	5
Congenital anomalies	1,141	9
Cancer	711	6
5 TO 14 YEARS	13,479	36
Accidents	**6,818**	**18**
Motor-vehicle	3,286	9
Drowning	1,300	3
Fires, burns	580	2
Other	1,652	4
Cancer	1,807	5
Congenital anomalies	742	2
15 TO 24 YEARS	47,545	119
Accidents	**24,121**	**60**
Motor-vehicle	15,672	39
Drowning	2,520	6
Poison (solid, liquid)	1,332	3
Firearms	758	2
Other	3,839	10
Homicide	5,493	14
Suicide	4,736	12

FIGURE 1.1 (continued)

	No. of Deaths	Death Rate*
25 TO 44 YEARS	104,732	196
Accidents	**22,877**	**43**
Motor-vehicle	11,969	22
Poison (solid, liquid)	1,853	4
Drowning	1,740	3
Fires, burns	961	2
Other	6,354	12
Cancer	16,645	31
Heart disease	14,922	28
45 TO 64 YEARS	450,066	1,034
Heart disease	160,384	368
Cancer	128,371	295
Stroke	25,789	59
Accidents	**19,643**	**45**
Motor-vehicle	7,663	18
Falls	2,449	6
Fires, burns	1,602	4
Drowning	1,120	2
Other	6,809	15
Cirrhosis of liver	18,235	42
Diabetes mellitus	8,238	19
65 TO 74 YEARS	442,496	3,189
Heart disease	183,667	1,324
Cancer	107,604	776
Stroke	42,056	303
Diabetes mellitus	10,432	75
Accidents	**9,220**	**66**
Motor-vehicle	3,047	22
Falls	2,148	15
Fires, burns	795	6
Surg. complications	785	6
Other	2,445	17
Pneumonia	8,915	64
Emphysema	7,127	51
75 YEARS AND OVER	774,976	9,087
Heart disease	355,004	4,163
Stroke	121,435	1,424
Cancer	107,725	1,263
Pneumonia	29,517	346
Arteriosclerosis	23,872	280
Accidents	**15,403**	**181**
Falls	8,510	100
Motor-vehicle	2,640	31
Surg. complications	976	12
Fires, burns	879	10
Ingestion of food, object	594	7
Other	1,804	21
Diabetes mellitus	14,865	174
Emphysema	6,722	79

* Deaths per 100,000 population in each age group. Rates are averages for age groups, not individual ages.
Source: Deaths are for 1975, latest official figures from National Center for Health Statistics, Health Services and Mental Health Administration, U.S. Department of Health, Education and Welfare.

[6] The Accident Problem

damage, and the money value of time lost by individuals who are either directly or indirectly involved in accidents.

The available accident information reveals that accidents are a major problem in the United States. Many safety education and accident prevention programs have been and are being implemented to help lessen the problem. However, accidents continue to plague people, and there is a continual need for first-aid and emergency care programs. These programs are designed to effectively prepare an individual to assist an injured person.

TYPES OF ACCIDENTS

In order to deal with the data of the accident problem, it has been helpful to classify accidents according to the places of occurrence or activity participated in by the individual. The National Safety Council organizes accident statistics into these major areas: motor-vehicle, work, home, and public. In this text another major area will be the school. The area of public accidents does not include those motor-vehicle and work accidents that happen in public places but does include recreational accidents such as boating, hunting, and swimming. Figure 1.2 shows the number of accidents in each state in the motor-vehicle, work, home and public classifications, while Figure 1.3 depicts the number of accidents by month and type.

Motor-Vehicle Accidents

The motor vehicle, a rather recent innovation in American society, has become a vital part of our way of life and has been involved in accidents responsible for over 2 million deaths since the early 1900s. In this country now, there are over 139.8 million licensed drivers driving over 142 million motor vehicles approximately 1,412 billion miles annually. These drivers are involved in more than 15.5 million motor-vehicle accidents each year, averaging about 1 accident for every 13 persons or 1 for every 7 drivers. In a recent yearly report, motor-vehicle crashes resulted in over 46,700 deaths, 2 million persons with injuries, and 15.6 million property damage accidents. It is possible that the foregoing statistics could be higher if all states used uniform accident reporting systems.

It is difficult to visualize the great loss of life and the vast number of injuries caused by traffic accidents; also many are not aware of the incurred economic loss. The cost of motor-vehicle collisions is computed to be over $24 billion annually. This amount will increase due to the rising medical and hospital costs, car repair costs, and vehicle insurance premiums.

According to the National Safety Council the motor-vehicle death rate (based upon the number of deaths per 100 million miles of travel) has been around 3.3 in recent years, dropping from a high of 12.0 in 1941.

The lowering of the motor-vehicle death rate must be credited to a number of accident countermeasures. Increased public interest in the safety of highway travel, the development of driver education programs, improved traffic law enforcement, the application of traffic engineering principles, the use of restraining devices, improved vehicle design, and the 55 mph speed law have assisted in lowering the traffic death rate.

An improved quality and a greater availability of emergency medical services are necessary to continue the lowering of the death rate among traffic victims. Primarily this requires improved transportation facilities of the injured and the wise use of first-aid and emergency care techniques.

Home Accidents

It seems difficult for some people to realize that accidents happen within the confines of their home and that each year the home is a major source of accidental death and injury. However, upon examination of the accident facts for a recent year it is noted that 24,000 accidental deaths occurred in the home, and during that same period of time 3.7 million disabling injuries happened there also. These totals represent both urban and farm homes. Thus, in the United States 1 person in 5.8 was disabled one or more days by injuries received in home accidents. Although these facts are staggering, a recent National Health Survey suggests that home injuries would be in excess of 20 million if all home accidents were reported.

Home accidents could be a financial drain upon a family. The national total cost of home accidents is reported to be approximately $6.3 billion per year, or $150 per year per family of four.

Figure 1.6 depicts the types of home accident deaths and injuries and their number as reported by the National Safety Council. It shows that the major cause of death in the home is falls, followed by fires, suffocation, poisoning, firearms, and poison gases. Home accidents are usually a problem of a nonschool-aged population, principally the very young and old.

Farm Home Accidents Today, the farm home is comparable in many aspects to the urban home, and accidents in each location are quite similar, but there are some differences. For example, the canning of vegetables, fruits, and other produce is still a common activity in farming communities. Farm chores, which by definition are household duties, subject the farm wife, husband, or child to various accident potentials. It is difficult to know the extent of farm home accidents because many are never reported. Many times farm injuries are neglected and medical attention never given to the injured person. Traditionally, farm families have learned to live with such problems. It is possible that new Occupational Safety and Health Administration (OSHA) regulations will require better data collection methods for farm accidents.

FIGURE 1.2 PRINCIPAL CLASSES OF ACCIDENTAL DEATHS BY STATES

State	TOTALS Deaths	TOTALS Rate*	Motor-Vehicle Deaths	Motor-Vehicle Rate*	Work Deaths	Work Rate*	Home Deaths	Home Rate*	Public Non-Motor-Vehicle Deaths	Public Non-Motor-Vehicle Rate*	Unclassified Deaths	Unclassified Rate*
Total U.S.	100,000	46.6	46,700	21.8	12,500	5.8	24,000	11.2	21,500	10.0	—	—
Alabama	2,201	60.1	1,112	30.3	105	2.9	414	11.3	293	8.0	277	7.6
Alaska	—	—	—	—	—	—	—	—	—	—	—	—
Arizona	1,427	62.9	775	34.1	64	2.8	281	12.4	310	13.7	21	0.9
Arkansas	—	—	—	—	—	—	—	—	—	—	—	—
California	—	—	—	—	—	—	—	—	—	—	—	—
Colorado	1,379	53.4	651	25.2	106	4.1	210	8.1	394	15.3	60	2.3
Connecticut	907	29.1	428	13.7	19	0.6	286	9.2	154	4.9	20	0.6
Delaware	201	34.5	116	19.9	2	0.3	48	8.2	35	6.0	0	0.0
Dist of Col.	226	32.2	74	10.5	13	1.9	105	15.0	31	4.4	9	1.3
Florida	4,153	49.3	2,086	24.8	—	—	—	—	—	—	—	—
Georgia	2,428	48.9	1,181	23.8	152	3.1	594	12.0	448	9.0	87	1.8
Hawaii	303	34.2	156	17.6	25	2.8	34	3.8	93	10.5	3	0.3
Idaho	570	68.6	295	35.5	58	7.0	83	10.0	130	15.6	4	0.5
Illinois	4,410	39.3	2,068	18.4	226	2.0	1,220	10.9	614	5.5	282	2.5
Indiana	2,747	51.8	1,449	27.3	135	2.5	605	11.4	539	10.2	19	0.4
Iowa	1,514	52.8	797	27.8	125	4.4	175	6.1	445	15.5	3	0.1
Kansas	1,192	51.6	574	24.8	117	5.1	261	11.3	231	10.0	41	1.8
Kentucky	1,782	52.0	872	25.4	192	5.6	268	7.8	249	7.3	244	7.1
Louisiana	2,320	60.4	1,004	26.1	152	4.0	338	8.8	419	10.9	407	10.6
Maine	523	48.9	244	22.8	37	3.5	133	12.4	112	10.5	8	0.7
Maryland	1,219	29.4	682	16.5	49	1.2	286	6.9	216	5.2	1	—
Massachusetts	—	—	—	—	—	—	—	—	—	—	—	—
Michigan	3,925	43.1	2,189	24.0	—	—	—	—	—	—	—	—
Minnesota	—	—	—	—	—	—	—	—	—	—	—	—
Mississippi	1,498	63.6	719	30.5	—	—	—	—	—	—	—	—

Missouri	2,338	48.9	1,177	24.6	105	2.2	431	9.0	617	12.9	8	0.2
Montana	593	78.8	308	40.9	71	9.4	101	13.4	140	18.6	10	1.3
Nebraska	789	50.8	398	25.6	91	5.9	122	7.9	194	12.5	5	0.3
Nevada	439	72.0	244	40.0	32	5.2	78	12.8	71	11.6	21	3.4
New Hampshire	290	35.3	149	18.1	20	2.4	69	8.4	53	6.4	0	0.0
New Jersey	2,451	33.4	1,050	14.3	79	1.1	568	7.7	407	5.5	347	4.7
New Mexico	991	84.8	572	49.0	60	5.1	130	11.1	257	22.0	5	0.4
New York	4,920	27.2	2,109	11.7	166	0.9	1,310	7.2	1,334	7.4	39	0.2
North Carolina	3,173	58.0	1,587	29.0	—	—	512	9.4	—	—	—	—
North Dakota	419	65.2	214	33.3	49	7.6	73	11.4	92	14.3	1	0.2
Ohio	4,033	37.7	1,864	17.4	102	1.0	902	8.4	1,143	10.7	22	0.2
Oklahoma	—	—	—	—	—	—	—	—	—	—	—	—
Oregon	1,282	55.0	670	28.8	89	3.8	230	9.9	259	11.1	63	2.7
Pa. (10 mos.)	3,769	38.1	1,708	17.3	196	2.0	1,197	12.1	366	3.7	323	3.3
Rhode Island	285	30.7	137	14.8	19	2.1	77	8.3	54	5.8	5	0.5
South Carolina	1,780	62.5	875	30.7	—	—	—	—	—	—	—	—
South Dakota	439	64.0	243	35.4	36	5.2	68	9.9	86	12.5	15	2.2
Tennessee	2,359	56.0	1,253	29.7	128	3.0	447	10.6	391	9.3	178	4.2
Texas	5,792	46.4	2,893	23.2	323	2.6	971	7.8	1,019	8.2	586	4.7
Utah	569	46.3	286	23.3	59	4.8	114	9.3	126	10.3	11	0.9
Vermont	189	39.7	89	18.7	18	3.8	32	6.7	48	10.1	2	0.4
Virginia	2,437	48.4	1,058	21.0	186	3.7	546	10.9	678	13.5	33	0.7
Washington	1,824	50.5	878	24.3	149	4.1	369	10.2	479	13.3	8	0.2
W. Va. (8 mos.)	682	56.2	318	26.2	76	6.3	112	9.2	185	15.2	8	0.7
Wisconsin	2,003	43.5	960	20.8	129	2.8	438	9.5	427	9.3	79	1.7
Wyoming	425	109.0	259	66.4	57	14.6	49	12.6	87	22.3	1	0.3
P. R. (11 mos.)	847	31.3	474	17.5	40	1.5	128	4.7	199	7.4	6	0.2
Virgin Islands	64	77.5	8	9.7	4	4.8	6	7.3	49	59.3	0	0.0

Source: Provisional reports of vital statistics registrars; deaths are by place of occurrence. U.S. totals are National Safety Council estimates.
* Deaths per 100,000 population, adjusted to annual basis where less than 12 months reported.

[9]

FIGURE 1.3   ACCIDENTAL DEATHS BY MONTH AND TYPE

Month	1976 Totals	All Types	Motor-Vehicle	Falls	Drown-ing †	Fires, Burns *	Ingest. of Food, Object	Fire-arms	Poison (solid, liquid)	Poison by Gas
All Months	100,000	103,030	45,853	14,896	8,000	6,071	3,106	2,380	4,694	1,577
January	7,800	8,162	3,191	1,442	260	745	290	237	368	237
February	7,250	7,306	2,949	1,253	250	651	272	167	366	203
March	8,100	8,124	3,405	1,244	400	685	276	185	451	157
April	7,900	7,870	3,412	1,145	480	645	262	176	382	108
May	8,850	9,387	4,145	1,255	1,200	419	243	162	407	100
June	9,100	9,556	4,190	1,198	1,430	343	235	165	416	73
July	9,950	10,093	4,437	1,302	1,590	286	243	158	444	62
August	9,000	9,620	4,460	1,234	1,120	280	270	190	391	61
September	8,100	8,285	4,059	1,184	490	325	223	177	375	109
October	8,200	8,433	4,016	1,336	320	440	240	236	394	91
November	7,750	8,160	3,896	1,096	270	525	284	311	351	173
December	8,000	8,034	3,693	1,207	190	727	268	216	349	203
Average	8,330	8,586	3,821	1,241	667	506	259	198	391	131

1975 Details by Type

Source: National Center for Health Statistics and National Safety Council.
* Includes deaths resulting from conflagration regardless of nature of injury.
† Includes drowning in water transport accidents. Some totals partly estimated.

Types of Accidents [11]

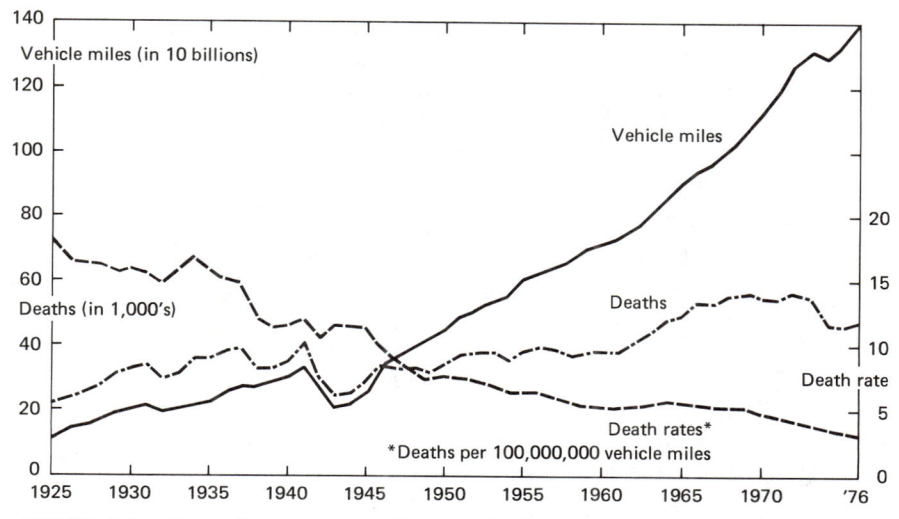

FIGURE 1.4 The traffic situation in the United States. (National Safety Council)

Public Accidents

There are various types of accidents that come under this classification. They are identified as either transportation or nontransportation. The collection of information in this classification is difficult, especially the recreational accidents. Yet the National Safety Council reported approximately 15,000 public accidents resulting in death during a recent year. Thus, in these accidents 1 person is killed about every 26 minutes, while some 500 are injured during the same time period. Figure 1.7 shows the number of deaths resulting from public accidents in recent years.

Public accidents result from a variety of occurrences related to buildings, transportation, and recreational activities. Falls are the first and drownings are the second most common type of public nontransportation deaths. Concerning public accidents, for the under 25 age group, drowning is the most frequent cause of death, and firearm accidents are a major cause of death and on the increase at this time. For the senior citizen falls are the most frequent cause of death and injury. Railroad accidents are one type of public accidents that have decreased in number in recent years. This may be due to the use of fewer trains, improved safety programs, and elimination of railroad crossings.

An encouraging fact is that the number of public accidental deaths has remained stable in recent years. Perhaps this is a result of the improved use of public transportation and the development of public safety education programs by the U.S. Coast Guard, National Rifle Association, and American National Red Cross.

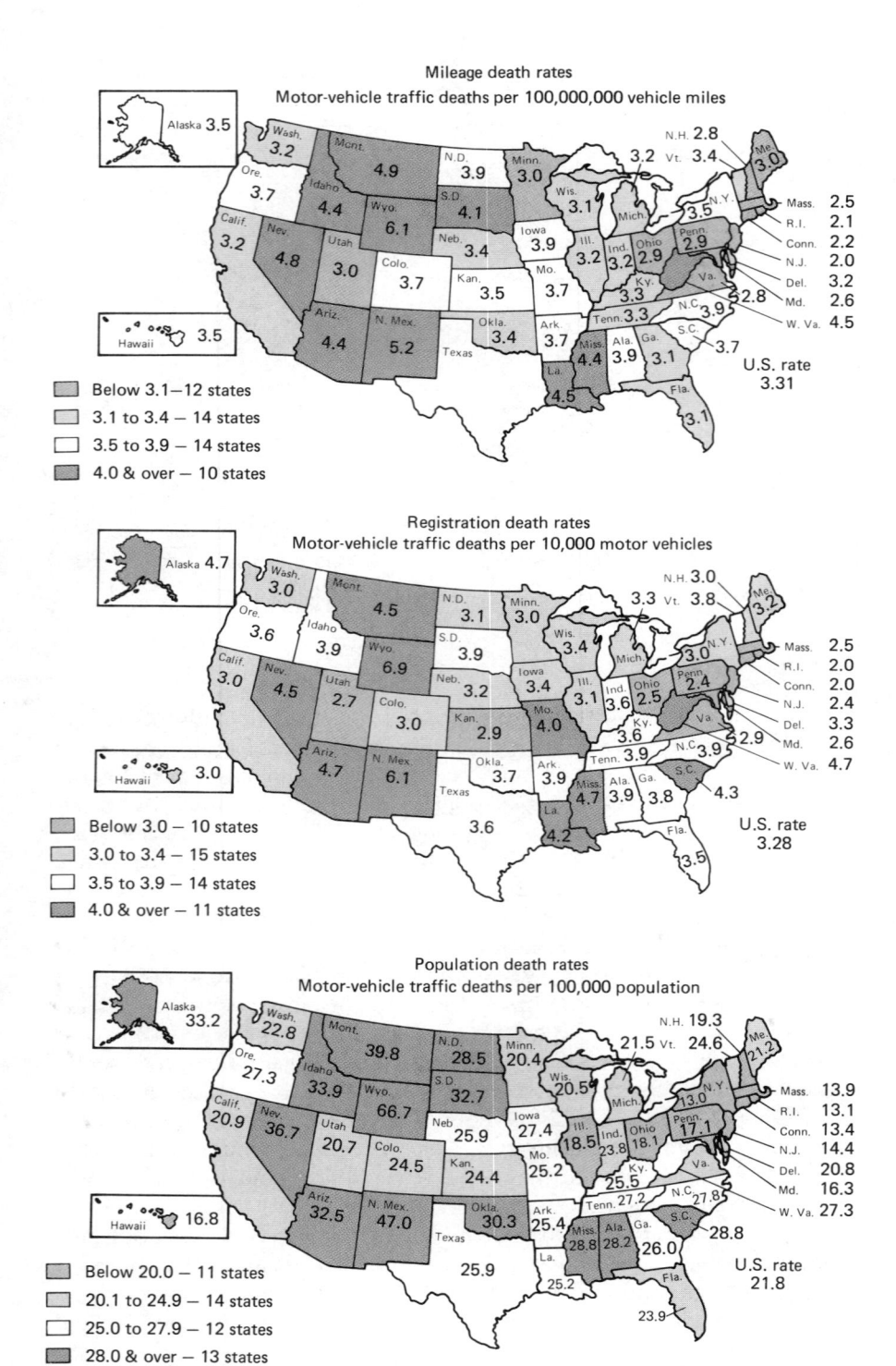

FIGURE 1.5 Motor vehicle death rates by states. (National Safety Council)

[12]

Types of Accidents [13]

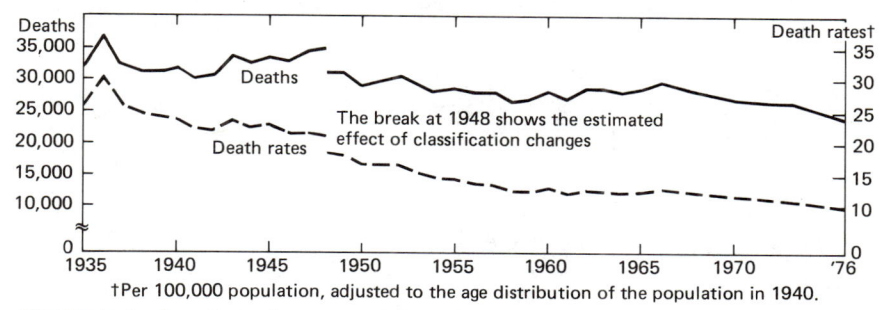

FIGURE 1.6 Trends in home accidental deaths and death rates. (National Safety Council)

Work Accidents — *lowest*

Approximately 12,500 persons are killed and 2.2 million sustain disabling injuries annually in work accidents. Thus, there were fewer deaths caused by work accidents than public, home, or motor-vehicle accidents. Both the frequency and severity rates have been lowered by about 50 percent during the past 35 years. Certainly significant progress has been made in the industrial community in the implementation of accident reduction programs. Federal and state laws have been the foundations of much of what has been accomplished in the lowering of frequency and severity of industrial accidents. However, the organized safety movement has been the most important factor in this progress to date. It has been demonstrated that industries with safety programs have fewer accidents than those with no programs. The passage of the Occupational Safety and Health Act has also had a serious impact upon the curtailing of work accidents.

Prevention of financial loss is a motivating force behind the development of safety programs in industry. Industries have a primary interest in reducing economic costs of accidents in their production processes.[4] The time lost due to work injuries amounted to about 2.45 million mandays annually. Compensation paid to injured workers during a recent year exceeded $6.52 billion. Of the total cost some $7.9 billion were visible costs (loss of wages, administration costs, medical costs), whereas $7.9 billion were indirect costs (money value of time lost and investigation and reporting time). There were approximately $2 billion accountable to fire losses. Basically it cost industry about $200.00 per injured man.

Off-Job Accidents Accidents to workers on the job have been steadily decreasing since World War II. However, off-the-job accidents have been on the increase and are a source of much concern to industry management.

[4] M. K. Strasser et al., *Fundamentals of Safety Education*. New York: Macmillan, 1973, p. 17.

FIGURE 1.7 TOTAL PUBLIC DEATHS, 1975 (Excluding motor vehicle and persons at work)

Year	Total Public	Transport Total	Air	Water Drowning	Water Other	Rail	Nontransport Total	Falls	Drowning	Firearms	Fires, Burns
1950	15,000	3,950	1,050	1,000	100	1,450	11,050	2,750	3,750	1,150	500
1952	16,000	3,900	1,350	900	150	1,200	12,100	2,900	4,450	1,200	500
1954	15,500	3,650	1,300	1,000	150	950	11,850	3,150	4,300	1,050	450
1956	16,000	3,450	1,200	1,050	100	900	12,550	3,700	4,100	1,000	450
1958	16,500	3,400	1,150	1,150	100	800	13,100	3,600	4,300	1,000	750
1960	17,000	3,150	1,150	1,000	100	700	13,850	3,700	4,350	1,100	750
1961	16,500	3,050	1,050	1,000	100	700	13,450	3,600	4,300	1,000	700
1962	17,000	3,100	1,100	1,000	100	700	13,900	3,900	4,200	1,000	750
1963	17,500	2,900	1,000	1,000	100	600	14,600	4,300	4,100	1,000	800
1964	18,500	3,200	1,200	1,000	100	700	15,300	4,800	4,400	900	800
1965	19,500	3,200	1,200	1,000	100	700	16,300	5,300	4,400	900	800
1966	20,000	3,300	1,200	1,100	100	700	16,700	5,400	4,600	1,000	800
1967	20,500	3,400	1,400	1,000	100	700	17,100	5,500	4,600	1,100	800
1968	21,500	3,500	1,500	1,100	100	600	18,000	5,400	4,800	900	700
1969	22,500	3,600	1,400	1,300	100	600	18,900	5,100	5,000	800	700
1970	23,500	3,300	1,200	1,200	100	600	20,200	5,000	5,200	900	700
1971	23,500	3,100	1,200	1,100	100	500	20,400	5,100	4,800	900	700
1972	23,500	3,200	1,200	1,200	100	500	20,300	5,100	4,900	900	700
1973	24,500	3,400	1,200	1,300	100	600	20,100	5,000	5,700	1,000	700
1974	23,000	3,200	1,200	1,200	100	500	19,800	5,000	5,100	900	600
1975	23,000	3,000	1,100	1,200	100	400	20,000	4,800	5,200	900	600
1976	21,500	2,800	1,000	1,100	100	400	18,700	4,600	4,500	900	600

Source: National Safety Council.

Types of Accidents [15]

FIGURE 1.8 TRENDS IN ON-JOB AND OFF-JOB DEATHS AND INJURIES

	Deaths					Injuries		
	On-Job		Off-Job		Ratio			Ratio
Year	No.	Rate*	No.	Rate*	Off./On	On-Job	Off-Job	Off/On
1945	16,500	33	30,000	60	1.82	2,000,000	2,750,000	1.38
1950	15,500	27	31,500	56	2.03	1,950,000	2,500,000	1.28
1955	14,200	24	31,300	53	2.20	1,950,000	2,400,000	1.23
1956	14,300	23	31,700	52	2.22	1,950,000	2,500,000	1.28
1957	14,200	23	31,700	52	2.23	1,900,000	2,450,000	1.29
1958	13,300	22	29,000	48	2.18	1,800,000	2,250,000	1.25
1959	13,800	23	29,000	47	2.10	1,950,000	2,200,000	1.13
1960	13,800	22	29,200	47	2.12	1,950,000	2,250,000	1.15
1961	13,500	21	28,900	45	2.14	1,950,000	2,200,000	1.16
1962	13,700	21	30,000	46	2.19	2,000,000	2,250,000	1.13
1963	14,200	21	31,700	48	2.23	2,000,000	2,350,000	1.18
1964	14,200	21	34,600	51	2.44	2,050,000	2,500,000	1.22
1965	14,100	20	36,500	52	2.59	2,100,000	2,700,000	1.29
1966	14,500	20	39,600	55	2.73	2,200,000	2,900,000	1.32
1967	14,200	19	40,000	54	2.82	2,200,000	3,000,000	1.36
1968	14,300	19	41,900	54	2.93	2,200,000	3,100,000	1.41
1969	14,300	18	43,300	55	3.03	2,200,000	3,200,000	1.45
1970	13,800	17	43,700	55	3.17	2,200,000	3,250,000	1.48
1971	13,700	17	41,500	52	3.03	2,300,000	3,200,000	1.39
1972	14,000	17	42,500	52	3.04	2,400,000	3,200,000	1.33
1973	14,300	17	43,700	51	3.06	2,500,000	3,300,000	1.32
1974	13,500	16	39,400	45	2.92	2,300,000	3,200,000	1.39
1975	13,000	15	37,800	44	2.91	2,200,000	3,200,000	1.45
1976	12,500	14	38,200	44	3.06	2,200,000	3,100,000	1.41
Change 1945-76	—24%	—58%	+27%	—27%	+68%	+10%	+13%	+20%

Source: National Safety Council.
* Deaths per 100,000 workers.

Management is devoting a great deal of time to the development of off-the-job safety programs. Figure 1.8 shows the relationship between on- and off-the-job deaths and injuries for one year.

School Accidents

Accidents, the primary cause of death and disability of school age youth, are a major concern of the people of all the nation's schools—elementary, secondary, and college. Accidents claim more lives of children 1 through 14 years of age than the six leading diseases combined and claim more lives of youth 15 through 24 years old than all other causes.

Studies show that there are numerous schools housing thousands of students in areas that have little medical assistance to offer in time of need.

[16]   The Accident Problem

In some of our wealthiest states there are rural counties without hospitals and with only one or two medical doctors to cover many square miles and a great many people. This is one of the major social and health problems facing this nation. How long does it take to get medical help when it is needed? This is a question that each school should consider as emergency care plans are developed.

Elementary Schools   Children in the elementary school are involved in a great number of accidents on the playground and upon play apparatus. About three fourths of such accidents occur on the school grounds. Boys and girls in the elementary grades are also involved in numerous accidents in classrooms, in auditoriums, on steps, and as pedestrians going to and from school. Because of the differences in the accident experiences of boys and girls, accident information is summarized according to sex by the National Safety Council. Figures 21.2 and 21.3 show their total accident experience for a recent year.

Senior and Junior High Schools   Accidents involving junior and senior high school youth occur mainly in physical education classes. Apparatus incidents rank very high in this age group, as do accidents related to interscholastic sports. Many accidents take place in the industrial arts classes also.

Colleges and Universities   The American College Health Association reports that students sustain injuries as a result of a variety of accident experiences. Principal causes relate to recreational, residence, and building incidents. A more complete summary of the accident experience of college-age youth is presented in Chapter 21.

Suicide and Homicide

Today some deaths are classified as accidental when in fact they are murders and suicides. Deaths by violence are inadequately investigated in many parts of the nation. Therefore, it is extremely difficult to ascertain the extent to which such occurrences are misclassified. Some motor-vehicle accidents are suicides, but without thorough examination of the events leading up to the collisions, they are reported as single vehicle accidents. Police officers and emergency rescue squads should be trained to determine whether such events are accidental, suicide, or homicide.

ACCIDENT CAUSES

To understand the dimensions of the accident problem, knowledge as to "why people have accidents" is necessary. The answer to the question stated is not always found. Very often a reported accident cause is nothing more than a description of the physical evidence left as a result of the accident event. Because of the advancement of evaluation and research work in accident prevention, an effort is made now to determine the basic cause of an accident.

Fundamental accident causes are usually classified into two categories: (1) unsafe behavior or human failure and (2) unsafe environment. It is important to note that some scientists are classifying accidents medically by the type of physical and chemical energy released to cause the incident. This concept will be discussed later in the chapter.

Unsafe Behavior

Human failure is considered by many persons to be the primary cause of accidents. Car, industrial, home, and school injuries are many times the result of an individual's unsafe behavior patterns. These patterns of behavior that lead to accident-producing events are observed in children, junior and senior high school youths as well as adults. Unsafe behavior may be the result of a single factor or may result from a series or a combination of factors.

Attitudes The attitude of a person is usually thought of as being the most important cause of why people have accidents. A positive attitude, or the wanting to do something correctly in a socially acceptable manner, is ordinarily a sound approach for a person to use for self-preservation. Evidence today suggests a close correlation between a person's adjustment to his environment and his attitudes toward safe performance.

Physical Limitations A number of accidents occur each year because a person attempts to perform a task that is beyond his physical capabilities. Individuals with health problems should endeavor to match their ability to perform with the job or task attempted. An annual health examination should help a person understand any condition that might cause him to become involved in an accident.

Habits It is necessary for a person to learn correct habits in the performance of various tasks if he is to carry out these tasks safely. Suitable habits usually lead to correct responses, whereas improper habits lead to accidents. Therefore it is important that correct habits be established initially for safe performance.

Skill The performance of a task without the required skill may result in an accident. Skills and task requirements should be compatible for safe performance. People should understand this formula and strive to develop themselves in order to perform to the best of their abilities.

Knowledge To avoid accidents an understanding and knowledge of a task to be accomplished are necessary. Not recognizing the hazards in-

[18] The Accident Problem

volved in a particular task can lead to an accident. A basic knowledge of traffic, recreational, home, school, or industrial activities is essential for a person to live safely in the world of today.

Unsafe Environment

More and more accidents are said to be products of an unsafe environment. Highways, school plants, industrial facilities, farm machinery, and numerous pieces of equipment present a great many hazardous situations in today's society. Depending upon existing conditions and the equipment being used, approximately 15 to 20 percent of today's accident problems are related to an unsafe environment. There are those suggesting that as more research is conducted on the relationship between environment and accidents, a larger percentage of the total accident problem will be shown to be the result of an unsafe environment.

Equipment and Machines Equipment and machines became an integral part of the American way of life with the expansion of the Industrial Revolution. Hazards accompanied these innovations, and without proper safeguards and operation these machines and equipment are the sources of numerous accidents. Since the inception of these modern devices accident prevention safeguards have been introduced and are assisting in the control of these types of accidents. Protective equipment, such as hard hats, safety glasses, machine guards, and seat belts, is now in common use across the nation.

Specific pieces of equipment or a particular machine is intended to do certain tasks. When they are taxed beyond their limitations a hazardous situation exists. A child riding a bicycle too large for him, the sportsman overloading a boat, and a worker using the wrong tool are examples of the misuse of equipment.

Conditions A disorganized or cluttered environment is a conducive setting for an accident occurrence. Conditions such as this lead to many accidents. Such accidents can be said to be the result of a disorganized way of life. Engineering techniques to improve order and flow are being used extensively in schools, in industries, on highways, and on waterways in an effort to eliminate conditions that may cause accidents. Overall, conditions that bespeak orderliness are a sound accident prevention measure.

Energy Cause Theory

A recent approach to explaining accident causes suggests that it is more accurate to use injury description plus the physical and chemical agents released as a basis for determining cause. Haddon states that "it is convenient to regard all physical and chemical injuries, whether unexpectedly or deliberately initiated, as belonging to one of two classes."[5]

The first class includes injuries where damage is caused by the delivery to the body of an amount of energy in excess of the corresponding local or whole-body injury thresholds, whereas class two includes injuries caused by interference with normal whole-body or local energy exchange. This approach states that each injury sustained is specific and usually cannot be produced in another manner. Thus the problem in the curtailment of physical and chemical injuries is the prevention of such abnormal energy exchanges. Figures 1.9 and 1.10 outline this concept and cite examples of injuries in these two classes.

ACTIVITIES

1. Visit a local hospital and make an analysis of the emergency accident cases admitted for a one-week period.
2. Develop a term paper on the subject "Accidents Are a Major Problem Among Schoolchildren."
3. With two classmates organize and present a panel discussion on the topic "Attitudes Are a Major Cause of Accidents."
4. Develop a series of posters depicting the major types of accidents occurring in the United States during a typical year.
5. Analyze the accident experience of a local school or industry. Prepare a report to be given to the instructor.

QUESTIONS TO ANSWER

1. Briefly discuss the dimensions of the nation's accident problem.
2. Identify the major types of accidents as classified by the National Safety Council.
3. Discuss the statement "today there is a need for extensive programs of first aid and emergency care."
4. What are the two basic causes of accidents?
5. How do habits influence a person's accident experience?
6. Why should accidents be a concern of elementary and secondary schools?
7. Loss prevention is a primary force behind the development of accident prevention programs in industry. Explain the motivation behind such programs.

[5] D. W. Clark and B. MacMahon (eds.), *Preventive Medicine.* Boston: Little, Brown, 1967, p. 592.

FIGURE 1.9 ILLUSTRATIONS OF CLASS I INJURIES CAUSED BY DELIVERY OF ENERGY IN EXCESS OF LOCAL OR WHOLE-BODY INJURY THRESHOLDS

Type of energy delivered	Primary injury produced	Examples and comments
Mechanical	Displacement, tearing, breaking, and crushing, predominantly at tissue and organ levels of body organization	Injuries resulting from the impact of moving objects such as bullets, hypodermic needles, knives, and falling objects; and from the impact of the moving body with relatively stationary structures as in falls and plane and auto crashes. The specific result depends on the location and manner in which the resultant forces are exerted. The majority of injuries is in this group.
Thermal	Inflammation, coagulation, charring, and incineration at all levels of body organization	First-, second-, and third-degree burns. The specific result depends on the location and manner in which the energy is dissipated
Electrical	Interference with neuro-muscular function and coagulation, charring, and incineration at all levels of body organization	Electrocution, burns. Interference with neural function as in electroshock therapy. The specific result depends on the location and manner in which the energy is dissipated.
Ionizing radiation	Disruption of cellular and subcellular components and function	Reactor accidents, therapeutic and diagnostic irradiation, misuse of isotopes, effects of fallout. The specific result depends on the location and manner in which the energy is dissipated.
Chemical	Generally specific for each substance or group	Includes injuries due to animal and plant toxins, chemical burns, as from KOH, Br_2, F_2 and H_2SO_4, and the less gross and highly varied injuries produced by most elements and components when given in sufficient dose.

Source: D. W. Clark and B. MacMahon, *Preventive Medicine*, Boston, 1967. (Courtesy Little, Brown and Company)

[20]

FIGURE 1.10 ILLUSTRATIONS OF CLASS II INJURIES CAUSED BY INTERFERENCE WITH NORMAL LOCAL OR WHOLE-BODY ENERGY EXCHANGE

Type of energy exchange interfered with	Types of injury or derangement produced	Examples and comments
Oxygen utilization	Physiological impairment, tissue or whole-body death	Whole-body: suffocation by mechanical means. For example, by drowning, strangulation, and CO and HCN poisoning. Local: "vascular accidents." These also involve more than mere O_2 deprivation, since waste and nutrient exchange are also blocked.
Thermal	Physiological impairment, tissue or whole-body death	Injuries resulting from failure of body thermoregulation; frostbite; and death by freezing

Source: D. W. Clark and B. MacMahon, *Preventive Medicine*, Boston, 1967. (Courtesy Little, Brown and Company)

8   What are the first and second most common types of public non-transportation deaths?
9   Why are traffic accidents an economic drain upon the American public?
10 Briefly discuss the need for improved emergency medical services.

SELECTED REFERENCES

CLARK, D. W., and MACMAHON, B. (eds.), *Preventive Medicine*. Boston: Little, Brown, 1967, p. 592.

HAFEN, BRENT Q., and PETERSON, BRENDA, *First Aid For Health Emergencies*. St. Paul, Minn.: West Publishing Co., 1977.

HALSEY, MAXWELL N., *Accident Prevention*. New York: McGraw-Hill, 1961.

HEINRICH, H. W., *Industrial Accident Prevention*. New York: McGraw-Hill, 1960.

NATIONAL SAFETY COUNCIL, *Accident Facts*. Chicago: The Council, 1977.

STACK, HERBERT J., and ELKOW, J. DUKE, *Education for Safe Living*. Englewood Cliffs, N.J.: Prentice-Hall, 1966.

STRASSER, M. K., et al., *Fundamentals of Safety Education*. New York: Macmillan, 1973.

U.S. DEPARTMENT OF TRANSPORTATION, *Highway Safety Program Standards*. Washington, D.C.: National Highway Safety Bureau, December, 1968, pp. 18–19.

U.S. PUBLIC HEALTH SERVICE, *Accidental Death and Injury Statistics*. Washington, D.C.: U.S. Government Printing Office, Publication No. 1111, 1963.

2. SAFETY: PHILOSOPHY AND MOVEMENT

The desires to survive and to seek adventure have been basic human characteristics since the beginning of mankind. The thrill of the chase, hunting the wild beast, exploring uncharted waters, playing in a game with competing individuals, and searching outer space are examples of activities that have captured the imagination, interest, and time of countless persons throughout the years. People feel a need to do these things, and thus it is generally accepted that living is experiencing the unknown and entails adventure. However, people can participate in such activities without undue concern if the risks are recognized and appropriate measures are taken to eliminate or compensate for the hazards.

THE PHILOSOPHY

Every person has his own philosophy of life, which "is the integration of all the acquired knowledge and experiences into a pattern of human behavior."[1] Each person chooses what knowledge and experiences he wants and makes them a part of his personal behavior. Literally, philosophy is the love of wisdom. According to Webster's definition, philosophy, in actual usage today, is the science that investigates the facts and principles of reality and of human nature and conduct.

No one person seems able to absorb all of this world's knowledge, and thus all knowledge cannot be integrated into the life of any one person. Neither can one person hope to contribute much to the clarification of

---

[1] M. K. Strasser et al., *Fundamentals of Safety Education*. New York: Macmillan, 1973, p. 63.

ideas in a particular field of study if he is not a student in that field; one cannot hope to contribute much to the clarification of ideas in mathematics who is not himself a mathematician. Thus it seems inevitable that a number of philosophical disciplines should evolve corresponding to the various areas of study whose concepts need investigation.

In the past couple of centuries, mostly in this century, safety has been one of those areas of study and people began to hear of its philosophy. "In the field of safety, philosophy makes us aware of certain needs or shortcomings while science shows us how to remedy or overcome these needs." [2]

CONCEPT OF SAFETY

Perhaps a philosophy of safety as it is known today is relatively new compared to the centuries man has lived on this earth. But it has been developing over the centuries just as man has developed. The early man who avoided accidents lived longer, reproduced, and taught his children. He began to realize and understand that he lived to tell of certain experiences while others did not. The conclusion was that he avoided or eliminated certain aspects of some experiences that allowed him to live longer. Man of every century has had a love of wisdom and has used it to survive and progress. Man continued to learn about what experiences or aspects of an experience to avoid. Today the aspects of experiences that are found unsafe are referred to as hazards.

Many people of today, as did some in times past, find it difficult to determine the hazards and some choose to ignore them. However, to live and experience a full life, man must integrate safety into his human behavior. Thus, the prevention of accidents involves changing human behavior to eliminate or avoid the hazards.

Prevention of accidents also involves changing the physical environment so accidents will not occur or at least will decrease in number; and severity may be much less as a result of changes in physical environment and human behavior.

Positive Nature of Safety

Safety makes it possible for a person to expand the number of good adventures experienced during a lifetime. In a modern society the consideration must be safety for increased efficiency in day-to-day living and safety for an ordered world. Safety should contribute to the positive fulfillment of an adventure or experience. This applies to experiences at home, work, school, on the highway, and in recreational activities.

[2] Herbert J. Stack and J. Duke Elkow, *Education for Safe Living*. Englewood Cliffs, N.J.: Prentice-Hall, 1966, p. 14.

[24]   Safety: Philosophy and Movement

Safety should be a positive concept rather than a negative one. It is better to perform safely and think on the pleasant times ahead than to think on what has been escaped. For example, a person should learn to water ski in a safe manner and ski safely at all times in order to enjoy another day of skiing or some other future adventure. Also, in cutting a piece of meat, a person should cut it correctly with the knife going away from any body part. He should think of the pleasure of eating the meat or some activity that can be accomplished as a result of the nourishment provided rather than dwell on the thought that he has escaped without a cut.

Safety should not be thought of as a list of don'ts but rather as a list of do's performed in a safe manner. The old idea of "safety first" is a negative concept which would keep man from doing many things. Life would be very uninteresting and uneventful. If safety were put first before everything, in a sense, people could become slaves to anything and everything that threatened to endanger their lives. People should do what is to be done, but do it safely.

Risk Acceptance

Certain risks are essential if a highly industrialized society is to continue. There are many risks in the fields of medicine, industry, and technology. However, to overcome the risks and to experience safe adventures, persons must recognize the potential hazards and dispose of or learn how to live with them. "Life at its best is taking risks for the things worthwhile. The good life is adventuring in the creation of values. Safety has a rightful place when no greater value is at stake for which a risk should be taken." [3]

Safety for the Betterment of Society

It is not easy to determine what risks should be made. Science sometimes finds some products and innovations harmful after they have been in use, though their use has been beneficial to man in some ways. Our ecology movement today is related to this idea. Farmers use commercial fertilizers and insecticides in order to produce more food. This food is not as healthy for people as food grown without commercial fertilizer, and the insecticides can be harmful. However, it would be disastrous if there were not enough food for our people. Sometimes the removal of a hazard can create more or greater hazards. Man has the responsibility to control innovations for the betterment and enrichment of life.

It is essential to try to teach and influence all people to incorporate safety into their philosophy of life so that their lives and the lives of others

[3] Ibid., p. 17.

are not endangered. An unsafe act on the part of one person can destroy or injure many, even safe-minded, strong, intelligent individuals. When accidents are caused by another person, the accident is no respecter of others.

Safety education helps people to plan their activities to avoid or eliminate hazards. People will react involuntarily to immediate danger or hazards, but they must learn to plan voluntarily against these in order to ensure safe living.

People should teach the correct way to do something rather than teach by saying, "Do it this way because it is safer." In most all activities the correct way is determined by its safeness. The safe way is accepted as the correct way as long as it is good for society and the individual.

Safety Objectives

Often a philosophy is expressed in terms of planned objectives. Four safety objectives that follow express the contribution that safety can make in developing in people an awareness of the twentieth century and in helping to equip people with appropriate accident prevention methods to overcome the hazards: [4]

1. Develop an awareness of the scope and nature of the accident problem.
2. Promote research and evaluation to gain greater understanding of the scope and nature of the problem, and develop methods of accident prevention.
3. Develop safe attitudes which will promote accident prevention in both old and new activities.
4. Integrate safety and accident prevention into the value structure and personal philosophy of each member of society.

EMERGENCY CARE

Emergency care is protecting an emergency incident victim and keeping him safe from further injury, from shock, from another accident. In putting emergency care in this perspective it seems it can be called a concept of safety. Certainly there is a need to teach emergency care in schools, industry, etc., along with accident prevention.

The Need

During the past fifty years the number of accidental deaths has risen from 72,400 to around 100,000, annually. A National Health Survey reports that over 63 million persons are injured each year.[5] A problem

---
[4] Strasser et al., op. cit., p. 68.
[5] National Safety Council, *Accident Facts*. Chicago: The Council, 1977, p. 2.

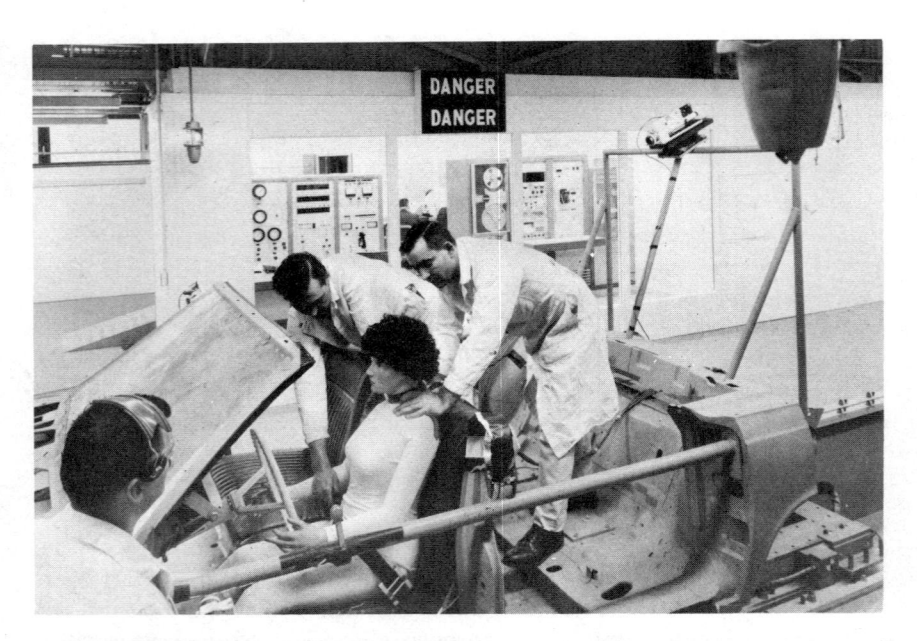

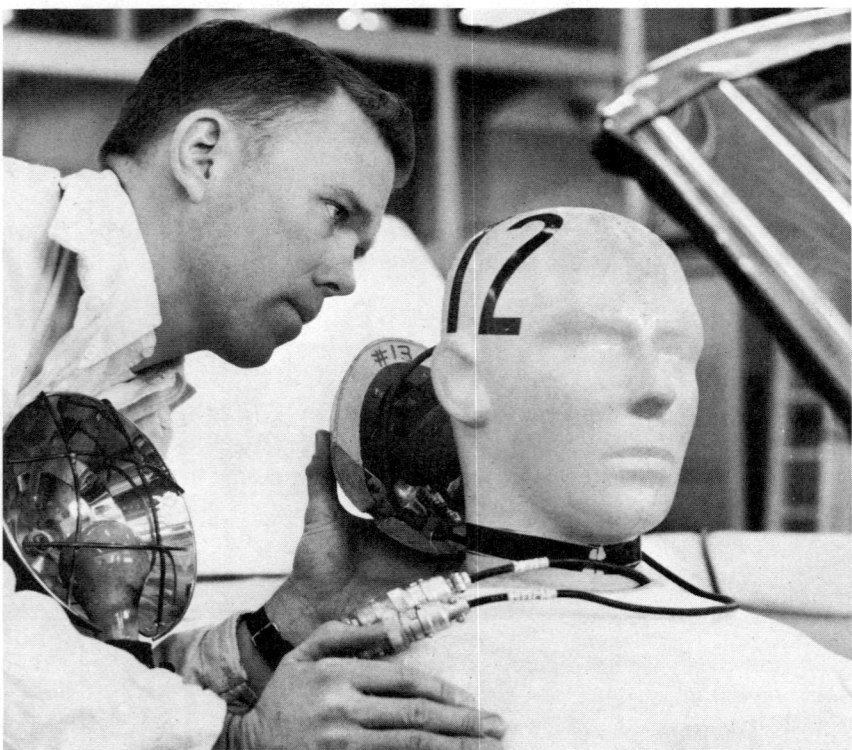

FIGURE 2.1 Research provides a greater understanding of the nation's traffic accident problem. (Ford Motor Company, Public Relations, Engineering Staff)

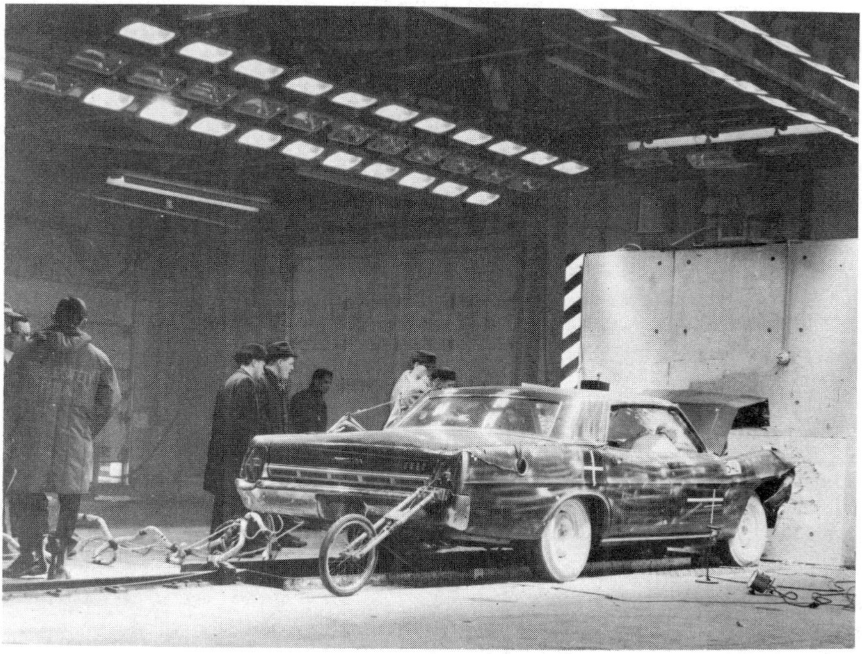

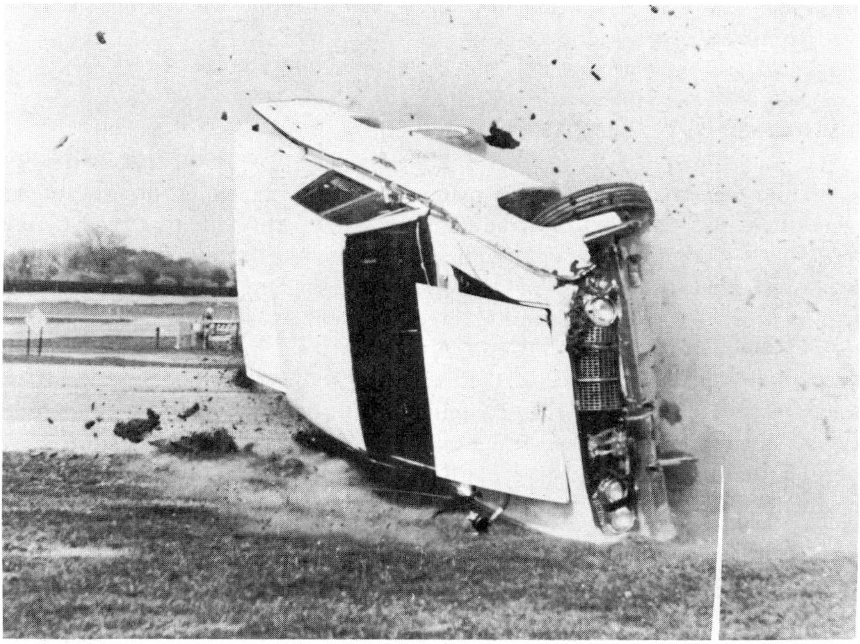

FIGURE 2.1 (Continued)

with these dimensions needs to be given serious attention by all agencies concerned. Also it would be helpful if all accident victims could be protected by persons with adequate training.

Many accidents occur where medical assistance is not readily available. Obviously this suggests the need for many trained first-aiders to protect the accident victim. Through the American National Red Cross it has been demonstrated that laymen including teachers, police, parents, civil defense personnel, and rescue squad members can provide first aid until medical help is available. Although the American National Red Cross has offered countless first-aid courses, far too few people are prepared to give emergency care to the injured. Consequently many persons die each year or are permanently disabled because of inattention or lack of proper emergency care.

The Goal

Ideally, all adults and teen-agers should be trained in first aid. A more practical and immediate goal would be to have one member of each family competent in first-aid protection. To accomplish this would require the expansion of the number of first-aid courses far beyond the level of current offerings. As discussed in Chapter 25, a goal of the Department of Transportation's Highway Safety Program Standard, Emergency Medical Services, is to have first-aid training programs available for all emergency service personnel, with the general public also being encouraged to enroll in such courses.

ORGANIZED SAFETY MOVEMENT

While society was basically primitive, accidents were thought of as events that just happened. Certainly there was no thought that man could prevent or control such occurrences. It was not until industrial states developed that the safety of the individual became a concern of the people. Increased hazards to industrial employees and the increased number of accidental deaths and injuries stimulated public interest in the curtailment of this problem. Within the industrial society that emerged out of the Industrial Revolution, the accident prevention movement of the nation had its beginning. The fundamental principles of safety education that were applied in the early days of the safety movement are essentially the same concepts of accident prevention that are in use today.

Forces Behind the Safety Movement

Successful programs of accident prevention have been the result of much planning. It should be understood that a number of factors have influenced the safety movement. Without these forces behind the movement, progress in dealing with the vast majority of the nation's accident problems would have been much slower.

The forces that have assisted most in the evolution of the accident prevention movement are

1. *Legislation.* Standards for improved safety conditions in factories, fire protection, licensing of drivers, driver education in secondary schools, and workmen's compensation have all emerged from legislative acts.
2. *Disasters.* Concern is always present after a major disaster strikes the nation. Legislation, improved standards, and control programs usually are implemented while public attention is high and focused upon the disaster.
3. *Economic Measures.* Accidents cost money; therefore industries, states, and business concerns welcome the implementation of loss prevention programs. Such measures have been very influential in the advancement of accident prevention programs.
4. *Social Mores.* People from all avenues of life have joined together from time to time in the betterment of mankind. Conferences, public forums and workshops have been conducted to influence the development of the safety movement.
5. *Protective Equipment.* Equipment such as seat belts, hard hats, radar, safety glass, and guards for industrial machinery have contributed significantly to the safety of people engaged in all types of activities.

ORGANIZATIONS IN THE SAFETY MOVEMENT

Similar interests and backgrounds tend to join hands in a common cause. Thus as the safety movement grew, people that devoted their time and talents to accident prevention began to organize themselves into professional groups. These professional organizations have been a major force behind the safety movement of the nation.

American National Red Cross (ANRC)

The American National Red Cross was organized in 1909 with its principal objective "the conservation of human life through the prevention of accidents."[6]

Throughout the years the ANRC has attempted to attain its objective through the development of programs to reduce accidents on highways, in homes and industries, on farms, and on or about water. Basic programs are concerned with first-aid training and various accident prevention activities. The ANRC is chartered by Congress to help carry out obligations assumed by the United States under certain international treaties. At both the local and national levels the ANRC activities are performed by

---

[6] American National Red Cross, *First Aid Program Planning for Chapters.* Washington, D.C.: American National Red Cross, 1966, p. 1.

[30] Safety: Philosophy and Movement

volunteers. The national headquarters of the American National Red Cross is maintained at 17th and D Streets, NW, Washington, D.C. 20006.

National Safety Council (NSC)

The National Safety Council is a voluntary, noncommercial, nonprofit membership association. The Council has as its primary objective the reduction of the number and severity of all kinds of accidents. Founded in 1913, the NSC has served as the organizing framework of the safety movement in America.

Chartered by Congress in 1953, the NSC is a national and international clearinghouse for the collection and distribution of information and materials related to safety education and accident prevention. The staff of the Council exceeds 350 full-time members who work in their headquarters office. In addition there are regional offices with staff services available. The NSC is organized into conferences to work on accident problems related to schools, industry, traffic, home, public, religious activities, youth, farm, labor, and women. The National Safety Council maintains its headquarters office at 444 N. Michigan Avenue, Chicago, Illinois 60611.

American Society of Safety Engineers (ASSE)

The American Society of Safety Engineers was formally organized in 1911. For a period of time the Society operated as a section of the National Safety Council, but since 1947 it has functioned as an independent organization.

Although the objectives of ASSE are related to the development of the safety engineering profession, the members of its various local chapters contribute their talents in the development of numerous safety projects in the interest of accident prevention.

American Association for Health, Physical Education, and Recreation (AAHPER)

AAHPER, an affiliate of the National Education Association, has programs related to health, general safety, recreation, physical education, and athletics. Interest in first aid and emergency care is an integral part of all their programs. The Association was organized in 1885 and today has a membership in excess of 60,000. AAHPER provides leadership in the areas mentioned as they relate to schools and colleges. Conferences, workshops, and numerous publications are sponsored by them annually. A headquarters office is maintained at the NEA Center, 1201 16th Street, NW, Washington, D.C. 20036.

American Driver and Traffic Safety Education Association (ADTSEA)

A group of state driver education association officers met and organized the ADTSEA in 1956. The Association was granted departmental status within the National Education Association in 1960. Today it operates independently of the NEA. The Association serves as the unifying force for educators with a professional interest in driver and safety education. Its membership is served through an annual conference, publications, and scholarship opportunities. The headquarters is at the NEA Center, 1201 16th Street, NW, Washington, D.C. 20036.

National Congress of Parents and Teachers (PTA)

The National PTA has had vital interest in health and safety for many years. Founded in 1897, the PTA gives approximately 30 percent of its legislative platform to matters pertaining to safety and accident prevention. In addition, a strong statement concerning health is included in their total legislative statement. Owing to their concern for the welfare of all children and youth, child-related activities receive much PTA attention annually. Materials relative to health and safety may be obtained from their national headquarters located at 700 North Rush Street, Chicago, Illinois 60611.

DEFINING BASIC TERMS

Throughout this text a number of basic terms are frequently used. To assist the student in the understanding of these terms they are defined from the point of view of common usage.

Accident

An accident is defined as "that occurrence in a sequence of events which usually produces unintended injury, death, or property damage." [7] It is usually an unwanted, unplanned, and undesirable occurrence.

Disabling Injury

The National Safety Council defines a disabling injury as "an injury causing death, permanent disability, or any degree of temporary total disability." [8] Such an injury requires a great deal of medical attention and hospitalization.

---

[7] National Safety Council, op. cit., p. 97.
[8] National Safety Council, op. cit., p. 97.

First Aid

First aid is the immediate care given to a person who has been injured or has been accidently taken ill.[9] Basically, this is the protection that a layman can provide the injured to ease suffering or save a life. It is not considered as medical treatment.

Emergency Care

Emergency care is the first aid, handling, and transportation provided an injured person from the time he is first discovered at the site of the accident until definitive treatment is instituted."[10] This is a broader concept than first aid because it goes beyond temporary protection to include the prevention of further deaths. In other words, consideration is given to possible complications that may develop at a later time, along with the steps to prevent the complications from occurring.

Protection

Protection involves the steps taken by the first-aider to ensure the comfort, safety, and well-being of an injured person. It includes the application of basic first-aid techniques but does not imply medical treatment of the injured.

Safety

For purposes of this text, safety is defined as "a condition or state of being resulting from the modification of human behavior and/or designing of the physical environment to reduce the possibility of hazards, thereby reducing accidents."[11] This definition includes the two primary causes of accidents—unsafe behavior and unsafe environment.

Treatment

Treatment is limited to those tasks and services performed by medical doctors, nurses, and trained hospital personnel. First-aid and rescue persons do not treat the injured. They perform protective measures until the aforementioned people take over.

---

[9] American National Red Cross, op. cit., 1973, p. 11.

[10] Maxwell N. Halsey (ed.), *Accident Prevention*. New York: McGraw-Hill, 1961, p. 278.

[11] Strasser et al., op. cit., p. 66.

ACTIVITIES

1. Write a 500-word essay on your philosophy of accident prevention.
2. Visit a local American Red Cross office. Interview the director and analyze the local ARC program. Develop a report to be given in class as assigned by the instructor.
3. Write to all the organizations discussed in this chapter requesting sample copies of their first-aid and safety materials. Organize the materials to be retained as a permanent reference library.
4. Plan and give with three other class members a panel discussion on the subject "The Forces Behind the Safety Movement."
5. Make a survey of the emergency care services available in a selected community. Determine the adequacy of the services and make recommendations for improvement.

QUESTIONS TO ANSWER

1. Define the concept of risk acceptance.
2. Outline the scope of the National Safety Council's accident prevention activities.
3. What is the purpose of the American National Red Cross?
4. Explain what it means to "integrate safety into one's philosophy of life."
5. What are the objectives of safety in the development of appropriate accident prevention methods?
6. Why should one's concept of safety be positive in nature? Explain the difference between a positive and negative approach to safety.
7. What role did industry play in the safety movement of America?
8. How did legislation influence the development of the accident prevention movement?
9. Defend the statement "One member of each family should be trained in first aid."
10. Explain the difference between first aid and emergency care protection.

SELECTED REFERENCES

AMERICAN NATIONAL RED CROSS, *First Aid Program Planning for Chapters.* Washington, D.C.: American National Red Cross, 1966, p. 1.

AMERICAN NATIONAL RED CROSS, *Standard First Aid and Personal Safety.* New York: Doubleday, 1973.

[34] Safety: Philosophy and Movement

CLARK, D. W., and MACMAHON, B. (eds.), *Preventive Medicine*. Boston: Little, Brown, 1967, p. 615.

HALSEY, M. N. (ed.), *Accident Prevention*. New York: McGraw-Hill, 1961, p. 278.

NATIONAL SAFETY COUNCIL, *Accident Facts*. Chicago: The Council, 1977.

STACK, HERBERT J. (ed.), *Safety for Greater Adventures—The Contributions of Albert Wurts Whitney*. New York: Center for Safety Education, New York University, 1953.

STACK, HERBERT J., and ELKOW, J. DUKE, *Education for Safe Living*. Englewood Cliffs, N.J.: Prentice-Hall, 1966, p. 16.

STRASSER, M. K., et al., *Fundamentals of Safety Education*. New York: Macmillan, 1973.

3. PRINCIPLES AND PROCEDURES IN THE ADMINISTRATION OF EMERGENCY CARE

In accident and emergency cases, the application of the principles and procedures of emergency care may be a matter of life or death, permanent or temporary disability, or the severity of an injury or illness. The practical application of these principles might save the child next door who is strangling, a person who is hemorrhaging in an automobile collision, or a close friend in insulin shock. The first-aid knowledge required to protect the injured in the foregoing situations is not great. However, the action taken must be prompt and accurate.

There are a few basic first-aid principles that apply to most emergency care situations. The first-aider has the obligation to use these principles regardless of where the accident occurs.

CONCEPT OF PROTECTION

In Chapter 2 protection was defined as those steps taken by the first-aider to ensure the comfort, safety, and well-being of an injured person. It includes the protective measures needed to attend to the accident victim's emergency care needs, but does not include any medical treatment.

The application of the protection concept must be constantly kept in mind by the person administering first aid. In view of the fact that the first-aider is not a trained medical person, he should be concerned about the limits to which he may go. Primarily he should perform first-aid tasks considering the question, "What would a normal prudent individual do under similar circumstances?"

In the final analysis the concept of protection may be summarized in the basic reasons for first aid as stated by the American National Red Cross:

[36] Principles and Procedures in the Administration of Emergency Care

A. First aid knowledge and skill often mean—
1. The difference between life and death
2. The difference between temporary and permanent disability
3. The difference between rapid recovery and long hospitalization

B. First aid training is of value in—
1. Preventing and caring for accidental injury or sudden illness
2. Caring for persons caught in a natural disaster or other catastrophe
3. Equipping individuals to deal with the whole situation, the person, and the injury
4. Distinguishing between what to do and what not to do

C. First aid training is needed because—
1. Statistics show that among persons from age 1 to age 38, accidents are the leading cause of death, and thereafter they remain one of the leading causes.
    a. The death rate is twice as high among males as females.
    b. The annual cost of medical attention, loss of earning ability due to temporary or permanent impairment, and direct property damage and insurance costs amount to many billions of dollars each year.
    c. Accidents take their toll in pain and suffering, disability, and personal tragedy.
    d. Motor vehicle accidents account for approximately half of all accidental deaths.
2. The concept of massive numbers of casualties has become a reality with the advent of the nuclear age.
3. The pattern of medical care has changed.
4. The growing population and expanding health needs have not been balanced by a proportional increase in numbers of doctors, nurses, and allied health workers.
5. The limitation of *time* in case of an accident or sudden illness may be so critical in terms of *minutes* or even *seconds* that only a person with first aid knowledge and skills who is on hand has any opportunity of preventing a fatal outcome.

D. First aid training promotes safety awareness in the home, at work, at play, and on streets and highways. In the promotion of such awareness, it is important to closely relate three terms: cause, effect, and prevention.
1. Cause
   When in-depth study of an actual or hypothetical accident situation identifies all the causative factors, it becomes possible to determine what can be done to eliminate, control, or avoid the hazards.
2. Effect
   When analysis carefully considers both immediate and long-range, or permanent, effects of injury or sudden illness, it becomes obvious why every possible effort should be taken to eliminate, control, or avoid a situation that is hazardous to oneself or to others.

General First-Aid Principles   [37]

3. Prevention
A better understanding of the overall accident problem is developed if all the circumstances surrounding various types of accidents are carefully studied. Preventive measures should include consideration of *how* accident-causing conditions and activities can be eliminated, controlled, or avoided.[1]

The concept of protection further implies that in the attempt to comfort the injured or save a life the first-aider must guard against making any fundamental errors. Errors may cost a life. These are some common emergency care errors that need to be prevented:

1 Improper use of the tourniquet.
2 Improper bandaging technique—either too tight or too loose.
3 Improper transportation of the injured.
4 An attempt to be too courageous.
5 Too much time spent on minor problems when there are critical situations that need immediate attention.

GENERAL FIRST-AID PRINCIPLES

By definition a principle may be thought of as a rule of conduct, especially of right conduct. Further implied is the adherence to the principle in the performance of certain tasks. Basically, principles are guidelines to follow.

There are a number of general principles for the first-aider to learn and use as basic guides when administering first aid. By adhering to these principles the first-aider can be reasonably assured that he is performing in a satisfactory manner.

Here are a number of general principles for giving protection to the injured. A person should

1 Remember that he is a first-aider.
2 Send for medical help and if necessary an ambulance.
3 Keep himself under control—calm if possible.
4 Do first things first—protect the most seriously injured, then the others.
5 Expect the worst—protect the condition.
6 Keep the victim quiet and comfortable. (a) Keep victim in lying position unless other positions are best. (b) Don't let victim walk. (c) Raise head, turn head, or elevate head or feet if necessary to make victim comfortable.
7 Check for bleeding, breathing, poisoning, burns, fractures, and dislocations, and remember: (a) Pain is an important indication. (b) Talk to

[1] American National Red Cross, *Standard First Aid and Personal Safety*. New York: Doubleday, 1973, pp. 11–13. (Excerpt from *Standard First Aid and Personal Safety*, Copyright © 1973 by The American National Red Cross, reprinted with permission.)

Keep the injured person lying down

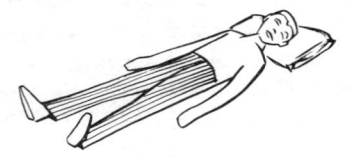

Do not give liquids to the unconscious

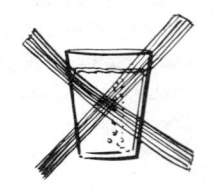

Control bleeding by pressing on the wound

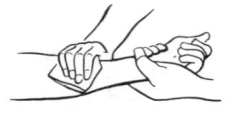

Restart breathing with mouth-to-mouth artificial respiration

Dilute swallowed poisons

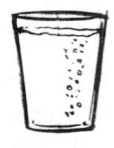

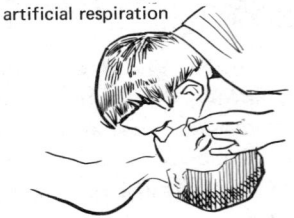

Keep broken bones from moving

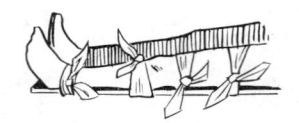

Cover burns with thick layers of cloth

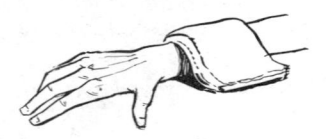

Keep heart attack cases quiet

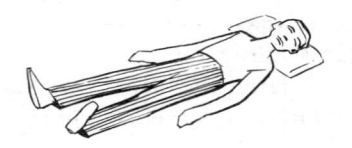

Fainting: Keep head lower than heart

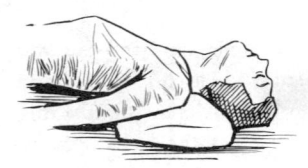

Cover eye injuries with gauze pad

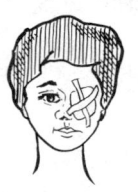

ALWAYS CALL A DOCTOR

FIGURE 3.1 General directions for giving first aid. (American Red Cross Poster)

[38]

General First-Aid Principles [39]

victim if conscious. (c) Remove clothing if necessary. (d) If victim is unconscious or semi-conscious, suspect a head injury. (e) If victim is bleeding from ears, nose, and mouth, suspect a head injury.
8   Keep victim warm—insulate from weather.
9   Never give food or water to the unconscious.
10 Give water, which is preferred for the injured over tea or coffee—never alcohol.
11 Keep onlookers away.
12 Improvise—don't waste time.
13 Loosen tight clothing.
14 Splint fractures and dislocations before moving.
15 Protect victim from vomitus and other secretions by turning head, etc.
16 Not be in a hurry to move victim.
17 Reassure the victim—keep him cheerful.
18 Not let victim see his injury; shock may result or his condition may become more severe.
19 Not touch wounds with hands or mouth.
20 Notify parents or others.

Traffic

Even the best of drivers can have automobile collisions. Therefore one should know the steps to take immediately following the accident to protect the life, property, and legal rights of those involved. Giving the appropriate protection, in the correct manner, at the right time, may save a life.

In most states there are basic principles to follow in the event of a traffic collision. Most states mandate by law the following guidelines if involved in a traffic accident:

1   Stop immediately in a safe place.
2   Assist the injured if aid is necessary or requested. Protect the victim from traffic. In case of serious injury get a doctor or call an ambulance—whichever will arrive sooner. Try to make the victim comfortable, but don't move him unless absolutely necessary. *Don't* attempt first aid unless you know something about it.
3   Warn traffic. This will help prevent another accident. Stationing someone at a safe spot to warn approaching drivers is a good idea. Use flares when they are available.
4   Stay at the scene of the accident until you have exchanged names, addresses, and license numbers with the other parties involved.
5   Notify the nearest police station as quickly as possible.
6   Report the accident to the Illinois Department of Transportation.[2]

[2] State of Illinois, *Rules of the Road*. Springfield: Office of the Secretary of State, 1977, p. 48.

School

The number of accidents involving school-age youth in recent years has been increasing, so that there are more occasions when the school nurse, teacher, or administrator must administer first aid or emergency care. In most states the school is responsible for the welfare of its students. Therefore it is wise to have some written board of education policies that establish the basic procedures to follow in case of accident or sudden illness. Such policies should be known by the faculty and students alike. By having these policies the guesswork is taken out of determining what to do during such emergencies. The following is one example of procedures in the event of a student injury or illness at school:

1. Do what needs to be done for the pupil. The school must act as it is determined by law: in loco parentis. This conceivably can mean giving artificial respiration, applying a pressure bandage or even more severe measures to control critical bleeding, emergency treatment for shock, or other measures for which there is not time to receive parental permission. The teacher or principal will normally feel parent permission should be obtained first. However, where life and death are at stake, the responsible person on the scene must assume parental authority. Of course, parents should be contacted as soon as possible, preferably while first aid is being given or the pupil is being taken to doctor or hospital.
2. If the emergency is less critical, follow the emergency procedure as indicated on Form P117 or P118 on file in the school office for the pupil.
3. If Form P117 or P118 is not on file for the pupil, attempt to contact a parent for instructions. If neither parent can be reached, the school must assume parental authority and do what needs to be done for the pupil, contacting parents as soon as possible.
4. Teachers and principles should give only such emergency treatment as is necessary to preserve life and limb and prevent undue suffering until hospital and/or medical care can be obtained.
5. In all cases, usual first-aid procedures should be followed.
6. In the absence of good evidence to the contrary, anything that happens to a pupil in the public shools that potentially endangers the life or limb of the individual should be considered an emergency.
7. Realizing that frequently much damage can result from too enthusiastic first-aid treatment, it is wise to administer first-aid measures with a degree of restraint. As quickly as possible have the patient transferred to a doctor's office or one of the local hospitals.
8. The proper procedures and delineation of responsibility in cases of emergency illness or injury have been set forth in items 1–5.[3]

[3] Lansing School District, *Emergency Procedures and First Aid*. Lansing, Michigan: The District, 1965, pp. 2–3.

General First-Aid Principles [41]

Teacher's Role The teacher must remember that it is his responsibility to assume the role of the parent or guardian as far as the schoolchild is concerned (in loco parentis). This means that if a child becomes sick or is injured at school and the parent cannot be found or contacted, the teacher is expected to do what the parent would do under similar circumstances.

Administrative Role School boards and administrators are responsible for the health and safety of the children at school; provisions must be made to take care of all school emergencies, including accidents, injuries, and illness. Schools should have a written plan for disaster and emergencies. Teachers, students, and staff should know this plan well if it is to function effectively.

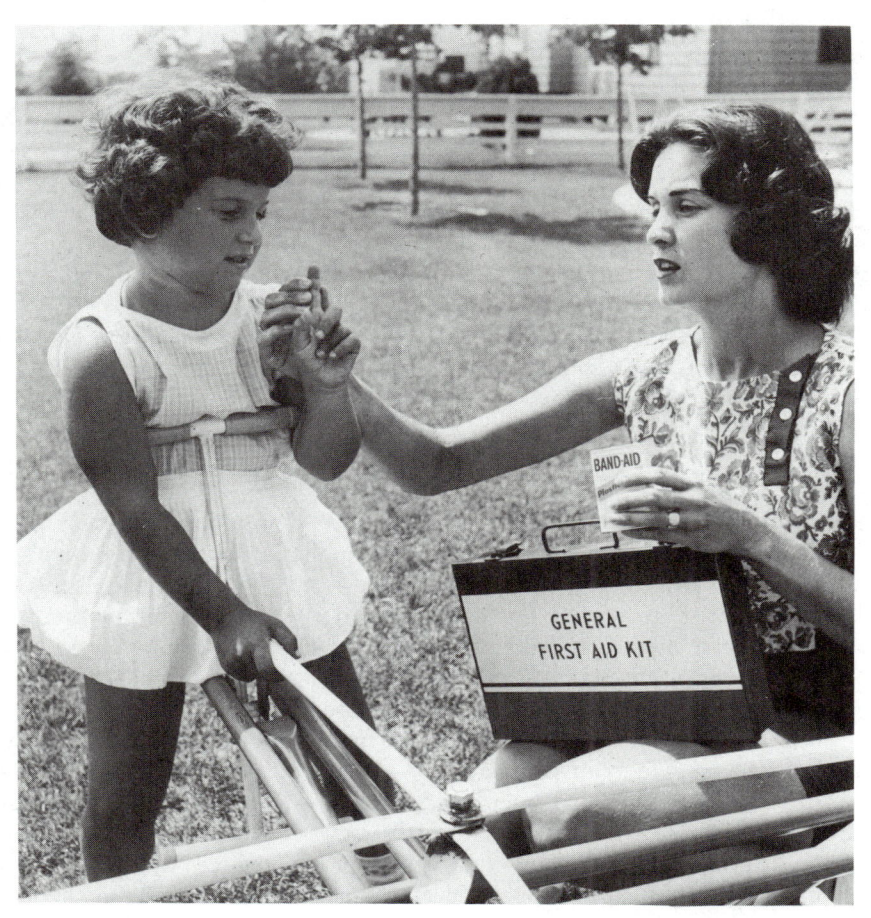

FIGURE 3.2 Being prepared at home means having a handy, well-stocked first-aid kit. (Johnson & Johnson)

Home

Accidents occur in the home at an alarming rate. In a recent year 1 person in 58 was disabled one or more days in injuries received in home accidents. The opportunities to use first-aid skills in the home are frequent. Falls, fire burns, suffocation, and poisoning are the most common types of accidents involving persons around the home. Thus first-aid knowledge concerning a variety of accidents is desirable. Those techniques discussed in Parts II, III, and V of this text may be used to gain knowledge necessary to apply appropriate first aid and emergency care to those injured at home. Also refer to the general principles on page 37 to support those that follow:

1 When necessary, immediately get a doctor or ambulance or obtain medical advice by telephone. When summoning professional help it is important to ask what can be done until the doctor gets there.
2 Stop profuse bleeding.
3 Determine whether artificial respiration is necessary.
4 Never give fluids to an unconscious or partly conscious person. They may enter his windpipe. Never attempt to arouse such a person by shaking him or talking to him.
5 Keep the person lying down and protect him from handling or disturbance by others about him.
6 Try to keep the patient's body temperature from falling but do not apply excessive heat. Cover with a blanket.
7 With indoor accidents, be cautious about opening windows. Make sure the patient has enough air, but avoid chilling him.
8 Loosen the clothing about his neck if the patient is unconscious.[4]

Industrial

Although industries have sound programs of industrial accident prevention, occupational health services, and industrial hygiene, the number of accidental deaths and injuries suggests a need for the development of extensive programs of first aid and emergency care. Frequently there is a medical staff including a doctor and industrial nurse employed to care for the serious injuries that occur. In most cases the nurse will determine the need for prompt medical attention. Also she will make a tentative diagnosis of the worker's condition and if necessary employ the necessary resuscitative and first-aid protection.

In view of the fact that many industries do have professional medical staffs, it is usually a requirement that all injuries be reported immediately to the health services. It is felt that such a policy reduces the possibilities of infection and disability. Further, such a policy assists in the avoidance

---

[4] Doris Ruslink, *Family Health and Home Nursing*. New York: Macmillan, 1967, pp. 393–394.

of false claims of injury and disability. Also OSHA regulations require accurate reporting systems.

In the establishment of an adequate first-aid and emergency care program for industries the following guidelines could be used:

1 Properly trained and designated first-aiders on every shift.
2 A first-aid facility and supplies, or first-aid kit.
3 A first-aid manual.
4 Posted instructions for calling a physician and notifying the hospital that the patient is en route.
5 Posted instructions for transporting ill or injured employees and for calling an ambulance or rescue squad.
6 An adequate first-aid record system.
7 First-aid procedures, approved by the consulting physician, should embrace the type of medication, if any, to be used on minor injuries, such as cuts and burns.
8 The equipment and supplies should be in accordance with the recommendations of the physician, and service should be rendered only as covered by written standard procedures, signed and dated by him.
9 Since unwise care might involve the company in serious complications, the first-aid attendant should be duly qualified and certified by the Bureau of Mines or American Red Cross.[5]

Public

Accidental public deaths occur at a rate of about 21,000 each year. Falls, drownings, firearms, fire burns, and water transport account for the greatest percentage of these. Because of the scope of public-related accidents it is difficult to know exactly how many persons are injured annually. For example, the total number of recreational deaths and injuries is unknown. But it is suspected that the number represents a substantial percentage of those identified as public-type accidents.

There are millions of people engaged in recreational activities, so that the opportunities for the use of first-aid skills are considerable. A basic recommendation is that all persons involved in recreational-type activities complete a first-aid course.

Although it is difficult to establish principles that cover all situations where recreational accidents occur, the following are suggested as a series of sensible guidelines:

1 *Cessation of breathing.* There should be a clear air passage from the mouth or nose through the throat to the lungs.
2 *Control of bleeding.* Immediate pressure should be applied on the bleeding area with sterile or clean cloths and, if possible, the part of the body with the bleeding area should be elevated.

[5] National Safety Council, *Accident Prevention Manual for Industrial Operations*. Chicago: The Council, 1976, pp. 1232.

[44] Principles and Procedures in the Administration of Emergency Care

3. *Minor wounds, cuts, and scratches.* Bleeding should be controlled by direct pressure on the wound surface. Then prevent contamination.
4. *Internal poisoning.* The ingested poison should be diluted as quickly as possible by giving fluids, just plain water or milk. Generally, vomiting should not be induced.
5. *Fractures.* The broken ends and adjacent joints should be immobilized.
6. *Burns.* The pain should be relieved and further contamination prevented.
7. *Shock.* The injured person should be kept lying down in a comfortable position.
8. *Transporting the injured.* The injured part should be prevented from twisting, bending, and shaking.
9. *Foreign body in the eye.* The most common place for foreign bodies to lodge is on the inner surface of the upper lid. It is important that a person should not rub the eye. If the speck is in the eye, he should look down, then hold the edge of the upper lid firmly, and pull it over the lower lid.
10. *Plant poisoning.* Most common are poison ivy, oak, and sumac. Certainly, the best first aid is prevention. The exposed part should be washed with soap and water and then sponged with rubbing alcohol. The blisters should not be broken. Calamine lotion or wet compresses should be applied.
11. *Bites and stings.* Some people have violent allergenic reaction to the bites of bees, wasps, mosquitoes, and other insects. Most victims can be helped by the application of ice or ice water, which will give some relief and may even slow the absorption rate. The placing of a constricting band around the part (extremities) may be of further help.[6]

RECORDS AND ACCIDENT-REPORTING SYSTEM

In order to know the scope of an accident problem it is advisable to have an adequate accident records and reporting system. This is a basic principle in the development of all accident prevention programs related to schools, industries, police, driver licensing agencies, and public safety departments. The information collected from such a system provides the primary data upon which these agencies can organize and conduct effective accident prevention programs. It is essential that the authorities involved understand the conditions and unsafe acts that are contributing to their agency's accident experience.

Organization

A successful accident reporting system functions best when it is well organized and an integral part of a well-administered accident prevention

---

[6] Earl Breon, *Family Recreation and Safety.* New York: Center for Safety Education, New York University, 1961, pp. 72–75.

program. When a system is organized it should be implemented throughout the school system, industry, or agency.

Policy   Accident reporting systems usually function best when established upon written policy. The school administration, industry management, or police superintendent should give their support and see that guidelines are developed and used. In the establishment of such a policy OSHA standards should be considered.

Staffing   For an accident reporting system to be useful, someone must be assigned the responsibility of overseeing the program. In the school this person should be the supervisor of driver and safety education. A nurse would assume this task in industry, while a trained records man would be the logical staff person in a police department.

Budget   An adequate budget is needed to assure the effectiveness of a records and reporting system. Funds are needed for supplies, file cabinets, printing, publications, and general overhead costs. In some instances the budget may not be very large, but it must be sufficient for a sound program.

Reporting Procedure

There needs to be an established procedure for the reporting of all accidents. This eliminates confusion and expedites the care necessary to protect the injured person. The procedure should be carefully studied and thought out before implementation. Published copies should be posted in appropriate places and file copies sent to all related personnel. For schools the principles discussed on page 40 could be used as a guide in the development of such a procedure. Industry personnel may wish to organize a safety committee to work toward the formulation of a procedure. And police departments may wish to rely upon the administrative staff and their trained first-aiders to establish suitable guidelines.

AVAILABILITY OF TRAINED PERSONNEL

In the administration of first aid and emergency care, trained personnel are desirable. As discussed in Chapter 2 such persons are not to be found in great numbers. Therefore, many accident victims do not receive proper attention and their condition is made more serious.

First-Aid Personnel

The American National Red Cross makes available standard and advanced first-aid courses to all communities. As a basic principle it would be well for all schools, industries, and other organizations to recommend

[46] Principles and Procedures in the Administration of Emergency Care

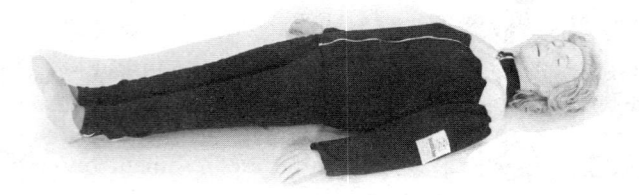

FIGURE 3.3 Resusci-Anne, used in preparing first aid personnel. (Dyna-Med, Inc., Carlsbad, California)

that all personnel enroll in a first-aid class periodically. Each school should have several persons qualified to render first-aid protection in the interest of student and teacher welfare. The same principle should apply to industries, civil defense workers, police, and recreational workers.

Parents should take advantage of first-aid training opportunities. Since the greatest number of injuries occurring each year are related to home accidents, such a background might save the life of a son, daughter, or neighbor.

Ambulance Service

Every community should have adequate ambulance service available on a 24-hour basis. The results of an accident can be influenced by the type and quality of the ambulance service available. In each instance the ambulance should be properly equipped and manned by trained medical paraprofessionals or first-aid personnel. Such persons may continue or initiate the care of the injured person in the ambulance en route to the hospital.

Emergency Care Facilities

Each hospital should have a facility designed, equipped, and stocked for emergency cases. The facility should be supervised by a senior physician with assistance from a trained nurse. Easy access should be provided to the facility and admittance should be automatic when the victim arrives.

Poison Control Centers

Many states are now designating Poison Control Centers on a geographic basis. Such a center can provide the care necesary for poison victims. In addition the center should be prepared to give information on emergency cases when contacted. Because of the high incidence of poison cases, the development of these centers should be encouraged.

ACTIVITIES

1 Organize an accident records and reporting system for a school of 1,200 students. Include the types of record forms and policies required to institute the program.
2 Contact the nearest OSHA office and request a copy of first aid and emergency care requirements. Summarize for your class in a ten-minute presentation.
3 Develop a set of procedures that a school could use in the handling of emergency injuries and illness. Check the state's school code for any laws that might apply to the procedures.
4 Make a survey of the county to determine the availability of emergency care services. Develop a detailed report for presentation to the class.
5 Contact ten State Departments of Public Health to determine the number and functions of the Poison Control Centers. Summarize the information received and make a ten-minute presentation to the class.

QUESTIONS TO ANSWER

1 Why is it difficult to ascertain the scope of the nation's public accicidental injury problem?
2 What is the difference between first-aid protection and first-aid treatment?
3 Identify five general principles of first aid that could apply to most emergency cases.
4 In a typical year how many persons are killed or injured in work-related accidents?
5 When a person is involved in a traffic accident, what are the basic steps to follow in satisfying the state's legal requirements?
6 Briefly discuss why trained first-aid personnel are necessary in the prevention of accidents.
7 Why is it important for parents to have a knowledge of first aid?
8 What contribution does a good ambulance service make to a community's emergency medical service program?
9 What is the definition of a "principle"? Of what value are principles in administering first-aid protection?
10 Who should assume the responsibility for the supervision of a school's accident records and reporting system? Explain why.

SELECTED REFERENCES

AMERICAN NATIONAL RED CROSS, *Standard First Aid and Personal Safety*. New York: Doubleday, 1973.

GRANT, HARVEY, and MURRAY, ROBERT, *Emergency Care*. Bowie, Md.: Robert J. Brady, 1971.

HENDERSON, JOHN, *Emergency Medical Guide*, 4th ed. New York: McGraw-Hill, 1978.

NATIONAL SAFETY COUNCIL, *Accident Prevention Manual for Industrial Operations*. Chicago: The Council, 1976.

NATIONAL SAFETY COUNCIL, *Family Camping*. Chicago: The Council, 1968.

NATIONAL SAFETY COUNCIL, *Student Accident Reporting Guidebook*. Chicago: The Council, 1966.

NEW YORK UNIVERSITY, *Family Recreation and Safety*. New York: Center for Safety Education, 1961, pp. 72-75.

RUSLINK, DORIS, *Family Health and Home Nursing*. New York: Macmillan, 1967, pp. 393-394.

STATE OF ILLINOIS, *Rules of the Road*. Springfield: Office of the Secretary of State, 1977, p. 48.

4. INDIVIDUAL RESPONSIBILITY AND LEGAL IMPLICATIONS IN EMERGENCY CARE

Never have all people found it convenient, pleasant, worthwhile, or satisfying to help an injured person. And in recent years the desire to fill the role of a "good neighbor" seems to have grown weaker. Perhaps this is due in part to the fact that liability suits for negligent acts, real or accused, have been on the increase. As a result, many people have assumed the position, "I don't want to become involved."

The person giving first aid and emergency care must be alert to his responsibility and make certain that he does not place himself in a position where he might be deemed negligent. This is why the first-aider should understand the difference between the concept of protection discussed in Chapter 3 and medical treatment.

TRENDS IN PERSONAL LIABILITY

The possibility of a person becoming involved in a legal action resulting from an injury involving a schoolchild or an employee or relating to a public-place accident is greater today than ever before.[1] In general, courts are requiring schools, industries, state agencies, doctors, and individuals to be more responsible for their negligent acts. This means that suits are more frequent because of a more liberal interpretation of liability laws.

As a result of these recent trends the general populace has been more concerned over the question, "Can I be sued for this action?" "No" usually is the answer if the person has acted in the best interest of that person in trouble. Further, if the individual has assisted as a prudent person, no

[1] Dennis J. Kigin, *Teacher Liability in School-Shop Accidents.* Ann Arbor, Mich.: Prakken Publications, 1963, p. 1.

[49]

[50] Individual Responsibility and Legal Implications in Emergency Care

court should rule against him. This is especially true where first aid has been given to an injured person. The American National Red Cross reports that no person has ever been held liable for the rendering of first-aid protection.

Application of Protection Concept

If the first-aider keeps in mind that there are limitations placed upon his role, there should be no question about his performance in caring for the injured. The concept of protection discussed in Chapter 3 clarifies this role. In summary the concept suggests that the first-aider is to provide immediate first-aid protection in an effort to comfort, to reduce the possibilities of a person dying due to lack of some basic attention, and to see that all is done that can be done for the injured prior to the arrival of medical help. Only in extreme emergencies when medical help is not available does the first-aider ever attempt to give medical treatment. If this approach is kept in mind the first-aider can perform without fear of being accused of giving medical treatment for which he has no preparation.

BASIC DEFINITIONS

To assist the reader in a better understanding of this chapter, a number of the basic legal terms are defined. These are common definitions and are acceptable to most authorities.

Negligence

Negligence is defined as "the failure to act as a reasonable person, guided by ordinary conditions, would—or doing something which a prudent and reasonable man would not do."[2] Fundamentally it is any conduct that falls below the standard established by law to protect others against unreasonable risk of harm.

Tort Liability

Usually tort liability is defined as "a wrongful act consisting of the commission or omission of an act by one, without right, whereby another receives some injury, directly or indirectly, in person, property, or reputation."[3] Tort cases always involve a personal claim rather than a criminal prosecution.

[2] NEA Research Division for the National Commission on Safety Education, *Who Is Liable for Pupil Injuries?* Washington, D.C.: National Education Association, 1950, p. 4.

[3] M. K. Strasser et al., *Fundamentals of Safety Education.* New York: Macmillan, 1973, p. 54.

Foreseeability

Most often the best means for determining whether a person's conduct was proper or negligent is that of foreseeability. "In situations where a reasonable and prudent person could have foreseen the harmful consequences of his action or inaction, an individual who disregards the foreseeable consequences is liable for negligent conduct."[4]

Assumption of Risk

Frequently a defense lawyer will raise the theory of assumption of risk in an effort to acquit his client of liability for negligence in an accident case. By definition, "assumption of risk is a legal doctrine which presupposes that despite a relation or situation known to be dangerous, a person appreciating the danger involved voluntarily chooses to enter upon and remain within the area of risk."[5]

BASIS FOR LIABILITY

There are many reasons that a person, school, industry, state agency, or physician might become the victim of a liability suit. This situation would apply most frequently to tortious acts, defined previously. The act does not need to be intentional. Very few instances can be identified where the wrongful act has been committed by intent. In all cases, a tortious act involves one of the following situations:

1. An act or omission causing harm which the person did not intend to cause, but which should have been foreseen and prevented.
2. An act in itself contrary to law or an omission of a specific legal duty, which causes harm not originally intended.
3. An act that is intended to cause harm and is successful.[6]

Negligence

In all cases of tort liability, negligence must be proven. Negligence is a legal determination that can be established only by the courts. Usually courts study and evaluate three factors in deciding whether a person is guilty of negligent behavior. These three factors are as follows:

1. *Test of foreseeability.* When a reasonable person could have foreseen the result of his actions or omission of action, and disregards this knowledge, he

---

[4] NEA Research Division for the National Commission on Safety Education, op. cit., p. 13.
[5] Ibid., p. 14.
[6] Ibid., p. 5.

is liable for negligent conduct. At the same time, if the danger could not be foreseen by a prudent person or was beyond the knowledge expected of the person, he is not liable.
2. *Contributory negligence.* When the plaintiff's own action contributes to his injury, and when this action or omission of action is determined to be negligent, the plaintiff is guilty of contributory negligence. In these cases, the plaintiff normally cannot recover damages. When both parties are at fault, neither can recover from the other for resulting harm.
3. *Comparative negligence.* This is a relatively new concept in legal judgment, one that attempts to weigh the extent of liability and to modify the possible harsh effect of the plaintiff's contributory negligence upon his right to recovery. In this concept, the courts will assign the degree of fault between the defendant and the plaintiff, and apportion the amount of recovery possible for the plaintiff. This type of decision permits the court to assign degrees of liability rather than a judgment based on full or no liability.[7]

SCOPE OF LEGAL RESPONSIBILITY

Over the years courts and legislative bodies have attempted to clarify responsibility for injuries that have occurred due to negligent acts of commission or omission. Such decisions by the courts influence the attitude of an industry toward its employees, of a school system toward students, and of the extent of the first-aider's role in rendering aid to the injured. The scope of the legal responsibility involved should be understood in order to avoid acts that might result in a liability suit. See Appendix for state-by-state EMS survey.

School System and Administrator

Usually it is a general rule that school systems and administrators are immune from tort liability for injuries involving students. However, this immunity has been challenged, and in many states the school system is liable for negligent acts that have been responsible for student injuries. In addition some states have seen fit to adjust the law to their own situations. By doing this the state becomes an exception to the theory of sovereignty, which is the basis for most common-law immunity statutes. A few of the states that have enacted laws to void, under various circumstances, immunity are California, Connecticut, Illinois, New Jersey, and New York.

In some states, school systems are required to employ school nurses, who in turn are responsible for administering first aid to injured students. The administrative officers of each school should work very closely with the nurse in locating an adequate emergency care office. Each facility

[7] Strasser et al., op. cit., p. 55.

Scope of Legal Responsibility [53]

should be adequately stocked, as discussed in Chapter 24. In addition a written policy or procedure should be established regarding the handling of student injuries and illnesses. The combination of a school nurse, well-equipped facility, and established first-aid procedures will assure a court that the school board and administration have done everything possible to take care of student needs in time of emergency.

Teacher

The legal status of the teacher will vary from state to state. Also the possibility of his liability will be influenced by the subject taught; e.g., physical education and science have greater liability potential than English and mathematics. The basic point to keep in mind is that no teacher is immune from tort liability. The courts have determined that a teacher is not a public officer, is not immune from liability as an employee of a governmental agency, and can be held liable for negligent acts as he performs in the role of teacher. There are approximately 41 states that do not permit suit against school systems, but in each instance the teacher is vulnerable.

Usually the law requires that a teacher perform and exercise the care and prudence any reasonable prudent individual would have exercised in the same or similar situation. If this guideline is followed, the teacher should never be overly concerned about being held liable for a negligent act.

In the situation where first aid is required for an injured student, the teacher should apply the basic principles of protection discussed throughout this text. It would be wise for all teachers to take a refresher first-aid course periodically.

State Agencies

Persons employed by state agencies usually fall under the common-law immunity statutes. Therefore such persons cannot be held liable. However, there are exceptions to this rule.

Police State and local police frequently are called upon to render emergency care and first-aid protection. If the basic principles presented in this text are followed, usually there is no need to be concerned over the probabilities of being held liable. Because of the diversity of state statutes and police agency policies, it is suggested that the basic first-aid principles be carefully evaluated and applied in all cases where first aid is given to an injured person.

Other Agencies There may be occasions when personnel of driver's license, highway, or public health departments are called upon to give first-aid protection. Common sense and the use of the concept of protection as presented in Chapter 3 are the best guides for such persons to follow.

In order to avoid being involved in an emergency situation without the proper knowledge to handle the injury, it would be well for all state agencies to sponsor first-aid courses on a regular basis for staff training purposes. This should be the policy especially of those departments where the potential for accidents is great.

Industries

Usually state workmen's compensation laws cover accidental injuries arising out of and during the course of employment. Such laws are either compulsory or elective. No workmen's compensation law covers every employer and every type of employment. In some 25 percent of the states, compensation laws apply primarily to identified hazardous or extra-hazardous jobs.[8] Further, not all employees in the nation are covered by compensation laws. Numerous workers still have only the common law as a means of recovery for personal injury.

In many instances, because of the requirements of workmen's compensation laws, industries provide excellent health services for their employees. Such programs are designed to take care of the emergency care needs of the individual on the job. As mentioned previously, this type of program also relieves the employer from numerous compensation claims because notice of accidents must be filed by the employee within a specified period of time. Failure to comply with this requirement may cause a claim to be void.

Industrial plants usually employ a nurse to handle first-aid cases. By such action, plus having available a physician either as an employee or on call, liability cases tend to be rare. In small industries where the full-time services of a nurse or physician cannot be justified, provisions should be made whereby a well-trained first-aider is on the job all the time. Periodic first-aid course attendance should be encouraged for all employees, especially in hazardous industries.

Physicians

In a highly complex society such as that of the United States, physicians are subject to numerous legal ramifications. All doctors should have a basic knowledge of the principles of law that apply to the practice of medicine.

The most prevalent concern of the average physician is being accused of medical malpractice. By definition, "medical malpractice covers wrong-

---

[8] National Safety Council, *Accident Prevention Manual for Industrial Operation.* Chicago: The Council, 1976, pp. 11-3, 11-4.

ful acts committed by a physician in the course of practice that cause harm to a patient." [9] Usually malpractice cases are negligence cases. This involves the alleged failure of the physician to render legally proper care, which results in harm to the individual. It is very difficult to adequately define negligence in this doctor-patient relationship. Most often, community standards and the reputation of the doctor determine the outcome of negligence cases.

In most cases of alleged malpractice the patient must have a doctor serve as a witness in his behalf and be prepared to state that accepted standards of medical practice were violated by the defendant. There are some obvious gross negligence cases where the patient can determine the negligence without supporting testimony.

Since most doctors are capable and dedicated persons, it is unlikely that a great number of malpractice suits will be ruled in favor of the plaintiff. Usually the doctor does the best he can for the health and welfare of the individual.

Homeowners

In recent years homeowners have come under closer scrutiny of the courts for alleged negligence. In general, suits filed against homeowners are "attractive nuisance" claims. Usually a person (perhaps a child) has been lured into a yard because of the presence of a swimming pool, play equipment, or some other item that had an appeal to the person. There are other instances where a person may have been injured in a fall or an accident that occurred because a handrail was faulty or a sidewalk hole was not repaired. Homeowners should protect themselves through proper supervision of swimming pools or other things that may attract others. In addition, the home and yard should be kept in good repair and free of litter to avoid injuries to invited guests or intruders.

In order to be in a position to assist persons who may be injured in or around a home it is suggested that at least one member of each family be trained in first aid. With this capability the homeowner could avoid becoming involved in a liability suit.

GOOD SAMARITAN LAWS

In recent years physicians, police officers, and lay persons have become reluctant to give first aid and emergency care to the injured because of the potential of becoming involved in a liability suit. Recognizing that such action might cost the life of an automobile crash victim or someone

---

[9] D. W. Clark and B. MacMahon, *Preventive Medicine*. Boston: Little, Brown, 1967, p. 875.

injured at the beach, changes have been made in the laws of several states that give protection when rendering first aid during a time of emergency. Such laws are called "Good Samaritan laws" and protect basically the doctor from malpractice suits. The scope of such laws usully covers others who are acting in good faith and are providing care as a reasonable, prudent individual should.

In view of the impact that such laws could have upon the saving of lives, many additional states are considering the enactment of such statutes. Certainly this would assure the first-aider that what he does for an injured person will not be held against him.

EMERGENCY CARE PROCEDURE

All persons are concerned over their responsibility and legal implications in the rendering of first aid and emergency care to the injured. In addition to those matters discussed in this chapter relative to this topic, it is suggested that Chapter 3 be reviewed. The principles presented in that chapter will assist a person to a better understanding of his role and of legal implications relative to first-aid and emergency care protection. The procedures outlined are basic to the avoidance of personal negligence.

ACTIVITIES

1. Contact a lawyer in the community. Make arrangements for him to attend class for purposes of discussing your state's personal liability laws.
2. Develop a research paper on the subject of "Good Samaritan laws." Attempt to obtain as much information as possible with reference to all state statutes.
3. Organize a class panel discussion with the assistance of two other persons on the topic "Recent Trends in Personal Liability."
4. Develop and keep a scrapbook of liability cases reported in local newspapers. Analyze each case and determine what each defendant could have done to have avoided such litigation.
5. Construct a questionnaire relative to the liability of school systems. Send it to ten school administrators with the request that the questionnaire be returned within a week. Evaluate the replies and make a short oral report to the class.

QUESTIONS TO ANSWER

1. Define negligence. How does this compare with comparative negligence?
2. Briefly discuss what is meant by "test of foreseeability."

3   What factors are usually examined in the determination of negligent behavior?
4   Why is the teacher most often the victim of tort liability suits?
5   How can the concept of protection help a person avoid a liability suit?
6   In what ways can state agencies protect themselves from tort liability suits?
7   Discuss workmen's compensation laws and how they protect both the employer and the employee.
8   Why is it wise for a homeowner to be concerned about personal liability?
9   How many states rule that a school system may not be sued but at the same time have statutes that permit suit of the teacher?
10 In what way can stated emergency care procedures help a teacher from becoming a victim of a tort liability suit?

SELECTED REFERENCES

AMERICAN ACADEMY OF ORTHOPAEDIC SURGEONS, Committee on Injuries, *Emergency Care and Transportation of the Sick and Injured*. Chicago: The Academy, 1971.

CHAYET, NEIL L., *Legal Implications of Emergency Care*. New York: Appleton-Century-Crofts, 1969.

CLARK, D. W., and MACMAHON, B., *Preventive Medicine*. Boston: Little, Brown, 1967, pp. 875–877.

ELLIOTT, H. (ed.), *Medical Aspects of Traffic Safety*. Montreal: The Traffic Accident Foundation for Medical Research, 1955.

GARBEN, L. O., and SMITH, H. H., *The Law and the Teacher in Illinois*. Danville, Ill.: Interstate Printers and Publishers, 1965.

KIGIN, DENNIS, *Teacher Liability in School Shop Accidents*. Ann Arbor, Mich.: Prakken Publications, 1963.

NATIONAL COMMITTEE ON UNIFORM TRAFFIC LAWS AND ORDINANCES, *Uniform Vehicle Code and Model Traffic Ordinances*. Washington, D.C.: The Committee, 1973.

NATIONAL SAFETY COUNCIL, *Accident Prevention Manual for Industrial Operations*. Chicago: The Council, 1976.

RESEARCH DIVISION FOR THE NATIONAL COMMISSION ON SAFETY EDUCATION, *Who Is Liable for Pupil Injuries?* Washington, D.C.: National Education Association, 1963.

WILSON, O. W., *Police Planning*. Springfield, Ill.: Charles C Thomas, 1972.

PART II
GENERAL EMERGENCY CARE PROBLEMS

This part of the book deals with general emergency care problems. Knowledge of these problems is fundamental in the rendering of adequate first-aid protection. The problems discussed are common to school, home, highway, and recreational environments. There are also applications to work and industrial accidents.

Included in Part II are the following chapters:

5 Cursory Examination: Physical Check of the Injured
6 Wounds
7 Shock
8 Respiratory and Cardiopulmonary Resuscitation (CPR)
9 Temperature Problems
10 Poisons
11 Bone, Joint, and Muscle Injuries

5. CURSORY EXAMINATION: PHYSICAL CHECK OF THE INJURED

In the United States a disabling injury occurs to some individual every three seconds; many others are injured whose injuries are not so severe or are not reported.[1] It is not reasonable for one to assume that there will be a trained medical person readily available or even present within an hour. When the injury-producing accident occurs, in most cases it will be an untrained person who takes care of the situation. Hopefully, the one providing emergency protection or first-aid care will be a person who has had some training in the care and recognition of injuries and other emergency problems, even though the training may be limited to a minimum first-aid course.

For two or three decades the American National Red Cross has emphasized the need for first-aid training and has indicated that there be a goal of training one out of every ten persons in the nation. In recent years through its program, Medical Self-Help, the Office of Civil Defense, has had as its aim the training of one person in each family—i.e., one out of every five or six persons. The Emergency Medical Services Highway Safety Program Standard discussed in Chapter 25 gives added emphasis to the need for well-trained first-aid and emergency care personnel. There is little danger that too many persons will be taught emergency care; such training is good basic education for everyone.

THE ACCIDENT ITSELF

The circumstances surrounding the accident can be most meaningful; consequently, the accident scene should be carefully studied. For the

[1] National Safety Council, *Accident Facts*. Chicago, Illinois: The Council, 1977.

[61]

[62] Cursory Examination: Physical Check of the Injured

person at the accident scene to best understand what has happened and to ascertain the nature of the accident, the possible injuries, and certainly the severity of the injuries, it is suggested that the area of the accident be carefully examined. If the injured person is lying on a street or highway and there are visible skid marks, it would be reasonable to assume that the victim had been hit by a motor vehicle. Likewise, if there is a bicycle, motorcycle, or scooter in the immediate area, then one could expect that an automobile or cycle had collided. From such accidents broken bones, abrasions, lacerations, head and neck and back injuries are quite likely. If at the scene there is evidence that one has fallen from a height—i.e., a ladder, steps, a tree, or a window—the first-aider should realize the possibility of broken bones. Each possibility should be carefully checked out. If it is at all possible, the accident scene should be secured. It may be necessary to ask other persons at the scene to help secure the location, to direct traffic, to go for help, and to give any other necessary assistance.

Witnesses at the Accident Scene

It can be most helpful to the person giving protection or aid to the injured if he can talk to a person who saw the accident or onset of illness. Such a person can tell how the accident happened, what the injured person was doing before the accident or emergency, how they reacted at the time of the incident, whether the person complained of pain, nausea, dizziness, headache, breathing difficulties, or any other symptoms.

The Injured Person

It is hoped that the injured person will be conscious. If he is, the person who is giving emergency care protection should carefully and reasonably ask the victim such questions as follows:

1 Do you have any pain? If so, where? Is it continuous or occasional? Is it local or general? Does it hurt to move?
2 Do you feel sick or nauseous? What have you eaten or drunk?
3 Do you have a headache?
4 Do you have a pain in your chest or down either arm?
5 Is it difficult or painful for you to breathe?
6 Can you move your arms or your legs? Is it painful to do so? Can you feel this pin prick?
7 Is your mouth dry? Are you thirsty?
8 Have you been drinking alcohol? How much did you drink and how long ago?
9 Are you taking medication? What do you take, and when did you last take it?
10 Is your vision clear? Is it double or blurry?

11 Are you under the care of a doctor? If so, what is your problem?
12 What is your name? Where do you live, and what is your telephone number? Are you wearing a medical information tag?

Answers to these questions by the injured will be of great assistance to the first-aider and will provide information for the ambulance crew or rescue team, the hospital, and the medical personnel.

If the injured person is unconscious the problem will be greatly magnified, and other checks will need to be made to help determine the nature of the problem. The first-aider should

1 Check for bleeding or hemorrhage.
2 Determine if the victim is breathing.
3 Check for a pulse or heart beat.
4 Examine the head and neck for possible injuries, such as bumps or possible depressions of the skull and malignment or position of the neck.
5 Examine the eyes to determine the condition and size of the pupils.
6 Smell the breath to determine its nature, e.g., alcohol, acetone, poisons such as kerosene or gasoline, and others.
7 Observe the color of skin as white, red, or blue. This will be discussed at some length later in connection with unconsciousness.
8 Observe for possible and severe internal injuries such as chest puncture and abdominal injury.

HURRY CASES

There are several types of injuries that have been referred to through the years as those which demand fast action. In these cases it is most important that protective measures be taken immediately if the life is to be saved. These hurry cases are hemorrhage, breathing stoppage, poisoning, shock, burns, snakebite, and bee and wasp stings.

Breathing Stoppage

Asphyxia in all forms demands the fastest possible emergency action. A life can be lost in a matter of a very few minutes if the cells and tissues of one's body are denied oxygen. Some of the causes of accidental asphyxia are

1 Too little oxygen in the air resulting from the presence of another gas, or not enough oxygen intake due to the presence of another gas.
2 The blood not being able to transfer oxygen because of too few red cells or heart failure.
3 The air passage being blocked by food, water, solids, other fluids or strangulation of the trachea.

[64]   Cursory Examination: Physical Check of the Injured

4 The respiratory center of the brain being paralyzed by drugs, electric shock, or a blow on the head.
5 The body being compressed by a great pressure as a cave-in or being pinned down beneath a motor-vehicle or some other heavy object.

Asphyxia will be dealt with at length in Chapter 8.

Hemorrhage

Hemorrhage or severe bleeding is an important hurry-case type of emergency. Bleeding from a major artery or vein is extremely serious. However, in a great majority of cases it is possible to control the bleeding until medical help is available.

Poisoning

There are several types of poisoning but internal poisoning—i.e., the taking of a poisonous substance into the mouth and digestive tract—is of primary consideration. This problem calls for speedy action because some poisons work very fast, are damaging and permanent. The victim should be examined carefully for the possibility of internal poisoning, which means checking the mouth, breath, and empty containers for poisonous substances, including medicines and drugs. Shock may be evident in poison cases; therefore, the condition should be checked for immediately or the result can be fatal.

Burns

Severe burns represent another hurry situation. There will be little difficulty in identifying the burns or burned area. Such victims need to be protected and taken to medical help as soon as possible. This problem will be covered in detail in Chapter 9.

Snakebite

The bite of the venomous snake is a problem that needs emergency care. There are several measures that can be taken. The most important factor to keep in mind is to get the snakebite victim to the hospital and/or medical help in the safest manner. Snakebite emergency care is one, if not, the greatest controversial area of emergency care. Several different methods will be presented in Chapter 13.

Stings—Bees, Wasps, Hornets, etc.

The speed at which the poison or venom works in the case of the stinging insect is most significant. If the victim of the sting is sensitive or allergic to this poison, he can be in a serious condition in a matter of minutes. This subject is discussed at length in Chapter 13.

The Cursory Examination [65]

THE CURSORY EXAMINATION

This is the physical check of the injured person at the accident scene by the first-aider. It is important to determine the nature of the injuries so the individual can be protected and information can be furnished to medical personnel later caring for the injured. Also, it will help if the hospital is prepared to receive the victim, especially in hurry-type situations such as hemorrhage, asphyxia, poison, shock, snakebite, and burns. In making the cursory examination, the first-aider should check

1. *For breathing.* This can usually be detected by placing the face close to the victim's mouth and nose, feeling the air escape, and by watching the movements of the chest and the nostrils of the nose. If breathing has stopped or is inadequate, this will probably be indicated by the bluish (cyanotic) skin, nails, and lips.
2. *For hemorrhage or bleeding.* This may be visible as a pool of blood or there may be blood-soaked clothes. There may also be bleeding from the mouth and other body openings.
3. *For poisoning.* The mouth and breath should be examined for odors, particles, stains, and burns and the abdomen checked for pain. The presence of alcohol or the sweet breath of diabetic coma may tend to mislead and give the impression that poisoning has not occurred.
4. *The neck and back.* If the victim is conscious, ask if there is pain in either area. The position of the head and neck should be observed. If he is positioned abnormally, and there is no effort to change or right the position, a neck injury should be suspected. Ask the victim to move his hands and feet. If he is unconscious, a pin or sharp-pointed object should be used to stick the palm and sole of his hand and foot for a reflex. If the conscious victim cannot move his hands or feet or if the unconscious victim fails to respond to the induced stimulus, it can be assumed there is an injury in this area and that the greatest possible protection must be given to prevent further injury here or injury to the spinal cord.
5. *The head.* The eyes, ears, nose, and mouth should be examined. The first-aider should look for bumps, bruises, soft places, or depressions on the head. Note whether the mouth is open or closed and note the alignment (occlusion) of the teeth. If the teeth do not meet this may indicate a fracture or dislocated jaw.
6. *The shoulder.* A person should gently palpate with his fingers the clavicles and the shoulder for tenderness and note any irregularity that could mean fracture or dislocation. If the victim tends to give way to his shoulder or clavicle by leaning or slumping to the injured side and tends to support that extremity, then one can suspect an injury to the shoulder or collarbone. An x-ray will confirm the suspicion but the first-aider can give some protection at the scene.
7. *The chest, or thorax.* The chest, or thorax, should be examined by gently feeling with the fingers. If the victim is conscious, ask if breathing is painful.

[66] Cursory Examination: Physical Check of the Injured

If the victim's breathing is fast and shallow and there was a blow to this area, then one can reasonably suspect a rib fracture or injury to the thorax.

8. *The abdomen.* The abdomen should be examined for muscular spasm. The muscles of the abdominal wall tend to contract if there is an injury in this area or internal bleeding.

9. *The arms and legs.* The extremities, arms and legs, can be carefully checked for position and also for possible abnormal motion when the victim attempts to move them. The first-aider can gently feel the arm and legs with his fingers, carefully following the bones. Sensitive areas and abnormalities can indicate bone or joint troubles and should be protected. In case of doubt, protect by splinting.

10. *The hips and pelvis.* Falls, automobile accidents, and other severe and crushing-type situations frequently involve the pelvis. The first-aider should check for extreme pain in this area and the abnormal position of the legs. If there is the possibility of an injured pelvis, the person must be kept off his feet. He should be protected before being moved. It would be far better to protect a person as though his pelvis were broken and be wrong than to let a victim with a fractured pelvis try to walk.

11. *The eyes.* The eyes of the victim should be carefully observed as there are several indications that can come from them which are helpful, as (a) The pupils of the eyes are dilated widely and equally. This is an indication of shock or fainting. (b) The pupils of the eyes are unequal in size, one dilated widely and the other small or smaller. This is an indication of a head or brain injury such as apoplexy, concussion, cerebral hemorrhage. (c) The pupils are very small in size, pinpoint. This is a strong indication of an overdose of a drug or narcotic. (d) The pupils of the eyes do not change in size when they are subjected to light (pupil reflex). This is an indication that too little blood is reaching the brain, that death is imminent. This is a most meaningful index to use in connection with heart failure to determine if the heart is beating. This check must be made before beginning external cardiac compression, which is discussed in detail in Chapter 8.

12. *The color of skin.* This observation can be made in a hurry and is helpful especially if the victim is unconscious. The skin color points to the following problems: (a) Blue skin (cyanosis) always indicates asphyxia. (b) White skin indicates bleeding, shock, heat exhaustion, fainting, poison, freezing, and convulsion. (c) Red skin indicates sunstroke, apoplexy, drunkenness, skull fracture and concussion, and epilepsy. It is quite evident that the skin and the eyes are good symptomatic indices in the evaluation of emergency situations.

13. *The pulse.* This can be taken better at the carotid, femoral, or radial artery. It is the indication that the heart is beating. Normally, the heart continues to beat for several minutes after breathing ceases.

14. *For vomiting.* Normally this suggests nausea or indigestion; however, it may also mean poisoning, heart attack, and alcohol.

Additional General Symptoms to Observe [67]

15 *The blood from body openings.* Blood from the ear canal could mean brain injury. Nasal bleeding is an indication more likely of a broken nose or a broken mucous membrane in the nose. Oral or mouth bleeding could be frothy blood (full of air) coming from the lungs due to a lung injury. Bright blood from the mouth could mean stomach injury such as a perforation of an ulcer. Dark blood appearing as coffee grounds from the mouth would indicate older blood. Blood in the urine which follows an injury to the back could indicate kidney injury. Bright red blood in the stool could indicate hemorrhoids and tarry black stools indicate a more serious problem such as cancer.

ADDITIONAL GENERAL SYMPTOMS TO OBSERVE

In addition to the symptoms just discussed, there are other general symptoms that the first-aider should be aware of

1 *Pain in the abdomen.* The appendix area is in the lower right quadrant of the abdomen. It should be checked if appendicitis is suspected.
2 *Sudden swelling of a joint or other part.* This could indicate a possible sprain, strain, or dislocation. If this is discolored, internal bleeding is quite likely.
3 *Severe pain at the site of an animal bite or sting.* There would be definite marks to indicate (a) snakebite by any pit-viper would leave two definite punctures; (b) bee, wasp, hornet, and yellow jacket would leave a definite single puncture, however, these insects are capable of stinging several times leaving as many punctures as stings or a multiple of stings; (c) spider bites usually indicate a single puncture, unless there is more than one bite; (d) dog and cat bites can leave puncture-type bites from the long canine teeth or can leave tearing-type lacerations depending upon the nature of the bite or attack; and (e) bites from rodents (squirrel, rat, or mouse) probably would be of the puncture type. The rat bite is especially dangerous from the standpoint of infection.
4 *Raised skin area filled with blood or fluid.* These are commonly known as blisters and the fluid content within can be blood or lymph, depending upon the type of blister.
5 *Painful and inflamed wounds.* These are the infected wounds that are characterized by swelling, red skin, and pus. Such wounds include boils, styes, pimples, and other skin infections.
6 *Discolored skin areas.* These may be red, bluish, or both with unbroken skin and called a bruise or contusion. There has been a severe blow, and internal bleeding is indicated. Emergency care is needed and probably medical attention.
7 *Reddened skin and blister.* Red skin and no blister is a first degree burn as in sunburn. If the blister stage is present, a second degree burn is indicated.

[68]   Cursory Examination: Physical Check of the Injured

8   *Convulsions in children and adults.* These may occur after a fever, or the person may be an epileptic.

When these symptoms occur, caution should be exercised and appropriate action taken. Certainly such information should be made available to the rescue and medical personnel.

RULES TO FOLLOW DURING AND AFTER CURSORY CHECK

The first-aider is not a physician; consequently, there is need for following a series of guidelines in giving emergency protection to the injured:

1. Call for medical help as soon as it is possible.
2. Keep one's self under control. Be positive in speech and action, and especially be careful about what is said.
3. Improvise and use the supplies at hand, even items of clothing if need be.
4. Keep the victim in the best position, usually down and flat on the back (supine). If he has breathing trouble, raise the head and shoulders. If he is unconscious, elevate the feet. The slogan "face red, raise the head, face white, raise the feet" has some merit and is good to remember.
5. Check carefully for bleeding, breathing, poisoning, wounds, broken bones, burns, and shock. Take appropriate action.
6. Be sure that the victim has an open airway and can breathe, otherwise put into the correct position by placing on the back (supine) and extending the chin as far up and the head as far back as possible.
7. If in doubt, do nothing more than protect by keeping the victim down and warm and by getting medical help at the earliest moment.
8. Splint a dislocation or fracture before moving the victim.
9. Protect the victim from his own vomitus and other secretions from the mouth which might block the breathing passage and make breathing difficult or impossible.
10. Give nothing by mouth to an unconscious person, and give nothing by mouth to a person suffering from abdominal pain. Anything placed in the mouth can cause muscular activity in the intestinal tract.
11. Keep the victim warm but not overly so. A person in shock can easily lose to much fluid if kept too warm.
12. Protect all open wounds by covering, if possible with a sterile dressing.
13. Never move the victim until his injury is determined. If needed the transportation should be correct, otherwise there might be additional injury.

It is important for the first-aider to have a definite and predetermined set of rules, guides, or principles to follow in making the cursory or physical check of the accident victim. Such a first-aider should prove beneficial to the injured person.

ACTIVITIES

1 Simulate an accident situation before the class and demonstrate how to conduct the cursory examination.
2 Consult experienced rescue and first-aid personnel in your community or area and find out how much training they have had. Inquire about specific training, refresher courses, and any new trends in the field of emergency care.
3 Discuss with the local or county civil defense director, the trauma program director, or the ambulance director how their programs differ from first-aid training.
4 Visit several accident scenes and determine the cause of the accidents. Attend the coroner's inquests in your county and listen and report on the proceedings.

QUESTIONS TO ANSWER

1 What are hurry cases?
2 Why is the sting of certain insects so dangerous for some people?
3 Why is asphyxia considered to be the number-one first-aid problem?
4 Why does the U.S. Navy consider asphyxia to be the foremost of the hurry cases?
5 Why are the eyes important to observe in making the cursory examination?
6 What can the rescuer learn from the accident scene?
7 What questions would a person ask a victim who had received a concussion or a hard blow to the head?
8 Under what conditions is there too little oxygen to sustain life? How would a person test a cave, well, or silo to find out about oxygen before entering?
9 How meaningful is the skin as an index or guide in making the cursory check?
10 Blood may leave the body through several natural openings. How does the blood differ in color?

SELECTED REFERENCES

AMERICAN NATIONAL RED CROSS, *Advanced First Aid and Emergency Care*. New York: Doubleday, 1973.
AMERICAN NATIONAL RED CROSS, *Standard First Aid and Personal Safety*. New York: Doubleday, 1973.

[70] Cursory Examination: Physical Check of the Injured

COLE, WARREN H., and PUESTOW, CHARLES B., *First Aid Diagnosis and Management.* New York: Appleton-Century-Crofts, 1965.

HENDERSON, JOHN, *Emergency Medical Guide*, 4th ed. New York: McGraw-Hill, 1978.

6. WOUNDS

Wounds are of two major types—the open, in which the skin is entered or broken, and the closed (contusion), in which the skin is not broken but the impact from a damaging object has injured or crushed tissues lying below the injury point. Needless to say, wounds can vary from a tiny pinprick or paper cut to an amputation. There can be bleeding, shock, infection, and other complications resulting from such bodily injuries. From the standpoint of emergency care or protection, one should not overlook the so-called minor wounds because a serious infection may result from such neglect.

OPEN WOUNDS

Open wounds are wounds in which there is an opening or break in the mucous membrane or skin; such wounds are known as abrasions, incisions, lacerations, avulsions, and puncture wounds. From the open wound, regardless of the nature or type of the wound, there is always the danger of bleeding (hemorrhage) and infection. It is the first-aider's primary task to control the bleeding and lessen or prevent the possibility of infection. Different types of wounds are shown in Figure 6.1

Abrasions

Abrasions can best be described as the scraping or rubbing off of the outside layer of the skin or mucous membrane. Abrasions are caused from falling and sliding on rough surfaces—e.g., the track man or runner falling and sliding on a cinder track; a bicycle, scooter, or motorcycle rider falling

[71]

[72] Wounds

and sliding on the pavement; or a basketball player receiving a floor burn from a fall and sliding on the gymnasium floor. Such injuries to the skin are common in baseball, track, football, and basketball. Certainly they can result from a wide variety of activities in which there is running and the possibility of falling or sliding.

Of the different types of wounds, the abrasion is the most superficial and probably not as serious as the other types; however, it is possible for the abrasion to cover a large area and for the scratches to penetrate well into the lower layers of the skin. Since the abrasion quite likely will occur on the street, gymnasium floor, sidewalk, running track, industrial plant, or other area which is heavily contaminated, infection as well as superficial bleeding is a likely possibility.

Abrasions can best be protected by controlling the bleeding, which usually is not a big problem because the wounds are not deep. Infection is a more serious danger in abrasive-type wounds than is bleeding. Consequently, it is suggested that the abrasions be carefully washed if possible with soap and water, using the cleanest possible dressing or cloth to do the washing. It is also suggested that the first-aider wash toward the outide of the wound and not toward the wound. As dirt quite likely will be ground into the wound, an effort should be made to remove the dirt. After the soap and water cleansing, it is helpful to bathe the wound with alcohol. It is not recommended that an antiseptic be put onto the wound, as some antiseptics may be injurious to the skin. The wound should be covered with a sterile dressing.

If the abrasion is large and does not respond to first-aid protection, then the service of a physician should be sought immediately. If the abrasion is deep and contaminated with dirt and other debris, a physician quite likely will administer tetanus protection. Tetanus protection will be discussed later in this chapter. School and recreation personnel should seek medical advice and have established procedures to follow concerning wounds. If the dressing sticks to the abrasion, hydrogen peroxide is helpful in removing it.

Incisions

The incised wound is usually caused by a can opener, sharp knife, razor blade, manila folder, piece of paper, glass, or some other sharp instrument. These breaks in the skin or mucous membrane are usually clean and they can go deeply into the underlying tissues and be especially dangerous from the standpoint of bleeding or hemorrhage. Veins, arteries, tendons, muscles, and other tissues can be severed or injured by such penetrating instruments. Infection is not a major concern from the incised wound; nevertheless, the skin has been broken and bacteria could have entered, thus the danger of infection may exist.

Incised wounds can be protected by washing them with soap and

Open Wounds [73]

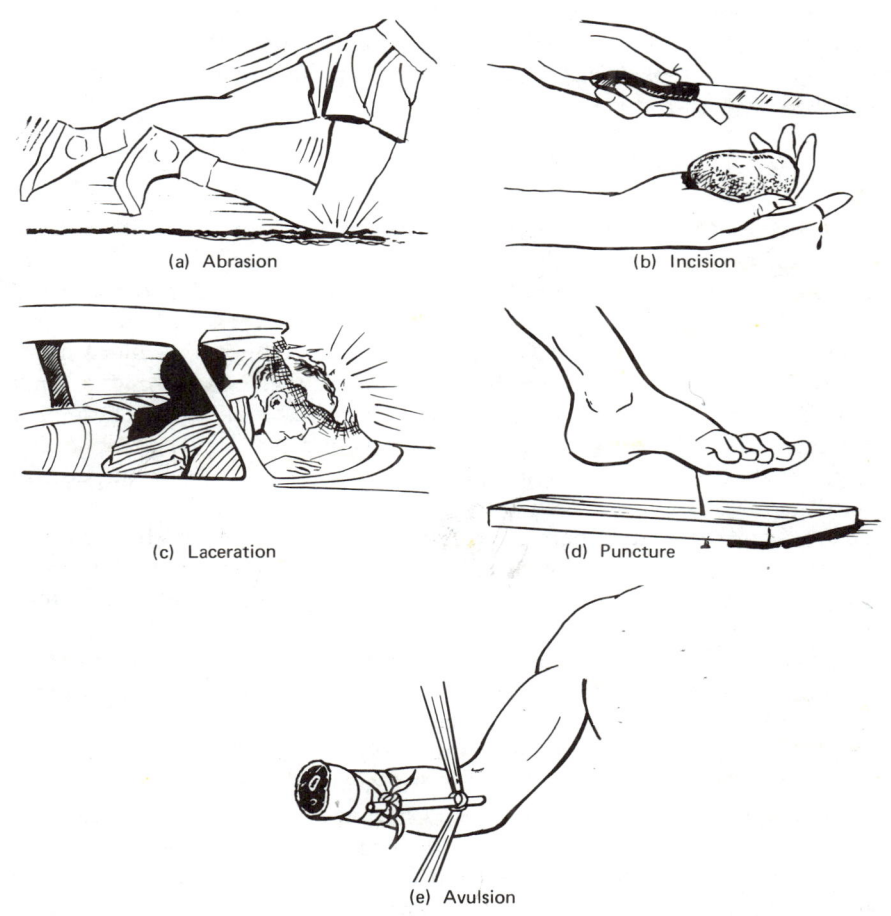

(a) Abrasion

(b) Incision

(c) Laceration

(d) Puncture

(e) Avulsion

FIGURE 6.1 Types of wounds.

water and by covering them with a sterile dressing. The small incision can be covered and protected after careful washing with a small compress known commercially as the adhesive compress or Band-Aid. There is some argument about the use of an antiseptic on incisions. It is suggested that this question be put to the family physician or the school's medical adviser for recommended procedures. There are several satisfactory antiseptics readily available. Many persons feel that washing the incision with soap and water, applying the recommended antiseptic, and covering with a sterile dressing or compress is the correct procedure to follow in caring for wounds.

If the incision is large, deep, and bleeding profusely, the first-aider should attempt to control the bleeding, cover the wound with a sterile dressing, and take the victim immediately to medical help. This is not a

[74] Wounds

first-aid problem. The first-aider only protects until medical help assumes responsibility. In the event that medical help is not obtainable, then the first-aider would of necessity use his very best judgment and do what he felt had to be done.

Lacerations

Lacerations are wounds in which the tissues are torn and have uneven and ragged edges. The Latin root *lacer* means to tear. Such wounds are most usually caused by blunt objects—e.g., a large piece of wood or metal driven or forced into the body tissue. The automobile and other vehicle accidents, with their great forces of impact upon collision, produce many such injuries as the victims are battered about during the collision. Many newspaper accounts state that "the victim received multiple lacerations of the face and body." The laceration is the wound that leaves an ugly scar. Usually the wound needs the attention of the physician or surgeon to neatly trim and suture it. Since a laceration can and often does penetrate deeply into the body, there is a danger of hemorrhage. When there is injury to deep tissues, the possibility of infection is enhanced because a variety of foreign substances, including infection-producing bacteria, may have entered the body.

Lacerations can be protected by carefully cleansing the wound. This should be done by the first-aider only in the event of a minor laceration. The laceration should be cleansed with soap and water. Minor lacerations can be closed by using adhesive tape strips, such as the "butterfly" tape strip which can be purchased at the drugstore or easily made.

After closing the wound, it should be covered with a sterile dressing. If the laceration is large and beyond the scope of the first-aider, the wound should be protected by covering with a sterile dressing, and the victim taken immediately to medical help. The avulsion type wound which is similar to the laceration will be discussed later.

Punctures

Punctures are wounds caused by the penetration of a sharp object into the deeper and underlying body tissues. Such a sharp object might be a nail, knife, splinter, ice pick, bullet, spear, or arrow. Such wounds may be small on the surface but may penetrate several inches into the body or, in the case of the bullet, may pass entirely through the body. Such penetrations and the accompanying foreign object may enter any organ of the body, depending upon the point of entry and the object's path. Consequently, the danger of punctures is great, and internal bleeding and shock are eminent dangers.

Puncture-type wounds are usually regarded as being the most serious. They do not bleed externally because the wound closes after the entrance of the object. There may be serious internal bleeding, and the chance of infection is significant because an infectious organism has entered and the wound is closed. If the wound is incurred in a location such as a garden, barn yard, pasture land, or street, which would make tetanus a possibility, steps must be taken to protect the victim from this very dangerous infection.

Other wounds that must be considered as puncture wounds are the bites of animals and reptiles and the stings of insects. These will be treated in Chapter 13 in some detail.

Avulsions

This tearing-type wound involves the separation of tissues. It may involve the loss of an arm, ear, leg, or finger from the body. Avulsion wounds may cause much blood loss and possible shock. Common causes of avulsion wounds include animal bites and the automotive, gun, and heavy machine accidents. With good care it is not uncommon for the severed part to be reunited with the body.

CLOSED WOUNDS: CONTUSIONS OR BRUISES

Closed wounds are wounds in which the skin or outside body covering is not broken. However, underlying body tissues have been injured by a sustained impact or blow, usually from a blunt object or great force. These wounds are commonly known as bruises, and the noticeable discoloration results from the rupturing of blood capillaries in the injured area. Such injuries are quite common in all physical activities, especially the so-called contact sports of football, wrestling, soccer, baseball, and basketball. Protective equipment and padding for the contestant help to lessen the chance of the contusion or bruise type of wound.

To protect the contusion after the injury has occurred, it is suggested:

1. That cold compresses be applied to constrict the blood vessels in the immediate area to lessen the internal or tissue bleeding.
2. That the injured person be placed in a prone position and the injured part be immobilized. It would also be helpful to elevate the injured part to reduce circulation to the area. This can easily be accomplished if the injury is to the leg or arm.
3. That heat, preferably hot and wet, be applied to the injured part starting at a reasonable period of time, 24 hours after the injury. The black eye is a bruise and should be protected in the same manner as other bruises.
4. That the person who has received such a wound be protected against shock by keeping him warm, giving him water, and also comforting words.
5. That the injured person be provided medical help (x-ray examination and

[76] Wounds

treatment) after 24 hours if the injury is massive and there are indications of little improvement. The first-aider should protect the victim and furnish suitable transportation.

SPECIAL WOUNDS

Several wounds have been classified as special wounds because they present unique problems. Nosebleeds related to certain kinds of conditions can be quite serious. Gunshot wounds can be most destructive with their blasting and penetrating power. The fishhook with its barbs can be very damaging, and it is important that fishermen and others know how to remove the hook and treat the wound. Because of the preciousness of the eye, any injury to it should be handled carefully. The fingers are in constant use and danger, and special caution should be given them. Splinters and thorns present special problems as they produce puncture-type wounds.

Nosebleed

Some persons have frequent nosebleeds, especially children. It is possible to rupture the tiny blood vessels in the mucous membrane of the nose by hard blowing, a blow to the nose, or a broken nose. Sometimes nosebleed occurs following severe infections and sickness. Persons suffering from high blood pressure may experience this problem. High altitudes may induce bleeding from the nose also.

To protect a nosebleed, the victim should be placed in a sitting position with the head tilted back. If this is not possible, then elevate the head and shoulders from the position of lying on the back (supine). Cold applications, ice pack or bag, should be applied to the head, face, nose, and neck. Some suggest inserting sterile cotton into each nostril and applying gentle pressure with the fingers. The victim should be quiet and not be permitted to blow his nose, walk, smoke, or drink coffee. If the bleeding is intense and persists he should be examined by a physician.

Eye Injury

The eye is the most precious of the special sense organs, and any injury or interference that affects the eyes should be handled with the greatest of care. If dust, dirt, or an insect becomes lodged in the area between the eye and the eyelid, it should be carefully removed. The first-aider should very carefully wash his hands and, with a clean cloth (never dry cotton), carefully locate and remove the foreign object. The victim can assist by moving his eyes upon request. If the eye is injured and the eyeball punctured, the first-aider should carefully cover the injured eye with a sterile dressing and take the victim to an ophthalmologist or physician. If

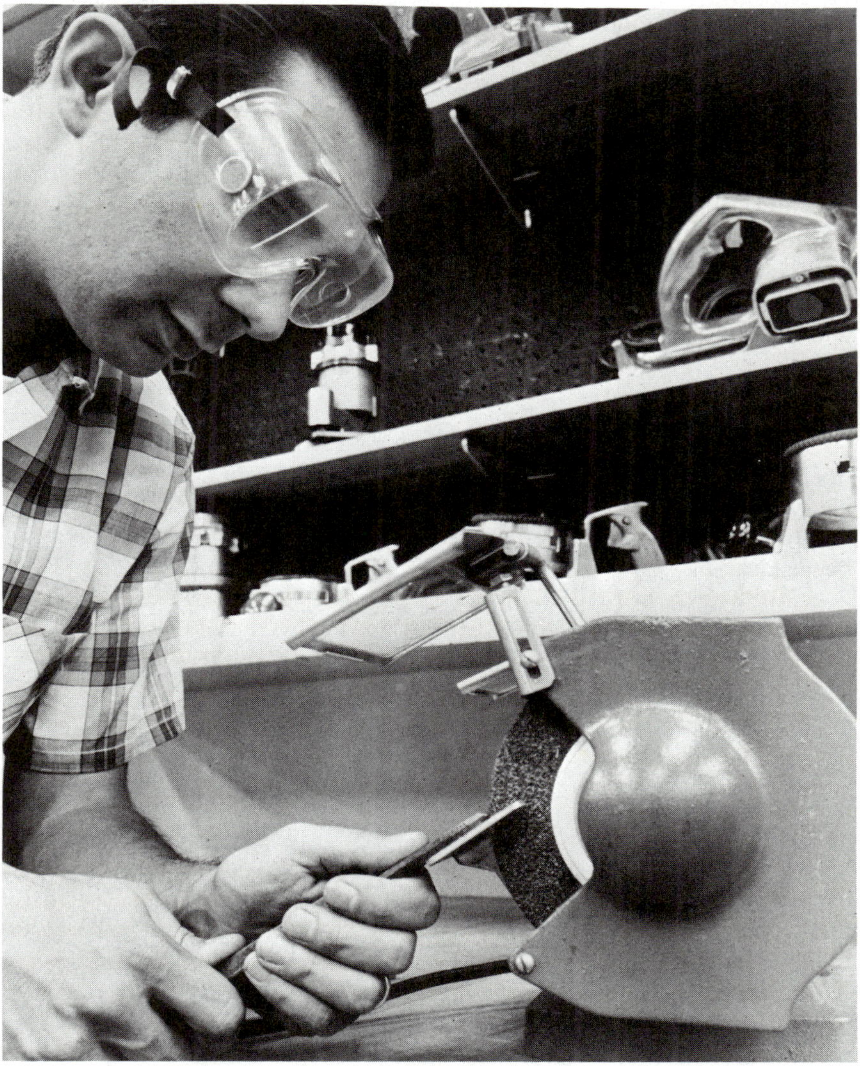

FIGURE 6.2 Safety glasses prevent needless eye injuries. (Power Tool Institute, Inc.)

a foreign body is lodged, no attempt should be made to remove it. The eye should be bandaged to avoid pressure, and medical help sought. If eye movement would enhance the damage, both eyes should be covered.

Gunshot Wounds

There are a variety of guns and ammunition, and the potential for bodily injury from them is great. The shotgun at close range is a most lethal weapon and is capable of tearing away massive areas. Slugs from

[78] Wounds

pistols and rifles vary from steel jackets capable of much penetration to lead slugs and hollow points. Their explosive action can do extensive damage.

The gunshot wound is a great producer of shock. Slugs from rifles and pistols can penetrate the liver, lungs, stomach, intestine, and other internal organs and cause massive and intense bleeding, both internal and external.

The victim of the gunshot wound should be kept down and warm. External bleeding should be controlled if possible and the victim should be delivered to a hospital or physician as soon as possible. Internal bleeding can be controlled only by the surgeon.

Such wounds must be reported to legal authorities. The first-aider should do nothing that might destroy helpful evidence concerning the gun incident, accident, suicide attempt, or suicide.

Finger Injuries

Many injuries occur to the hands owing to the variety of uses to which one puts the human hand. There are cuts, scratches, splinters, thorns, hangnails, and burns with the possibility of injuring blood vessels, nerves, tendons, and muscles, as well as skin. Fingers can be broken and joints can be dislocated.

The wounds of the hand should be cleansed with soap and water and covered with sterile dressings. Strong antiseptics should not be used. If there is an indication or likelihood that a finger is broken or out of place, it should be x-rayed and then protected by splinting so that it can properly mend. Unattended broken fingers and injured joints may leave permanently crippled fingers.

Fishhook Wounds

Fishhook wounds need special care. Most fishhooks are equipped with barbs to hold fish and to prevent the hook from backing out. When fishhooks become fast in one's body, the hook, if possible, should be forced forward through the flesh; the barbs removed with wire snips and then the remainder of hook should be backed out. This will prevent the tearing of tissues, including muscles, nerves, and blood vessels. The fishhook wound should be washed carefully with soap and water and covered with a sterile dressing. Since the bait was probably contaminated there should be protection against tetanus, and an antibiotic given by a physician to help resist infection. In cases of fishhook accidents, if possible medical help should be sought.

Thorns and Splinters

Small thorns and splinters should be carefully removed by the first-aider. It is advisable to disinfect the area by washing it with soap and water or by using alcohol. The instrument for removal should be sterilized

Hemorrhage and Bleeding [79]

over a flame, and the first-aider's hands should be washed. The thorn or splinter should be carefully removed and the wound protected with an antiseptic and covered with a sterile dressing. Large pieces of wood and other matter driven or forced into the body should be removed by a physician. Such injuries require medical action including suturing and protection against infection, tetanus, shock, and hemorrhage.

HEMORRHAGE AND BLEEDING

Hemorrhage usually refers to bleeding when it is profuse, and the loss of blood may be serious. The goal of the attendant is to control bleeding at the earliest moment possible because the human body does not have an excess supply of this precious life-giving substance.

Hemorrhage can be external or internal. The first-aider can respond physically in an effort to control or protect external bleeding. However, in the event of internal bleeding the first-aider can only keep the person quiet and warm, lessen shock, obtain suitable transportation, and deliver the victim to medical help as soon as it is possible.

Types of Bleeding

When there is external bleeding, the blood escapes from the capillaries, veins, or arteries. If the wound is large or deep, bleeding could come from all three sources. First-aiders should be able to recognize the type of bleeding in order to protect the victim.

Capillary Bleeding The most common type of bleeding is from the capillaries. Such bleeding is described as "capillary oozing." A Band-Aid or sterile pad will ordinarily control capillary bleeding. Also, cold application will hasten coagulation by constricting the blood vessels. With all minor cuts, scratches, and abrasions this type of bleeding is expected.

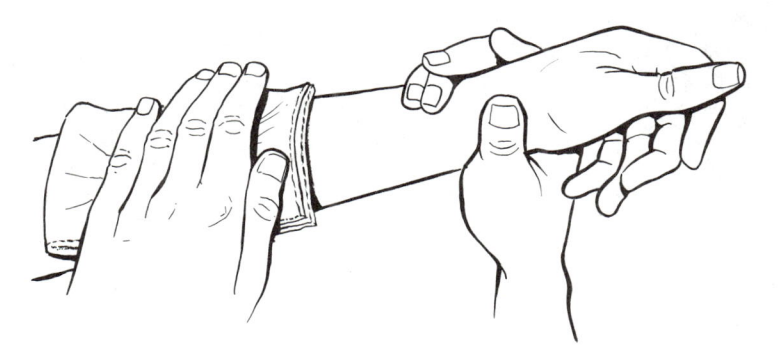

FIGURE 6.3 Direct pressure for hemorrhage control.

[80]   Wounds

Venous Bleeding   Venous bleeding occurs when a vein is severed or punctured, usually by a cutting instrument. Such bleeding will be characterized by an even flow of blood. There will be no pulsations as in arterial bleeding. Frequently it is said that the venous blood will be darker in color; however, this is a poor index, as there is usually no available arterial blood for making the comparison. The vein could be small or, on the other hand, could be large, as from the jugular vein in the neck.

To control venous bleeding, one should think first in terms of pressure. Pressure can be applied in several ways:

1. By placing a compress over the wound and grasping it firmly with the hand. As one compress becomes saturated, place the second compress over the first, then the third, etc. Do not remove the compress to disturb the clot formation, but continue to add one compress on top of another until bleeding is stopped.
2. By using digital pressure on the supplying vein or blood vessel below the wound. It is well to remember that veins carry blood toward the heart, so the supplying vessel will be below, or away from, the wound.
3. By elevating, as high as possible, the injured part from which the blood is escaping. Gravity can be a helpful factor in bringing the bleeding under control.

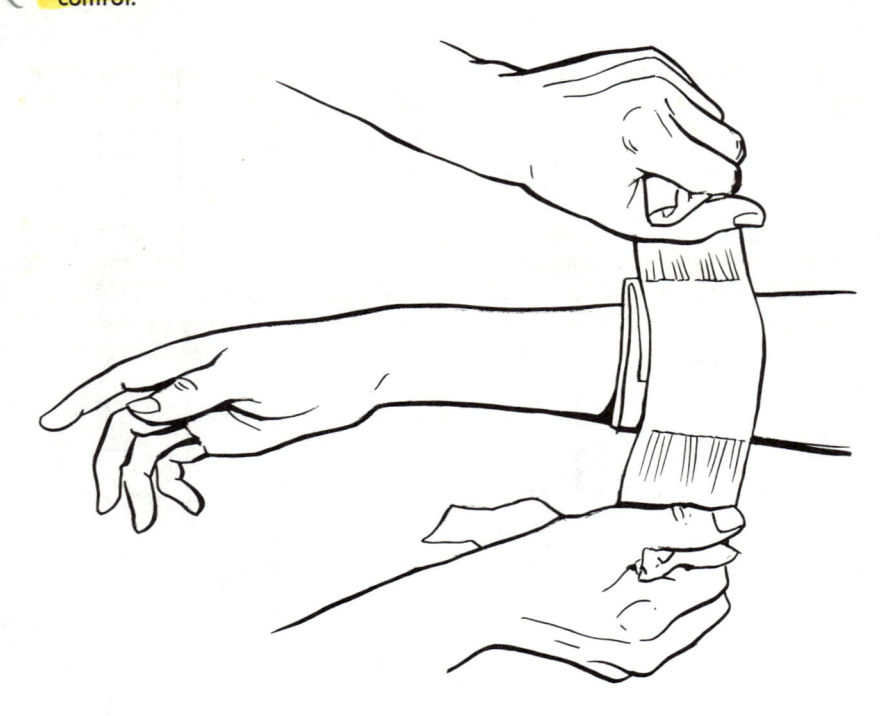

FIGURE 6.4   Large sterile compress used to control bleeding.

Hemorrhage and Bleeding [81]

4 By applying cold applications. The use of cold over the area, ice packs or cold packs, will cause the supplying blood vessels to constrict and thus lessen the supply and flow of blood, consequently helping to control the flow of blood from the wound.

Arterial Bleeding Bleeding from an artery will occur when the artery is severed or opened. Because arteries are more deeply located in the body, they are afforded the natural protection provided by the bones and other body structures. Injuries to the arteries are not common; however, when they are injured or severed, the condition is more serious and controlling the flow of blood is a matter of great concern to the first-aider and also to medical personnel.

Bleeding from an artery is characterized by the irregular spurting of blood. The arteries are always full of blood, and the pulsation caused by the contraction of the left ventricle of the heart, some 70 to 80 times per minute, results in the spurting. The blood may be a brighter red color, but without venous blood for comparison it would be difficult to distinguish. Some of the large arteries that can be involved in accidents are the carotids on either side of the neck, the brachials of the upper arms, the radials of the lower arm, and the femorals of the thigh. Fortunately, the great artery, the aorta or dorsal artery, is well protected. Any injury to the aorta would quickly take the life if it were severed. To control arterial bleeding, the following is suggested.

1 *Direct pressure and cold.* The wound should be covered with heavy compresses and direct pressure applied. This can be done by hand pressure or by binding the compress in place with a triangular bandage. Cold applications are worth trying to help constrict small blood vessels.
2 *Elevation.* Elevate the injured part and keep the victim as quiet as possible.
3 *Pressure points.* These pressure points refer to large arteries that are close to the surface and can be located easily with the fingers. The fingers can

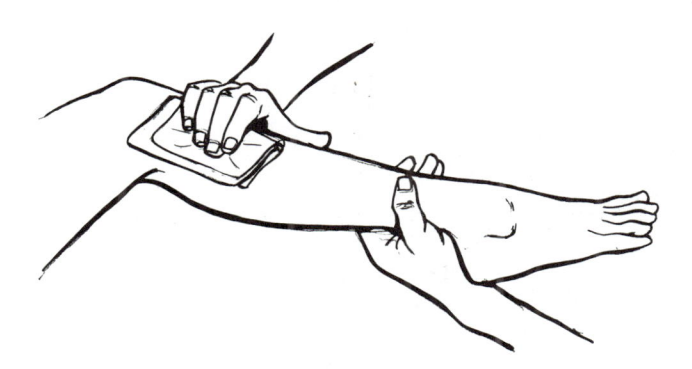

FIGURE 6.5 Direct pressure with compress to control bleeding.

Wounds

be used to apply pressure to the artery in order to lessen or control the flow of blood from the severed artery. The pressure points most commonly used and recommended to the first-aider are shown in Figure 6.6.

a. **Temporal artery.** This is a relatively small artery located in front of the ear. Pressure applied to this artery by the fingers can control arterial bleeding from arteries of the forehead and head.

b. **Facial artery.** This artery is found beneath the lower jaw. There is a notch in the lower jaw, and pushing up with the first finger behind this notch will locate the facial artery. Pressure against this artery can control arterial bleeding from the chin and lower face, including the upper lip.

c. **Carotid artery.** This is the large artery on either side of the neck, the arteries that supply the brain. The carotids can be located on either side of the neck by pushing in with the finger in the area of the trachea and larynx. When the carotid is severed, hemorrhage is severe, and the first-aider would be compelled to apply pressure to this area, first by placing a compress over the wound and then by using his four fingers to create pressure. Immediate transportation to medical help is mandatory, since a life could be lost in a short time.

d. **Subclavian artery.** This artery and the pressure point that it implies are well named. The subclavian artery is beneath the collarbone. Pressure can be applied to this artery by pushing down with the thumb behind

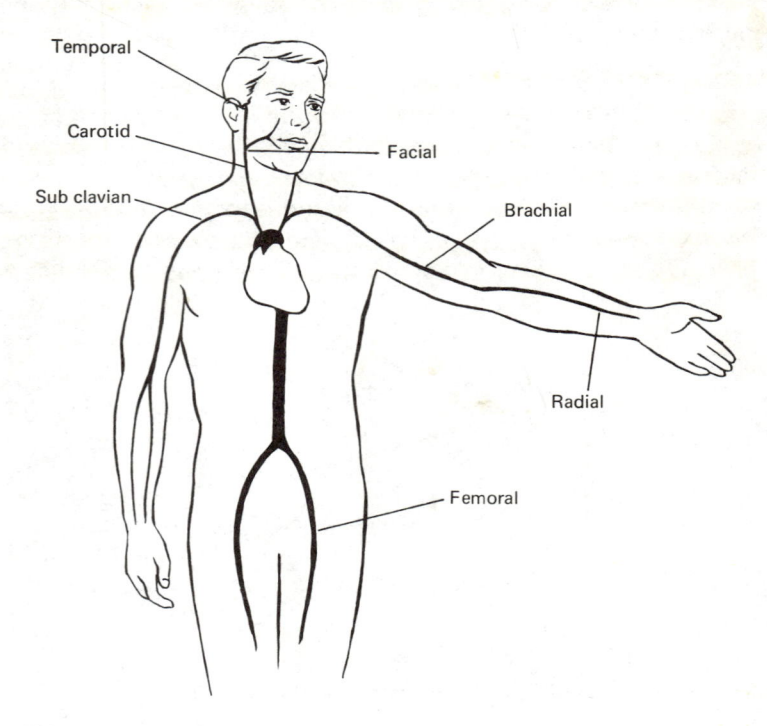

FIGURE 6.6 Pressure points.

Hemorrhage and Bleeding [83]

the collarbone or clavicle and against the top of the first rib where this artery crosses over. As the subclavian artery supplies the brachial artery, the best way to control bleeding when the arm is torn off at the shoulder is to use this pressure point and apply pressure against the subclavian artery with the fingers.

e. Brachial artery. This is the great artery of the upper arm. By applying finger pressure against this artery, bleeding can be controlled in the upper and lower arm. Because the brachial artery follows the humerus and is on the inside of the arm, it is suggested that the first-aider use all four fingers to apply the pressure. The arm should be raised, and the first-aider should reach around the back of the arm, placing the four fingers between the bicep and the tricep muscles and hold the artery against the humerus. The other hand and fingers can monitor the radial artery at the wrist.

f. Femoral artery. This is the major artery of the lower leg, and bleeding from the femoral can be controlled by pressure from the heel of the hand. The pressure should be applied where the femoral crosses over the pelvis at either groin, depending on the extremity that has been injured. The victim should be in a lying (supine) position. The first-aider can push upward with the heel of the hand against the femoral artery and the pelvis, extending the arm to apply pressure to control the bleeding. Considerable pressure may be required to control hemorrhage from the femoral artery. This is an easy artery to locate. The femoral is an important artery to monitor for the pulse when the victim of a heart attack is being given external cardiac compression.

In the event of a major injury with arterial bleeding in the leg, bleeding or hemorrhage can be controlled by maintaining pressure with the heel of the hand on this very important artery.

g. Other pressure points. For the first-aider, industrial nurse, police officer, coach and physical educator, the previously mentioned pressure points will serve them well; however, there are a number of other arteries that are close to the surface and can also be used for the control of bleeding.

Internal Bleeding Such bleeding refers to bleeding or the escape of blood inside one of the body cavities. There is little that the first-aider can do about internal bleeding other than keep the victim down and quiet, control shock, and obtain or provide the best transportation possible to medical help. Common causes of such bleeding are knife wounds, bullet wounds, crushing injuries, perforated ulcers, punctured lungs, ruptured kidneys, and other organ injuries. The following indications, which may prove helpful to the first-aider for making such a determination, are suggested by Henderson as basic symptoms:

1 Restlessness
2 Thirst
3 Faintness

4 Dizziness
5 Cold and clammy skin
6 Dilated pupils
7 Shallow and irregular breathing
8 Thin, rapid, weak, and irregular pulse beat
9 Great anxiety.[1]

USE OF THE TOURNIQUET

> Many physicians suggest that use of the tourniquet should never be taught in first aid courses. Organizations interested in first aid education indicate that the tourniquet may be used justifiably upon rare occasions, but there is general agreement that it is applied far too often and that harmful effects are common. Almost always, bleeding can be controlled by firm, direct pressure over the wound with a pad or cloth. The National Research Council advises that the tourniquet should be used only for a severe hemorrhage that cannot be controlled by other means. Use of the tourniquet might for example be the only effective way to stop bleeding in case of an extensive wound such as a partial amputation of the thigh or arm.[2]

The content of the preceding quotation should be taught in all first-aid courses—college, high school, police personnel, industrial nurses, and first-aid and rescue groups. Until emergency medical services are greatly improved and more readily available, it seems quite likely that people with too little knowledge may have to try as best they can to save a life by using the tourniquet in such trying situations.

Since one of the most common mistakes in emergency care involves the use of the tourniquet, at the present time it is recommended that it be used only in the most severe cases, such as amputations and other injuries involving massive bleeding from the extremities. Large compresses and pressure will control many cases of arterial bleeding and they should be used. The tourniquet is the last resort for the first-aider.

The tourniquet should be a flat, soft, and reasonably wide material such as a triangular bandage folded several times into a cravat about two or three inches wide. Preferably it should be placed halfway between the shoulder and elbow or midway on the thigh. If necessary a tourniquet may be placed close to the wound, always between the wound and the heart.

The tourniquet should be tightened sufficiently to stop the bleeding. If it is not tight enough it may encourage more bleeding. The twisting device should be strong enough to twist and to hold. After the tourniquet

---

[1] John Henderson, *Emergency Medical Guide*, 4th ed. New York: McGraw-Hill, 1978, p. 161.
[2] Carl J. Potthoff, "First Aid," *Today's Health*. February, 1966.

Use of the Tourniquet [85]

is in place and tightened, it should remain on the victim until he reaches medical help, a doctor, or the hospital. Only as a last resort should a rope or cord be used to control the bleeding.

The tourniquet should not be concealed, and if possible the victim should be attended continuously. It is suggested that the time of application of the tourniquet be indicated on the victim. Hemorrhage is a "hurry case" and even though a tourniquet is applied transportation to medical help is a first priority for the victim. This technique (Figure 6.7) should

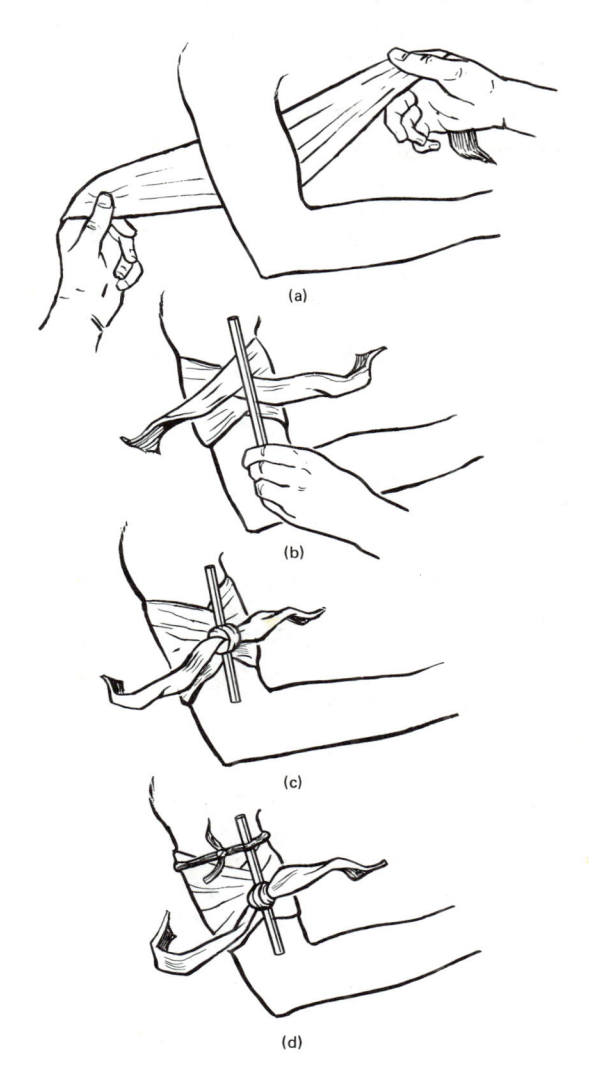

FIGURE 6.7 Procedure for applying tourniquet: (a) material wrapped twice around limb; (b) stick laid over half knot; (c) stick tied in place; (d) stick turned to stop bleeding and secured. DANGER: Secure the stick in this manner ONLY AS A LAST RESORT.

Wounds

be practiced until the first-aider can properly apply the tourniquet in one or two minutes.

INFECTIONS

Infections are caused by certain disease-producing organisms (pathogenic) which enter, grow, and multiply in the body. The causative organisms are pus-producing bacteria, the cocci, usually the staphylococci or the streptococci or both. Infection is indicated by redness, swelling, pus, temperature, pain, and, frequently, throbbing in the area. The skin and mucous membranes serve as the body's first line of defense against infection, so it must be remembered that when the skin or mucous membrane is broken, these germs enter the body. Consequently, the wounds need to be cleaned and covered carefully and the severely injured person needs to be transported to medical help. Infections are dangerous in any part of the body, especially in the area about the nose, eyes, and mouth. From this area, infection can quickly spread to the brain. Physicians are trained to treat infections; however, it is probable and possible that the physician will direct or prescribe the treatment for someone else to give or follow.

Boils, Carbuncles, and Pimples

These are infections about the hair follicles and are very common. They may occur on any area of the body but seem to have a preference for the head and neck, the arm, hand, buttocks, and leg. If there is a single core, it is known as a boil or furuncle; if there are several cores, it is called a carbuncle. Pimples are lesser skin infections with the characteristic pus pocket, and they too are caused by bacteria. The germ or organism that causes a boil is usually the staphylococcus. Because boils and carbuncles are caused by infectious organisms, it is possible for one boil to cause another, or for one person to infect another. The pus that comes from the boil should be carefully destroyed, as it is laden with organisms. The area about the infection should be carefully protected by soap and water and alcohol. The boil should be kept covered with a sterile dressing that is changed frequently. The common washcloth, towel, and garments are common means of infection. The following suggestions are made by Potthoff as how best to avoid this type of infection:

1. Prevention through cleanliness is best.
2. When boils develop, medical attention is needed. There are many dangers, often unappreciated. For example, boils may be a first sign of diabetes, and infections are serious for diabetics.
3. Don't squeeze boils. Opening a boil releases millions of germs upon the

skin. They may cause a crop of boils. If the boil does rupture, a most careful, gentle cleansing of the surrounding surface is needed.

4. Resolution of a small boil can be promoted sometimes by applying a hot, wet compress. But the measure has its risk unless done under medical direction.[3]

These skin infections are severe problems, and there is no better solution than keeping clean and giving the needed and necessary protection to skin injuries and disorders. It must be remembered that the skin is the first line of protection against infection.

Tetanus Infection

Tetanus is caused by a rod-shaped bacillus which is widely dispersed in nature. It is a spore-forming bacillus. The spores and organisms are found in the street, garden, barnyard, and any other area where domestic animals have been or where they have left their body wastes, especially their fecal matter. The tetanus organism can also be found on our bodies and our clothing. It is a very difficult organism to destroy or from which to escape. This organism is anaerobic and thrives best in the absence of oxygen. Deep puncture wounds are especially dangerous. They need attention and medical care.

The prevention of tetanus infection is assured through tetanus immunization—the toxoid vaccination. This is an active form of immunization and gives protection for a period of up to ten years. Initially two injections are given; a booster is given one year later and thereafter every ten years.

When someone is injured and tetanus is a possibility, he should be given the tetanus antitoxin, a passive form of immunization. Antitoxin is used in an emergency situation when the victim has not been protected by the toxoid vaccination. Since the antitoxin is prepared from horse blood or serum, it is important that a skin test for sensitivity be given before the injection of antitoxin. A reaction to the serum can be dangerous.

Although not in general use, a newer and safer immunization agent has been developed, tetanus immune globulin. It is a human blood product which has been hyper-immunized with tetanus toxoid. The physician will administer the globulin in the proper amount without testing for the specific wound and the possibility of tetanus infection from the wound.

The danger of tetanus is greatest in the summer. The increased incidence at this time seems to be associated with gardening and other activities involving soil and domestic animals and their wastes.

Tetanus is preventable. This has been well demonstrated in our more recent wars; the casualties from tetanus among our wounded soldiers have been exceedingly slight as compared with the Civil and Spanish-

[3] Carl J. Potthoff, "First Aid," *Today's Health*. August, 1968.

[88] Wounds

American Wars. Now all of our military personnel are immunized against this deadly disease. Tetanus remains a very dangerous infection. The solution to tetanus rests with the doctor and education concerning it. There is no need for anyone to have this deadly disease. It can be prevented.

ACTIVITIES

1. Consult your local and state health agencies concerning tetanus in your state and area.
2. Prepare a diagram or chart showing the major arterial pressure points and demonstrate and explain what is accomplished when pressure is applied to these particular locations.
3. Demonstrate to the class the correct application of the tourniquet; also indicate the dangers from the unwise and careless use of the tourniquet.
4. Demonstrate to the class the different techniques you would use to control venous bleeding, arterial bleeding, and internal bleeding.
5. Prepare and present a five-minute presentation on the cause and prevention of tetanus.

QUESTIONS TO ANSWER

1. What is the difference between a boil (furuncle) and a carbuncle? What do they have in common?
2. What can individuals do to prevent skin infections?
3. What are the five types of open wounds? Which is considered the most dangerous and why?
4. How do arterial and venous bleeding differ?
5. What are the indications of internal hemorrhage or bleeding in the victim?
6. What are the do's and don't's concerning the use of the tourniquet?
7. What is the source of the organism that causes the disease tetanus? What is unique about this particular organism?
8. How should a person attempt to control nosebleed? If nosebleed persists what should be done?
9. Why should first-aiders exercise great care in the use of antiseptics on wounds.
10. Demonstrate the application of the tourniquet on the arm and leg.

SELECTED REFERENCES

AMERICAN NATIONAL RED CROSS, *Standard First Aid and Personal Safety*. New York: Doubleday, 1973.

DOLE, WARREN H., and PUESTOW, CHARLES B., *First Aid Diagnosis and Management*. New York: Appleton-Century-Crofts, 1965.

HENDERSON, JOHN, *Emergency Medical Guide*, 4th ed. New York: McGraw-Hill, 1978.

MAHONEY, ROBERT F., *Emergency and Disaster Nursing*, 2nd ed. New York: Macmillan, 1969.

NATIONAL SAFETY COUNCIL, "Tetanus, What Your Family Should Know About It," *Family Safety*. Chicago: National Safety Council, Summer, 1966.

POTTHOFF, CARL J., "First Aid Nose Bleed," *Today's Health*. Chicago: AMA, May, 1968.

POTTHOFF, CARL J., "First Aid Tetanus Immunization," *Today's Health*. Chicago: AMA, May, 1963.

7. SHOCK

Many lives have been lost due to shock, the body's physiological reaction to a major physical or emotional insult. A tragic fact is that many of these deaths were needless because proper preventive measures can eliminate or lessen the danger of shock. In this chapter the different types of shock that may result from traumatic injury are discussed and the protective measures that can be taken to prevent shock or impede its progress are defined.

TRAUMATIC SHOCK

Traumatic shock, as defined by the American National Red Cross, is "a condition resulting from a depressed state of many vital body functions." The vital functions are depressed when there is a loss of blood volume, a reduced rate of blood flow, or an insufficient supply of oxygen.[1]

Shock is controlled by the autonomic nervous system and is a completely involuntary reaction without direction from the brain. It may result from any physical injury, such as a broken bone, puncture wound, crushing wound, burn, poisoning, or external or internal hemorrhage. The possibility of shock is present when there is an injury, no matter how slight the injury may be. Even though an injured person may not exhibit any of the symptoms of shock, he should be given protective care because shock may develop later. It can be repressed for as long as a day or two. Shock can be fatal, even if the injury is but a simple fracture. When

[1] American National Red Cross. *Advanced First Aid and Emergency Care*. New York: Doubleday, 1973, p. 59.

[90]

Traumatic Shock   [91]

```
                        TRAUMA OF ANY KIND
                                │
                                ▼
                       Depressed circulation by
                    1. Loss of blood externally
                    2. Pooling of blood in large vessels
```

11. Thirst increases

12. Unconsciousness often develops

3. Drop in blood pressure

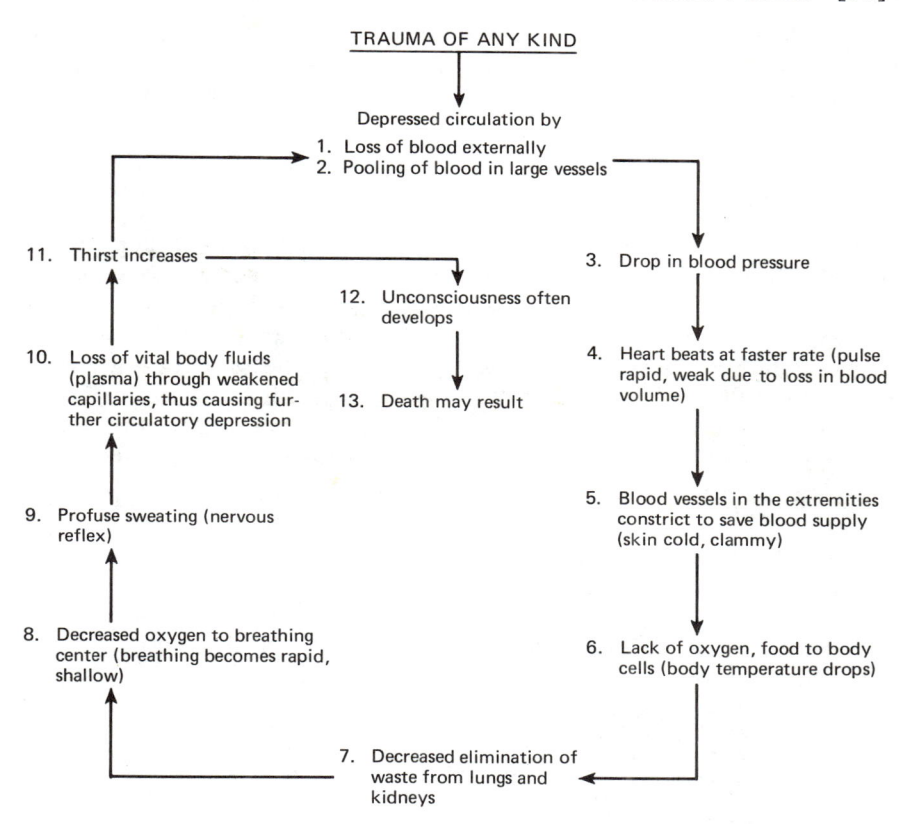

10. Loss of vital body fluids (plasma) through weakened capillaries, thus causing further circulatory depression

13. Death may result

4. Heart beats at faster rate (pulse rapid, weak due to loss in blood volume)

9. Profuse sweating (nervous reflex)

5. Blood vessels in the extremities constrict to save blood supply (skin cold, clammy)

8. Decreased oxygen to breathing center (breathing becomes rapid, shallow)

6. Lack of oxygen, food to body cells (body temperature drops)

7. Decreased elimination of waste from lungs and kidneys

FIGURE 7.1 Continuous cycle of traumatic shock. (From W. T. Brennan and D. J. Ludwig, *First Aid and Civil Defense*. Dubuque, Iowa: William C. Brown Company, Publishers, 1962.)

giving emergency care for injuries, shock should never be neglected or overlooked, for it can be as deadly as any injury.

The physiological effects of shock are the same for all injuries; however, shock may be hastened in the case of burns where there is direct loss of body fluid or in hemorrhage where large amounts of blood may be lost. In the event of an injury the body realizes the danger and takes action to keep functioning. The network of tiny blood vessels, or capillaries, that carry blood to the outer areas near the skin constrict greatly, reducing the amount of blood that can flow through them. The blood that is not allowed to flow to the extremities flows to the vital organs—the heart, kidneys, and liver. When the blood cannot circulate through the capillaries the blood plasma seeps through the capillary walls into surrounding tissues. The decrease in circulating blood volume causes a decrease in blood pressure. The heart beats furiously in an effort to circulate the limited supply of blood. As the blood pressure falls lower,

[92] Shock

the blood concentration increases, causing the oxygen level of the blood to decrease. Shock becomes more severe until death is imminent. From this discussion, shock can be viewed as a condition in which blood circulation is seriously disturbed.

Symptoms

One of the first signs that shock may be developing is a pale, cold, clammy skin resulting from blood rushing to the internal organs. After a period of time, the face may become cyanotic in color which indicates an oxygen deficiency resulting from reduced circulation. The pulse may be weak and rapid, or is sometimes absent as the heart strives to pump blood throughout the body. The eyes are vacant, dazed, lackluster, and the pupils dilated. There may be weakness, restlessness, and apprehension with a confused attitude. The victim may develop an excessive thirst and also feel nauseated with or without vomiting. The breathing will be

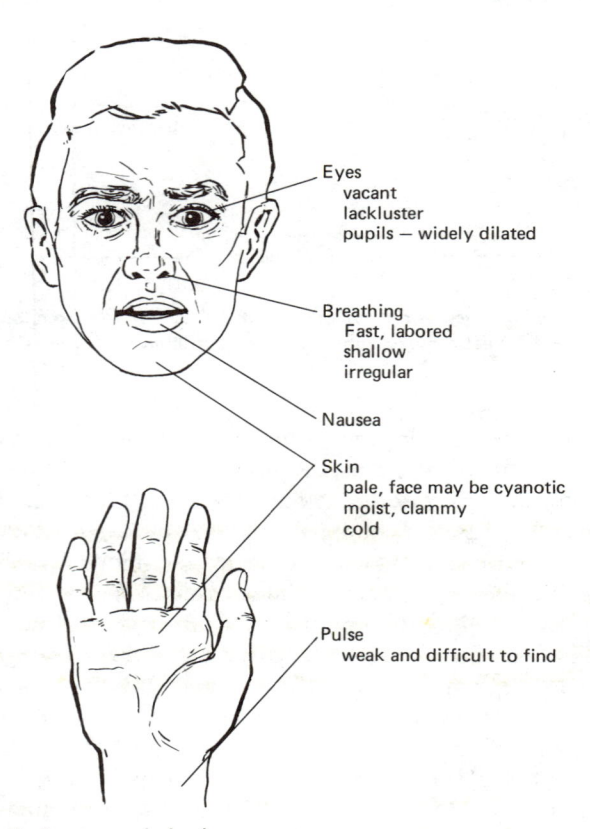

FIGURE 7.2 Indications of shock.

Traumatic Shock [93]

shallow and irregular, and in some cases the victim will lapse into unconsciousness. Any or all of these symptoms may appear, and protective measures should be taken immediately.

Protection

Emergency protection for shock should be given to all persons who are injured immediately after being assured that breathing is restored, that there is not a problem due to the injury, and that bleeding is stopped. The victim should not be moved before medical assistance arrives unless it is absolutely necessary.

The victim should be kept comfortably warm with a blanket over him and one under him when exposed to cold or dampness. He should not get hot or perspire, but his body heat should be preserved to keep him warm. If the temperature is warm, a light surface covering is enough; too much heat is harmful.

The position of the victim is very important. The victim should be kept lying down. If the person is unconscious, he should be placed on his side to prevent airway obstruction by allowing the drainage of fluids such as vomitus matter and blood. If there are no chest injuries and the victim has no problem breathing or feels no pain on being elevated, the legs should be lifted ten inches, thereby helping to improve the blood flow from the lower extremities.

If the victim has chest injuries, has difficulty in breathing, or has pain when his legs are elevated, it is best to raise his head and chest eight to ten inches. If the victim has head injuries, it is best to keep him lying flat (horizontal). Pain also affects the severity of shock, so it is important to perform whatever emergency measures are needed to relieve the injury and lessen the pain.

If an hour or more will elapse before medical assistance is available, liquids could be given. However, liquids should not be given if the victim is unconscious, vomiting or nauseated, or having convulsions. If the victim may require surgery, has a head injury, has an abdominal injury, or if medical assistance is readily accessible, liquids should not be given.

If liquids are given, a few sips of water should be given at first. Then the amount may be increased as the victim can tolerate it. It is important to replace fluid loss, and the victim probably will be thirsty. He should be given a solution of one teaspoon of salt, plus one-half teaspoon baking soda in a quart of water, if these are available. If vomiting or nausea occurs discontinue giving water. Under medical supervision, glucose and plasma can be administered; they effectively aid in restoring the volume of circulating blood in the body.

In the case of burns it is extremely important to begin giving the salt and soda solution for protection, as discussed in Chapter 9 on burns.

[94] Shock

When large amounts of blood are lost such as in hemorrhage, fluids must be administered to replenish the blood loss and help return circulation of blood.

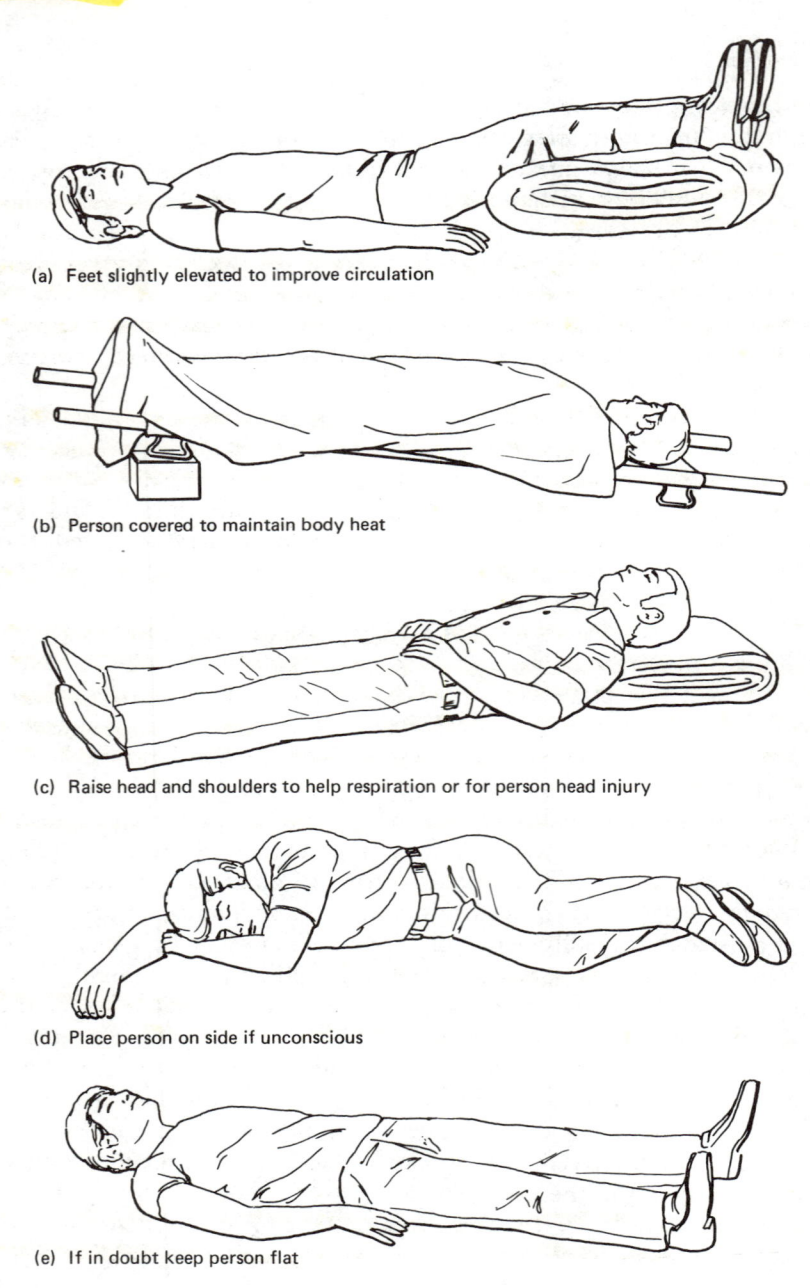

(a) Feet slightly elevated to improve circulation

(b) Person covered to maintain body heat

(c) Raise head and shoulders to help respiration or for person head injury

(d) Place person on side if unconscious

(e) If in doubt keep person flat

FIGURE 7.3 Normal positions for protection of shock victims.

Anaphylactic Shock [95]

PSYCHOLOGICAL SHOCK

Psychological shock results in the same physiological changes as take place in the body in traumatic shock. The one exception is that in psychological shock there is no direct loss of fluids from the body as in hemorrhage or burns. Also, there is no direct bodily injury to tissues. Psychological shock, just as serious as that resulting from direct bodily injury, can occur in the event of emotional jolts, such as the death of a loved one, or in cases of immense fear or tragedy. Some persons go into shock at the sight of blood, whereas others have died of shock resulting from imaginary injuries.[2] In psychological shock there is no physical injury, but emotional injury can be just as damaging.

When anyone has severe emotional trauma, the possibility of shock should never be overlooked. The symptoms and protection for psychological shock are similar to those of traumatic shock.

Fainting

Fainting is a quickly passing form of shock wherein the blood rushes from the brain to the internal organs, liver, kidney, and intestines. It may result from a variety of reasons—hunger, weakness, excitement, or terror —but it quickly passes. Protective measures include placing the head between the knees or placing the victim in a reclining position with the feet elevated to increase blood flow to the brain. (Read Chapter 15 for more information.)

ANAPHYLACTIC SHOCK

Anaphylactic shock is a severe, usually immediate response of the body to a foreign protein. It is an allergic reaction to sensitization by the foreign protein. It may be caused by (1) injection of drugs such as penicillin, (2) inhaled substances including dust and pollen, (3) ingested substances such as certain fish, shellfish, berries, and oral penicillin, and (4) insect stings from bees and wasps. It is believed that the allergic protein results in a sudden release of histamine into the blood, which allows plasma to flow through capillary walls and decreases the amount of blood for circulation.

Symptoms

The usual symptoms of traumatic shock develop also in anaphylactic shock, but in addition there may be itching skin particularly around the chest and face and hives over many body parts. The victim could be

[2] "Shock: The Killer Hardly Anyone Knows," *Family Safety*. Vol. 24, No. 2 (Summer, 1965), p. 23.

[96] Shock

restless with severe chest pains and congestion of the lungs, causing breathing difficulties. Also swelling of the vocal cords and cyanosis (bluish appearance) of the lips may be present. Unconsciousness may follow. Severe nausea, vomiting, and diarrhea may develop owing to swelling of the abdomen.

Protection

It is necessary in anaphylactic shock to obtain medical help immediately because an injection of epinephrine is imperative. It has been said that if the victim survives for 20 minutes after the allergic response, he has a good chance of recovery. Only medications can relieve this type of shock, so immediate medical care is essential. However, while transporting the person to medical facilities or waiting for an ambulance, the first-aider should

1. Give mouth-to-mouth or cardiopulmonary resuscitation, if necessary.
2. Place the person in a semi-reclining position if breathing.
3. Give protection for traumatic shock.
4. Scrape out the stinger if stung by a bee. Place a restraining band near the wound towards the heart. The stinger should be taken out with a scraping action making sure the stinger leaves the skin in the same direction it entered.

ELECTRIC SHOCK

Electric shock differs from traumatic or psychological shock in that the injury is the direct result of the passage of electric current through the body or parts of the body. The electric shock may paralyze the respiratory center in the brain, causing a cessation of breathing or ventricular fibrillation (irregularity or twitching of the heart), so that circulation of the blood through the heart is jeopardized.

There are several factors that influence the severity of electric shock. One factor affecting the severity is the amount of voltage and amperage of the current. Also the amount of moisture on the victim or the amount of the body's surface that is in contact with water will affect the seriousness of the electric charge. Water always increases the possibility and danger of electric shock. A third factor is the amount of insulation on the victim in the form of clothing or rubber shoes. The more insulation the less severe the shock will be. Lastly, the seriousness of an electric shock depends on what part of the body the current passes through. If it passes through the extremities, the less the severity; however, if it passes through the trunk of the body, the danger of severe shock is much greater.

The best way to prevent shock is to avoid the causes and make certain that none exist in the home. One cause of electric shock is lightning.

During an electrical storm it is precautionary to stay away from metal or electrical objects inside the home. If outside, never get under an isolated tree. It is best to lie in a depression in the ground or seek shelter where one will not be exposed.

A second cause of electric shock is contact with high-voltage wires. These can be extremely dangerous if they have fallen during a storm. Usually contact with a high-voltage wire is fatal. It is a good policy for children never to fly kites near such wires. Third, low-voltage household currents cause the largest percentage of shock incidences. Whenever any electrical appliance is used, the hands are separated from the electric current by some form of insulation which encloses wires and shields current-carrying parts. Any failure of the insulators can cause electrocution.

It is important that the Underwriters' Laboratories (UL) label be on any electrical material that is purchased. This gives a degree of assurance of the safety of the product. It is also wise to check and recheck any electrical product for deterioration. A defective appliance should never be used. A person in contact with water should never touch any electrical appliance. This type of shock causes many fatalities in the home.

Symptoms

In moderate shock there will be a dazed and confused condition for a period of time. There may be burns where the current came into contact with the skin.

In severe shock there is usually unconsciousness with a weak and irregular pulse or no pulse. The breathing may be shallow, irregular, or absent.

Protection

The victim should never be touched until he has been removed from the source of the current or until the current has been shut off. Without this procedure, a rescuer will be exposed to the same electrical charge. Any source of current in the home can be quickly shut off by throwing the main power switch. Every able person in the home should know the location of the power box and how to shut off the power in case of an emergency.

If the current cannot be shut off, the rescuer must free the victim from the source of power. There are several methods that can be used. The rescuer should stand on a dry surface of nonconducting material, such as rubber or a dry board. He should drag the victim from contact by looping some nonconducting material such as a dry rope or dry clothing over the victim's hand or foot and pull until the victim is freed from contact with the power source. If no loop can be made and successfully used, the rescuer can drag the victim away with one hand that has been heavily

[98] Shock

insulated with a material such as rubber, several layers of cloth, or heavy paper.

Another method of rescue is to push the victim away from the power source by, again, standing on a nonconducting material and pushing with a dry board or dry stick until contact is broken. Still another method of breaking contact with the current is to push or pull the source of current away from the victim with a dry board, stick, or roll of newspapers. The best method of rescue will depend on the circumstances.

After the victim has been freed from the source of electric shock, medical help should be sought immediately. Hospitalization is necessary if the shock is severe. Until a medical person can take over, cardiopulmonary resuscitation should be given to the victim. Continue the resuscitation until trained medical personnel can take over. The victim should be kept warm and lying down quietly. Some electrical shock victims react in a disoriented manner so protect the person from injuring himself and others.

INSUFFICIENT OR EXCESSIVE INSULIN SUPPLY

Insulin shock and diabetic coma are both attributed to the substance insulin. Insulin shock results when the level of insulin in the body is greater than the amount utilized, and diabetic coma results when a person does not receive the needed amount of insulin for the body to function properly.

Any diabetic should wear a medal stating the fact that he is a diabetic. When a diabetic is found unconscious or with unintelligible speech, the rescuer will realize these may be symptoms of diabetic coma or insulin shock.

Insulin Shock

Insulin shock may occur when the carbohydrate or sugar level in the body is too low for the amount of insulin in the body. Insulin shock may develop when a diabetic patient has not eaten enough food for the amount of insulin taken, when the patient has exercised more than usual and burned up more carbohydrates, or in the case of diarrhea or vomiting. Most diabetic patients always carry some candy with them in case of insulin shock. They know the conditions under which insulin shock can develop and can take some form of sugar to prevent it. They recognize the oncoming symptoms and the sugar will allay the condition.

Symptoms Insulin shock, or insulin reaction, may suddenly come on as a result of excessive insulin in the body. The diabetic person will feel very weak and dizzy. He will appear nervous and irritable, and his

Insufficient or Excessive Insulin Supply [99]

FIGURE 7.4 COMPARISON CHART FOR DIABETIC COMA AND INSULIN SHOCK

History	Diabetic coma	Insulin shock
Food	Excessive (Especially Carbohydrates)	Insufficient (Especially Carbohydrates)
Insulin	Insufficient	Excessive
Onset	Gradual Days	Sudden
Appearance	Extremely Ill	Very Weak
Skin	Dry and Flushed	Moist and Pale
Fever	Frequent	Absent
Mouth	Dry	Drooling
Thirst	Intense	Absent
Hunger	Absent	Intense
Vomiting	Common	Rare
Pain, Abdominal	Frequent	Absent
Respiration	Exaggerated Air Hunger	Normal or Shallow
Breath	Acetone Odor Usually Present	Acetone Odor May Be Present
Pulse	Weak and Rapid	Full and Normal
Tremor	Absent	Frequent
Convulsions	None	In Last Stages
Improvement	Gradual	Rapid—Following carbohydrate Administration
Suggested First Aid	Get Doctor Immediately	Get Doctor Immediately
	Keep Lying Down—flat or with head and shoulders raised.	Give Sugar (Orange juice, soft drinks, granulated sugar on tongue, sugar cubes or candy)—if conscious—if unconscious, and mouth can be opened—sugar cubes rubbed on tongue will work. Give retention enema.
	Keep Warm—Give fluids, except those containing sugar or starches.	
	Shock Solution May Be Given	

skin will be pale, moist, cool, and clammy. If the victim does not receive sugar and the insulin shock progresses unchecked, the breathing becomes slow and shallow and the pulse very rapid.

Protection A doctor should be called immediately. If the victim is conscious, he should at once be given orange juice, soft drinks, sugar cubes, or candy. This will help increase the carbohydrate level. If the

Shock

victim is unconscious, sugar cubes can be rubbed on his tongue. Only as much as can be absorbed should be given. If the victim does not regain consciousness, a retention enema could be administered by a physician. Sometimes it is necessary for a sugar injection to be given for the victim to retain consciousness. After consciousness is regained recovery is usually rapid.

Diabetic Coma

When a diabetic patient eats improperly or does not receive the necessary amount of insulin, he may develop diabetic coma. Fats and carbohydrates are not fully metabolized when the amount of insulin is insufficient. When fats are not used quickly enough by the body, they accumulate in the bloodstream, resulting in a condition known as acidosis. This causes an alteration of the body chemistry which leads to a coma.

Symptoms Diabetic coma results gradually from an insufficient amount of insulin. The victim will become confused, disoriented, and stuporous with a sweet acetone odor on the breath. The skin will be dry and flushed. Frequently there is a fever and the lips may be deep red. There may be intense hunger and thirst with frequent vomiting. Breathing will be weak and rapid, and the pulse may be absent. The victim will fall into a coma if no insulin is given, and the result could be eventual death.

Protection A doctor should be called immediately. The administration of insulin is necessary. If a doctor is not available, an insulin injection should be given by the victim with help from the first-aider. If neither the doctor or insulin is available, protection should be given as for traumatic shock, discussed earlier in this chapter. The victim should be kept lying down, flat or with head and shoulders raised, kept warm and given fluids except those containing sugar or starches. The solution of baking soda, salt, and water may be given until medical attention is possible.

ACTIVITIES

1. Suggest to all of your acquaintances who are allergic to some form of protein or who have diabetes that they get a medical tag stating their specific problem. This tag should be worn or carried at all times. Check with each person in three weeks to determine the number that have obtained medical tags.
2. Practice the different positions for shock, stressing the normal, chest injury, and head injury positions.
3. Write a paper on the similarities and differences between insulin shock

and diabetic coma. Emphasize symptoms and protein in the writing of this paper.
4 Check your home, place of work, recreational areas, and other places you may frequent and determine where the main power source can be turned off in case of an emergency involving electrical current.
5 Write a paper on the following topic: "Psychological Shock Is More Severe than Traumatic Shock."

QUESTIONS TO ANSWER

1 Define shock as it relates to a physical injury.
2 Why is it necessary to protect a person from shock even though no symptoms are present?
3 What happens to the blood in the body when traumatic shock is occurring?
4 Describe the symptoms of traumatic shock. How are they different from the symptoms of anaphylactic shock?
5 Describe the immediate and secondary protection or emergency care that should be provided for a person stung by a bee.
6 Describe the various methods that can be used to remove a victim from a source of high electrical power? What first-aid measures should be taken once the victim is removed from the electrical source?
7 Differentiate between the symptoms of insulin shock and diabetic coma.
8 How is the protection different for insulin shock as compared to diabetic coma?
9 Compare and contrast traumatic shock and psychological shock.
10 List and describe six ways of preventing electrical shock due to lightning.

SELECTED REFERENCES

AMERICAN ACADEMY OF ORTHOPEDIC SURGEONS, COMMITTEE ON INJURIES, *Emergency Care and Transportation of the Sick and Injured.* Chicago: The Academy, 1971, p. 72–79.
AMERICAN NATIONAL RED CROSS, *Advanced First Aid and Emergency Care.* New York: Doubleday, 1973, pp. 59–64.
BRENNAN, WILLIAM T., and LUDWIG, DONALD J., *Guide to Problems and Practices in First Aid and Emergency Care,* 3rd ed. Dubuque, Ia.: Wm. C. Brown, 1976, pp. 45–53, 126–127.
ERVEN, LAURENCE W., *First Aid and Emergency Rescue.* Beverly Hills, Calif.: Glencoe Press, 1970, pp. 45–54.

Shock

GRANT, HARVEY, and MURRAY, ROBERT, *Emergency Care*. Bowie, Md., Robert J. Brady, 1971, pp. 109–118, 216–218, 255–257.

GREEN, MARTIN I., *A Sigh of Relief*. New York: Bantam Books, 1977, pp. 150–151, 188–189.

KRANIK, ANDREW D., "Lightning Injuries." *Emergency Product News*, 7 October 1975, pp. 468–472, 474–475.

MAHONEY, ROBERT E., *Emergency and Disaster Nursing*, 2nd ed. New York: Macmillan, 1969, pp. 81–85.

8. RESPIRATORY AND CARDIOPULMONARY RESUSCITATION (CPR)

The material in this chapter is based upon the information resulting from the May 1973 National Conference on Standards for Cardiopulmonary Resuscitation (CPR) and Emergency Cardiac Care (ECC) cosponsored by the National Academy of Sciences-National Research Council and the American Heart Association. The standards that were derived were published on February 18, 1974 as a special supplement to *The Journal of the American Medical Association*, Vol. 227, Number 7.[1]

The exact procedures for cardiopulmonary resuscitation (CPR) seem to be continuously changing, and each first-aider must realize the need to keep abreast of these changes. It is advised that a first-aider get and maintain certification in CPR from a local Heart Association program and/or the American National Red Cross. Periodic training should be pursued in order to be up-to-date regarding CPR techniques. The information included in the following sections will give a first-aider an in depth look at the why, how, and when of performing CPR.

THE BREATHING SYSTEM

Breathing, or respiration, is the process by which the tissues of the body are supplied with oxygen and by which carbon dioxide, the chief waste product of oxidation, is eliminated from the body (see Figure 8.1). This exchange, which is accomplished between the blood and the cells of the body, is known as internal respiration; and the exchange that takes

[1] *Supplement to the Journal of the American Medical Association*, Vol. 227, No. 7 (February 18, 1974). Copyrighted by the American Medical Association.

[104]   Respiratory and Cardiopulmonary Resuscitation (CPR)

place between the air and the blood (in the lungs) is called external respiration. The chief organs of respiration in man are the lungs, and the chief muscle of respiration is the diaphragm. The diaphragm separates the chest cavity (thorax) from the abdominal cavity. For the air to get to the lungs from the outside it must pass through the nose, nasal passages, pharynx, larynx, trachea, bronchi, bronchial tubes, bronchioles, and finally into the thousands of air spaces of the lungs, the alveoli. In each of these tiny air spaces (alveoli) oxygen is exchanged for carbon dioxide. The process of breathing is controlled by the respiratory center of the brain.

The adult breathes some 15 to 20 times per minute, and the air volume measures from one-half to 1 liter or more in each inspiration. The inward movement of air is known as inspiration and the outward movement expiration. The fresh air that is inspired is approximately 20 percent oxygen and 80 percent nitrogen. The expired air is somewhat changed, as it is 16 to 17 percent oxygen, 3 to 4 percent carbon dioxide, and 80 percent nitrogen. In order for the air to pass from the outside into the

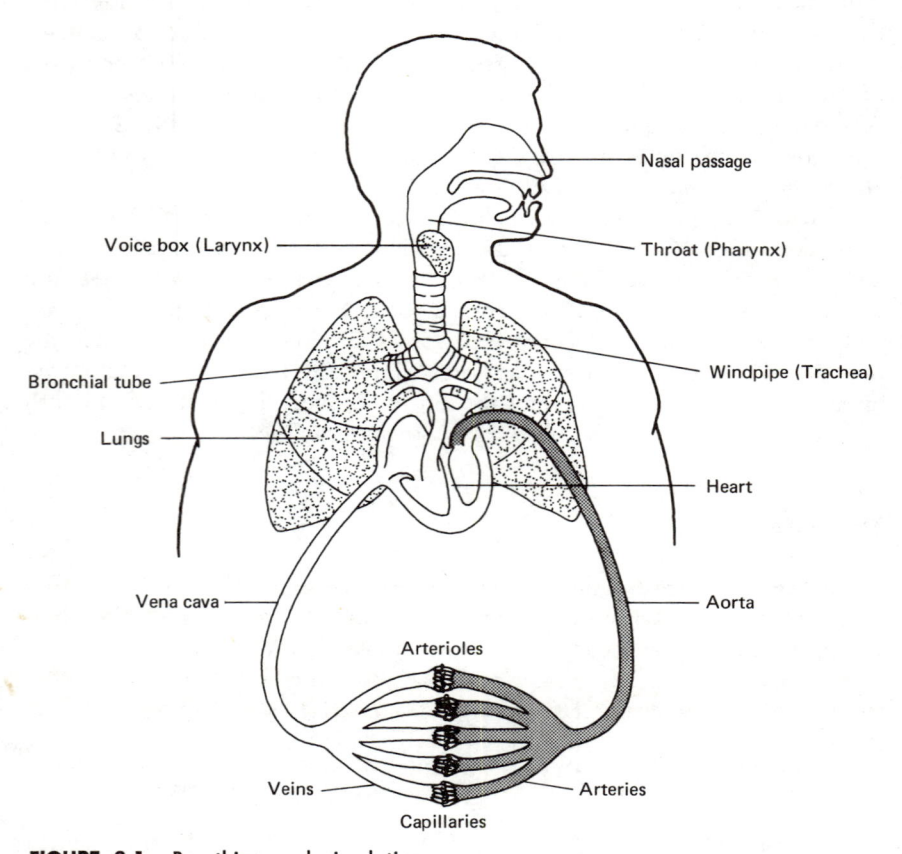

FIGURE 8.1   Breathing and circulation.

Cardiovascular System [105]

lungs, the chest or thorax must expand. This is accomplished by the intercostal muscles and the diaphragm. The intercostals cause the chest wall to move outward as they contract. The diaphragm pushes down and out; consequently the chest cavity is enlarged and the air moves inward. During expiration, the chest wall moves inward as the intercostal muscles relax, and the diaphragm moves up and inward. This combined action causes the thorax to become smaller, and the air moves to the outside. In compression-type asphyxiation accidents, the weight against the body prevents the enlargement of the thorax by the chest muscles and diaphragm. The victim cannot move air into and out of the lungs. This type of accident occurs in cave-ins, mines, and landslides.

The need for oxygen is continuous because our bodies can store little or none. It is said that athletes go in debt for oxygen during strenuous events such as the 400- or 800-meter run in track; i.e., oxygen is borrowed from other body tissues and is returned quickly during the recovery period. For example, if the brain is denied oxygen for four to six minutes, permanent damage can result. The brain is most susceptible to anoxemia, the reduction of oxygen. This emphasizes again the great importance of oxygen to our body cells and tissues and the need to begin artificial respiration at once should asphyxia occur.

CARDIOVASCULAR SYSTEM

The cardiovascular system is composed of the heart (*cardio*) and blood vessels (*vascular*) (see Figure 8.1). Knowledge of the heart and circulatory system is necessary for proper understanding of the various heart problems. The circulatory system of the body performs the following functions:

1   Regulates body temperature.
2   Distributes blood throughout the body.
3   Carries nutriments to the body cells.
4   Removes the waste products from the cells.

The heart, a muscular pump approximately the size of a fist, moves the blood throughout the body. It has been estimated that a drop of blood goes through the whole cardiovascular system every 90 seconds, even when the body is resting.

The blood moving to the different parts of the body from the heart is carried by the arteries. The arteries contain red blood, which carries the necessary nutrients and oxygen to the cells of the body. The blood exchanges the food and oxygen supply for waste materials and carbon dioxide through the walls of the capillaries. Then the blood returns to the heart through the veins and is dark bluish-red in color. Most of the waste products are removed from the blood by the kidneys. The carbon dioxide

[106] Respiratory and Cardiopulmonary Resuscitation (CPR)

is released in the lungs, where the blood receives a new supply of oxygen. Then the blood is carried back to the heart and the aforementioned cycle is repeated thousands of times a day.

If any component of the functioning parts of the heart and the circulatory system is inefficient, the blood supply to various parts of the body will be diminished. Damage to the lungs, kidneys, skin, and heart may result.

RESPIRATORY ARREST

When breathing stops for any reason, the condition is called respiratory arrest. The heart may continue to beat for several minutes after the breathing process ceases. Accidents involving water and electricity, too great a quantity of gases, smoke, compression depressants, along with heart attacks, and blockage of the air passage are the major causes of respiratory arrest. Each year in the United States some 8,000 persons drown; 1,600 persons are poisoned by gases and vapors such as carbon monoxide, while others suffocate because of choking, electric shock, or compressions. This is a needless loss of life, and many could have been saved had there been a person at the scene trained in first aid and artificial resuscitation to give protection. It is especially important that the many persons who fish, swim, boat, and ski be trained in artificial resuscitation. It is estimated that there are over one million swimming pools in the nation, and the number is increasing rapidly. This all points to the necessity of more and more people learning the techniques of giving artificial resuscitation.

The American National Red Cross reports that the chances for a recovery according to the time lapse between respiratory arrest and the beginning of artificial respiration is as follows:

98 out of 100 within 1 minute
92 out of 100 within 2 minutes
72 out of 100 within 3 minutes
50 out of 100 within 4 minutes
25 out of 100 within 5 minutes
11 out of 100 within 6 minutes
 8 out of 100 within 7 minutes
 5 out of 100 within 8 minutes
 2 out of 100 within 9 minutes
 1 out of 100 within 10 minutes
 1 out of 1,000 within 11 minutes
 1 out of 10,000 within 12 minutes [2]

---

[2] "Artificial Respiration," First Aid, Small Craft, and Water Safety Department. St. Louis, Mo.: American National Red Cross Mid-American Chapter, November, 1964.

Cardiac Arrest

The following are some problem situations where too little oxygen is present which may result in respiratory arrest:

1. The air containing too little oxygen, as in the case of old wells, silos, caves, and mines.
2. Possible blockage of the air passage caused by food, water, and other substances, hanging by the neck, and drowning.
3. Too little oxygen being circulated in the body because of heart failure or a great loss of blood.
4. An overdose of drugs, affecting respiratory center of the brain.
5. An injury to the brain.
6. An overdose of sleeping pills.
7. The red cells of the blood being too few or carrying too large a quantity of another gas such as carbon monoxide. Carbon monoxide unites with the blood many times (200 to 250) faster than oxygen; consequently the great danger from this gas. The production and distribution of carbon monoxide are quite common.

Symptoms of Respiratory Arrest

Without oxygen, breaths will become shorter and faster, a headache may occur, ears will probably pound, and memory will become fuzzy. The victim will appear to be under the influence of alcohol. He will become unconscious and his breathing will be arrested. Within a short time the heart will stop beating and death will follow. It is important to remember that as long as the heart is beating, or if the heart stops but starts beating again, it is possible for breathing to resume.

CARDIAC ARREST

Cardiac arrest refers to "the sudden and unexpected cessation of cardiac output."[3] Also, cardiac arrest can be viewed as any condition in which the circulation is either absent or inadequate to sustain life. When circulation stops, the pulse disappears and breathing stops at about the same time or soon after. When a victim suffers from cardiac arrest, artificial respiration and artificial circulation (cardiopulmonary resuscitation) are required to oxygenate the blood and circulate it to the brain. Cardiac arrest occurs as a result of one of the following: (1) heart standstill, which means that no blood is ejected from either the left or right heart circuit; (2) ventricular fibrillation, which is an uncoordinated jerking contraction of the individual heart muscles; or (3) a sudden deep circulatory collapse with not enough heart output to provide even circulation in the heart.

---

[3] James R. Jude, *Closed Chest Cardiac Resuscitation: Methods–Indications–Limitations.* New York: Distributed by the American Heart Association and its affiliates as a service to physicians, 1966.

[108]   Respiratory and Cardiopulmonary Resuscitation (CPR)

It is important to remember that although these three conditions are quite different, the same emergency care and protection is suggested for each.

There are many possible causes of cardiac arrest in addition to heart attack. These include drowning, electric shock, suffocation, strangulation, anaphylactic shock, or any other accident that causes the heart to come to a standstill. Some of these causes are discussed in other chapters.

Angina Pectoris

Angina pectoris is primarily a strangling or pain in the chest. Pain results because the heart muscle has received an inadequate supply of blood for a short period of time. The pain originates just under the sternum (breastbone), and may proliferate out to either one of the arms. Usually the left arm receives the pain. Depending upon the degree of deprivation of the heart's blood supply, the pain may be very mild or severe. Overexertion of the heart due to digesting a heavy meal, excitement, intense cold, effort, or worry may result in angina pectoris.

Occasionally, anginal pains are a precursor of a heart attack. If these pains have not occurred before, the person should see a physician as soon as possible. Many times the pain stems from other causes; however, the diagnosis should be made by a physician only.

Heart Attack

Heart attack is the common term for the condition physicians refer to as coronary thrombosis. Almost every minute during the day someone across the nation has a heart attack. Although heart attacks can be fatal, many are not. If given proper medical treatment, many a heart attack victim will lead a useful and productive life.

Heart attack is a sudden blocking of one of the heart arteries by a blood clot. A blood clot that remains stationary is called a thrombus. When a blood clot occurs in the heart's own circulation, a coronary thrombosis or heart attack results. The leading cause of heart attacks is atherosclerosis, which cuts off the blood supply to a particular part of the heart muscle.

Most heart attacks happen while a person is resting or working quietly. Working energetically may cause the blood clot in the heart artery, but the blood clot may have developed even though the person did not overwork. Thus, it would be difficult to say that a certain activity caused the heart attack.

Symptoms of a heart attack in many circumstances are difficult to identify. But if the following symptoms are present, the American Heart Association says a physician should be contacted at once:

1   Uncomfortable pressure, fullness, squeezing, or pain in the center of the chest for more than two minutes.
2   Pain may spread to the shoulders, neck, or arms.

Cardiac Arrest [109]

3   Severe pain, dizziness, fainting, sweating, nausea, or shortness of breath may also occur.
4   These signals are not always present. Sometimes they subside and then return.[4]

A physician is the only person who can diagnose whether or not a victim is having a heart attack. Therefore, an individual should not attempt to make such a judgment.

If the preceding symptoms are present, the first-aider should try to get the victim in the position that is most comfortable. This is usually in a semireclining or sitting-up position. A person who has had a heart attack will find it difficult to breathe if he is lying flat. The first-aider should try to reassure the victim because his condition may make him feel that he is dying. The name of the person's doctor should be obtained so he can be called. If the victim is under medical care, he might have on hand drugs that should be administered. These drugs include a nitroglycerine tablet which is placed under the victim's tongue.

The first-aider should try to maintain body heat by lightly covering the victim with a blanket. All tight clothing should be loosened. The victim should not be given anything to drink and no attempt should be made to move him without the physician's consent. If breathing stops, the first-aider should start mouth-to-mouth artificial ventilation, and if the heart stops functioning, cardiopulmonary resuscitation should be started.

Symptoms of Cardiac Arrest

The symptoms that occur with the three types of cardiac arrest (heart standstill, ventricular fibrillation, and circulatory collapse) are basically the same. The victim has the following indications:

1   Deathlike appearance or may be gasping for oxygen.
2   Skin may be pale or cyanotic.
3   Breathing is absent or gasping. Breathing sounds are noisy if they are present.
4   No carotid pulse.
5   Pupils of the eyes may or may not be dilated or enlarged.
6   Eyes are glassy looking.
7   Sudden unconsciousness.

Symptoms of Respiratory and Cardiac Arrest

Recognition of respiratory and cardiac arrest is important to the first-aider. Immediate performance of cardiopulmonary resuscitation is essential when one notices the following symptoms:

[4] American Heart Association, *Heart Attack*. Dallas, Texas: American Heart Association, 1975.

[110]   Respiratory and Cardiopulmonary Resuscitation (CPR)

1   Victim becomes unconscious. In some cases convulsions may be present.
2   No pulse is present.
3   Breathing is slowed and will discontinue within 30 seconds. During that time breathing will be labored, noisy, or effervescing.
4   Skin becomes pale or cyanotic.
5   Within 30 seconds, pupils will begin to dilate with full dilation in two minutes.

OTHER RESPIRATORY AND CARDIAC ARREST PROBLEMS

There are other conditions that may cause respiratory and cardiac arrest problems such as carbon monoxide, hanging, drugs, compression, electric shock, and gases. These conditions need to be known and understood by the first-aider.

Carbon Monoxide

Carbon monoxide is found in the exhaust fumes of cars, trucks, power mowers, outboard motors, and all gasoline and fuel oil burners. The burning of any fuel containing carbon can produce the gas. This is true of solids, such as coal, coke, wood, and charcoal. Carbon monoxide is present whether the burning takes place indoors or out. Charcoal grills, fireplaces, gas ranges, incinerators, and gas refrigerators are potential producers. Carbon monoxide kills over a thousand persons in the United States each year.

Two conditions are necessary to create a carbon monoxide poison situation—the lack of ventilation and improper burning. When both of these conditions occur at the same time the hazards are increased. A victim can be overcome and in serious trouble in a very short period of time.

Carbon monoxide unites with the blood very fast, and this greatly enhances the danger. When the gas is inhaled it combines with the hemoglobin of the blood's red cells and prevents the formation of oxyhemoglobin. This greatly reduces the blood's capacity to carry oxygen to the cells and tissues of the body.

The following are a number of precautions that can be taken to lessen the chance of carbon monoxide asphyxiation:

1   Gas stoves and refrigerators should be serviced carefully and regularly; an annual check or oftener.
2   No one should sleep in a poorly ventilated room where a coal or gas stove is the source of heat.
3   All gas- and oil-burning devices should be vented correctly.
4   Furnaces should be checked annually, and certainly the chimney and flue should be free of leaks.

Other Respiratory and Cardiac Arrest Problems   [111]

5   Fireplaces should have sufficient drafts.
6   Indoor grills should have suitable venting; they may be placed in a fireplace.
7   A car's exhaust system should be in good repair; it should be inspected annually.
8   No one should sit in a parked car with the motor running.
9   A gasoline-burning engine should not be indoors without sufficient venting and circulation of fresh air.
10 The tailpipe on a car should be checked to make certain it does not clog when backing into snow, sand, dirt, water, or any other substance. If the car stalls in water, the ignition should be turned off.
11 No one should breathe automobile exhaust gas, even for a short period of time.

Common symptoms of carbon monoxide poisoning are headaches, dizziness, sleepiness, nausea, vomiting, and muscular weakness which render the victim helpless. The victim's skin frequently turns to a cherry red.

Should such an accident occur, the victim should be moved from the area immediately. The rescuer should call a physician at once, give cardiopulmonary resuscitation, and keep the victim warm.

Other Gases

There are several gases that may lessen the amount of air getting to the lungs, including inhaled smoke, carbon dioxide, and natural gas. The symptoms differ according to the gas inhaled. Symptoms may vary from headache, vomiting, nausea, dizziness, and muscular weakness to unconsciousness, breathing stoppage, and death. Whether respiratory and/or cardiac arrest comes from one gas or another, the protection is the same as that indicated for carbon monoxide.

Hanging

The blockage of the air passage by hanging from the neck, whether on purpose or accidentally, is a common form of respiratory and cardiac arrest. Persons should be cut down immediately and cardiopulmonary resuscitation should be administered at once. If death results, it usually will be from the lack of oxygen—not a broken neck.

Drugs

The respiratory center of the brain can be depressed by overdoses of narcotics, which cause the breathing muscles to slow or to completely arrest breathing and cause heart failure. When there is such evidence, cardiopulmonary resuscitation should be started at once. Rescuers and

[112]   Respiratory and Cardiopulmonary Resuscitation (CPR)

medical help should be summoned, but the first-aider's task is to begin application of artificial respiration and not waste precious seconds or minutes. What he does before help arrives could well save a life. Drugs causing the trouble may be sodium amytal, phenobarbital, or Nembutal. These drugs and others should be taken only as directed by a physician.

Common symptoms resulting from a drug overdose are

1   Rapid and thready pulse.
2   Deep sleep and relaxed muscles.
3   Very shallow breathing.
4   White, cold, and clammy skin.
5   Pinpoint pupils which may not respond to light.

Compression

This is the cave-in type of accidental respiratory arrest. The weight of the dirt, sand, or object is so great that the muscles of respiration cannot expand the chest to allow air to enter. In this situation the weight must be eliminated, and the victim moved to safety; otherwise respiratory arrest is inevitable. The first-aider protects in this type of accident by giving cardiopulmonary resuscitation.

Measures to be taken during and after recovery are as follows:

1   This is a medical problem and the doctor should be called. He should come to the accident scene to direct the recovery and transportation.
2   An ambulance or suitable means of transportation should be summoned. The rescue operator should remain and continue giving aid at the scene; however, if the victim begins to breathe and is placed in a vehicle, a rescuer should be ready to resume artificial ventilation in the event that the victim stops breathing.
3   There should be no hurry to move the victim; the resumption of breathing is the important consideration at this time.
4   The victim should be kept warm to protect against shock. Also this will help to prevent pneumonia, which is another danger.
5   The victim should be taken to a hospital for treatment and observation by the doctors and hospital staff.

Electricity

Charges of electricity are capable of paralyzing the respiratory center of the brain causing the cessation of breathing and eventually cardiac arrest. A charge with that capability can come from 110 volts of electricity if the victim is grounded. Cardiopulmonary resuscitation is the best method for restoring breathing and heart circulation.

CARDIOPULMONARY RESUSCITATION (CPR)

Cardiopulmonary resuscitation (CPR) is an emergency procedure that assists a victim who has had respiratory and/or cardiac arrest until the person receives medical life support care. The procedures can be generally summarized as the A-B-C steps of CPR:

A Airway opened—by head tilt or other acceptable technique
B Breathing restored—by mouth-to-mouth or alternate method
C Circulation restored—by external cardiac compression

Clinical and Biological Death

At that time when breathing and circulation discontinues to function and there are no signs of life, a person is considered to be clinically dead. For approximately four to six minutes, brain tissue will survive. After such a period of time has elapsed, brain damage which is irreversible will begin to occur and the person is then considered to be biologically dead. This points out the need to begin CPR without delay.

Beginning and Terminating Cardiopulmonary Resuscitation

The first-aider, when the symptoms warrant it, should start cardiopulmonary resuscitation immediately. If one has any question as to when the victim collapsed, the first-aider should start cardiopulmonary resuscitation.

Once cardiopulmonary resuscitation has been started, the first-aider should continue until one of the following occurs:

1 Restoration of effective spontaneous ventilation and circulation.
2 Another responsible person takes over the cardiopulmonary resuscitation procedures.
3 A properly trained and designated EMT-A, paramedic, or allied health professional takes over responsibility of cardiopulmonary resuscitation.
4 A physician assumes responsibility.
5 Exhaustion of the first-aider takes place and he is unable to continue.

PROCEDURE FOR CPR

When a first-aider comes upon a victim who has respiratory and/or cardiac arrest, concern must be given to beginning CPR as soon as possible. The normal emergency procedures as discussed in Chapter 3 should be followed if other help is available. However, if no other assistance is available the first priority of the first-aider must be to start CPR immediately.

The discussion which follows presents CPR as a procedure that is a combination of many separately taught performances of the past. The

[114]   Respiratory and Cardiopulmonary Resuscitation (CPR)

FIGURE 8.2   CPR AT A GLANCE—ONE FIRST-AIDER

Procedure	Suggested time for performance
Establish unresponsiveness	4–8 seconds
Open airway	2 seconds
Establish breathlessness	3–4 seconds
Give 4 ventilations	3–5 seconds
Establish pulselessness	5–8 seconds
Locate landmark, positions hand(s) and compress sternum 15 times	10–12 seconds
Give 2 ventilations	3–5 seconds
Continue alternating 15 compressions and 2 ventilations	15 seconds per cycle
Every minute or so check pulse for no more than 5 seconds	3–5 seconds

procedure is viewed as one concept which has the potential for stopping at various steps and/or going to other techniques depending upon respiratory or circulatory problems. For example, mouth-to-mouth artificial ventilation is viewed initially as a step in CPR. In some circumstances, mouth-to-mouth artificial ventilation may be the prime step in the CPR procedure. Various options will be discussed in the steps that follow:

1. *Establish unresponsiveness.* This first step in CPR is to see if that a seemingly unconscious person is responsive or unresponsive to the first-aider's actions. The first-aider should shake the victim's shoulder and shout loudly, "Are you OK?" or "Speak to me." If the person responds affirmatively, the first-aider at the time does not have to proceed further, but should observe the person for additional problems. If there is no response to the actions of the first-aider then the airway must be opened. As a part of this step, the victim should be placed on his back on a hard surface (if not already in that position).

2. *Open the airway.* Opening the airway indicates tilting the head in a backward direction so the tongue does not block the airway thereby permitting air to reach the lungs. With an unconscious victim lying on his back, the muscles become relaxed thereby allowing the lower jaw to fall back. Since the tongue is attached to the lower jaw, the tongue also falls backward obstructing the air passage.

With the victim on his back, the first-aider places his hand, which is nearest the lower end (feet) of the body, palm up under the neck and gently lifts up while simultaneously placing the other hand, palm down, on the forehead and applies light tilting pressure downward. Maintain the head in this position as much as possible. There are many times when the breathing process can be restored merely by tilting the head.

Procedure for CPR [115]

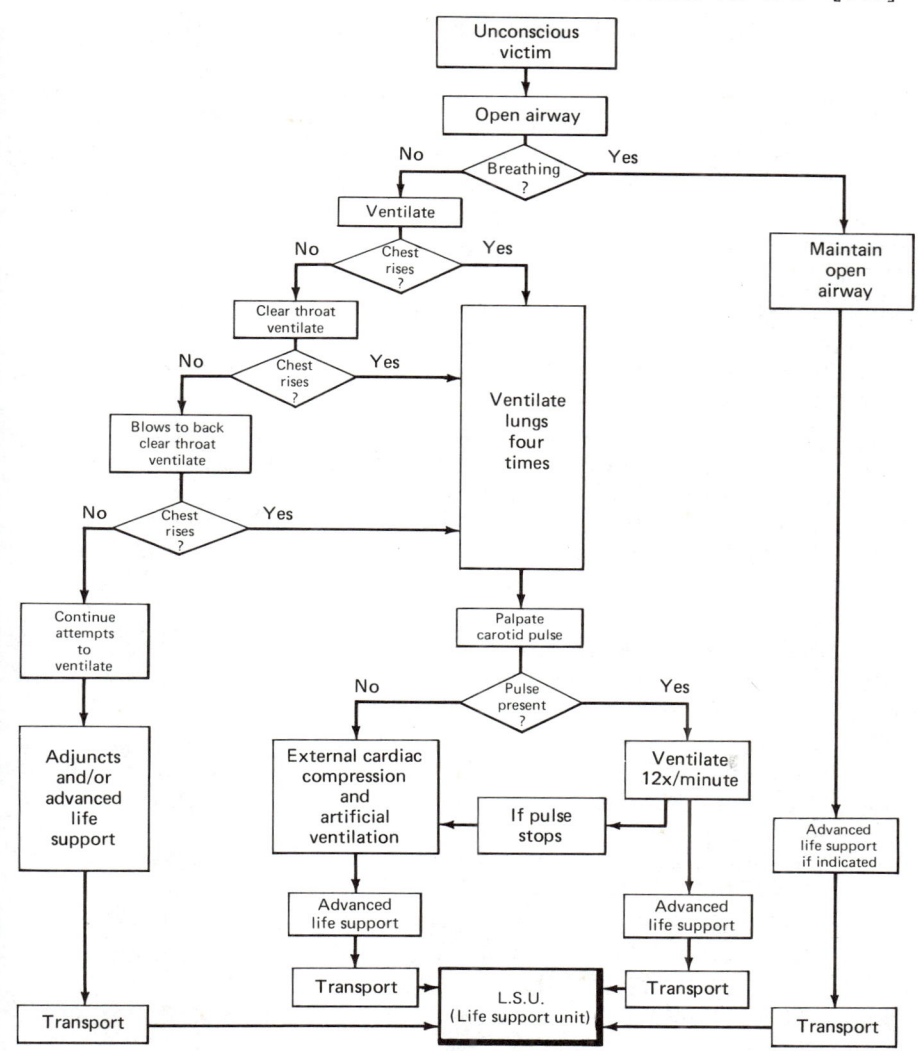

FIGURE 8.3 Life support decision tree—sequence of CPR procedure. (American Heart Association)

If the victim has a suspected cervical spinal injury, the technique of opening the airway must be used with caution. If the victim was involved in a diving or automobile accident, particularly where lacerations of the face and neck occur, then a neck fracture should be suspected. As much as possible, the head and neck should be kept in a fixed, neutral position avoiding all forward, lateral, and turning movements. The first-aider must place his hands on either side of the head and fixate it. The lower jaw is

[116] Respiratory and Cardiopulmonary Resuscitation (CPR)

then moved forward using the index fingers without head movement backward or to the sides.

3. *Establish breathlessness.* After opening the airway, the first-aider must establish if the person is breathing or not breathing. With the head tilt being provided, the first-aider places his ear near the victim's mouth and nose, feeling and listening for outgoing air, while watching the chest to determine if it is rising and falling. This procedure is known as the "look, listen, and feel" method of determining absence or presence of breathing.

4. *Give four (4) ventilations.* While maintaining the head tilt and after establishing breathlessness, the first-aider must provide four (4) quick, full breaths allowing no time for lung deflation between ventilations. While pressure is applied to the forehead, that same hand is so rotated to allow the thumb and index finger to pinch the nostrils of the nose together. The first-aider covers his mouth over the victim's mouth maintaining a tight seal. He blows a sufficient volume of air into the mouth so the lungs can inflate and the chest can expand. The first four (4) ventilations will help provide maximum inflation of the lungs and give optimal oxygen exchange. If an airway obstruction is noted the proper techniques should be followed. These are reviewed in a later part of this chapter.

In some cases the first-aider may decide to use mouth-to-nose artificial ventilation. While maintaining the head tilt with the one hand, the other hand lifts the underneath side of the lower jaw thereby sealing the lips. He takes a deep breath, covers the victim's nose completely, and blows sufficient volume of air to inflate the lungs. Four (4) ventilations must be given with this technique. The first-aider may have to open the lips to allow some of the air to escape.

Direct mouth-to-stoma artificial ventilation should be used for a victim who has had his larynx (voice box) removed. A permanent stoma connects his trachea directly to the skin of the front of the lower neck. The head tilt must not be done with mouth-to-stoma resuscitation, because airway blockage may develop as a result. After sealing the victim's stoma with his mouth, the first-aider blows air into the mouth until the chest rises. The victim's nose or mouth does not have to be closed.

In the situation where a cervical spinal injury is suspected, the first-aider should use either mouth-to-nose or mouth-to-mouth-and-nose following the airway opening described in step 2. If it is still impossible to ventilate the lungs, then the head should be tilted back enough to inflate the lungs, and the procedure described for mouth-to-mouth should be used. The head should not be moved to the side.

5. *Establish pulselessness.* The purpose of this step is to determine whether or not blood is circulating. The carotid pulse on the neck is the most reliable indication of blood circulation. After the fourth ventilation has been given and the head tilt maintained by the one hand on the forehead, the first-

Procedure for CPR   [117]

aider uses the index and middle fingers of the other hand to find the larynx (Adam's apple) of the victim. The rescuer then rotates the fingers toward himself into the groove between the trachea (windpipe) and the muscles on the side of the neck. If a pulse is present it should be found here.

If a pulse is present, then the first-aider must continue the artificial ventilations started previously. He should breathe deeply, place his mouth over the victim's mouth, and blow air into the mouth and lungs. He will watch the victim's chest expand and then remove his mouth from the victim's mouth. The first-aider will listen for and feel the air as it escapes from the victim's mouth and keep his face close to the victim's nose and mouth. This process should be repeated every four or five seconds or 12 to 15 times per minute for an adult. The procedure should be continued until adequate breathing has been restored. Even in this situation, the pulse must be checked every minute or so to determine the extent of blood circulation.

6. *Provide artificial circulation.* If no pulse is present or there is some doubt as to its presence, artificial circulation combined with and followed by artificial ventilation must be performed.

   a. Preparation for artificial circulation. The victim must be in a horizontal position on a hard firm surface. The chest of the victim must be bared to help in locating landmarks for hand placement for compressions and to reduce injuries from objects on and around the wearing apparel.

   b. Locate landmark and position hands. In order to avoid damage to the internal organs under the rib cage, the first-aider must realize that the ribs are fragile and are fractured when too much pressure is applied to them. Also, the lower end of the sternum (the xiphoid process) can cause damage to the liver and stomach if the xiphoid tip is broken. Therefore it is important to know how to locate the correct spot for applying external cardiac compression. Compression must be applied on the sternum about 1 to 1 and one-half inches (25 to 38 mm) from the tip of the xiphoid.

   The procedure for locating this correct area to apply the compressions is as follows. The first-aider kneels next to the victim (near the lower chest) and slides the fingers of the hand nearest the lower end (feet) of the victim up the rib cage until the ring finger comes in contact with the groove in the center of the chest. This groove can be viewed as the depression where the sternum and xiphoid process come together. Once the groove is found, the first-aider places the middle and index fingers against the ring finger. If this is done correctly the index finger will be lying across the lower edge of the sternum. At this point the heel of the other hand should be placed just above the index finger with the heel of that hand on the midline of the sternum. The first-aider then places the other hand on top of the hand located on the bottom part of the sternum. The fingers may be interlocked if preferred. In any case the fingers must be kept off the ribs.

[118]   Respiratory and Cardiopulmonary Resuscitation (CPR)

c. **Compress sternum 15 times.** After the two hands are placed one on top of the other, the first-aider holds the arms stiff, elbows straight, and exerts force directly down onto the sternum depressing it approximately 1 and one-half to 2 inches (38 to 51 mm). The hip joints should be the parts of the body that rock forward and backward.

The pressure on the sternum must be released completely after each compression and be of approximately equal duration. The heel of the first-aider's hand must not lose contact with the skin on the sternum during relaxation.

With one first-aider, 15 chest compressions must be given followed by two quick artificial ventilations. For most efficient use of the 15 to 2 ratio, the single first-aider must provide the compressions at a rate of 80 compressions per minute. If the 15 compressions are given in 10 to 12 seconds followed by two ventilations, the first-aider will be able to give approximately 60 compressions each minute. In order to achieve the rate of 80 compressions per minute, mnemonic (count) used is "one, and two, and three, and four, and five, and one, and two, and three, and four, and ten, and one, and two, and three, and four, and fifteen." For each number said a compression is made at the same time.

7. **Give two (2) ventilations.** After 15 compressions have been given, two lung ventilations must be given in quick succession, not allowing complete lung deflation between ventilations. From the time of the last compression on the sternum, a maximum of five seconds should be used to give two ventilations, locate the landmark, and have the hands in position again on the sternum.

8. **Continue alternating 15 compressions and two ventilations.** A steady continuous rhythm must be achieved to provide the maximum blood circulation and basic life support.

9. **Check for pulse every minute or so.** After the initial four cycles of 15 compressions and two ventilations, the first-aider must check the carotid pulse for spontaneous return of heart circulation and the mouth for return of respiration. No more than five seconds should be used for checking respiration and circulation. The first-aider then returns to 15 compressions and two ventilations.

Two First-aider CPR

The previous material was concerned with the techniques of one first-aider performing CPR. Two CPR trained first-aiders can perform CPR more efficiently and effectively. When two CPR trained first-aiders are available at a situation where there is a possible cardiac arrest victim, one of the first-aiders should conduct the steps to establish unresponsiveness, open airway, establish breathlessness, give four ventilations, and establish pulselessness. Once pulselessness has been determined, the first-aider conducting the preliminary steps will motion the second first-aider to start chest compressions at the required number and rate. The two first-aiders must be on opposite sides of the victim.

The required compression rate for two first-aiders is 60 compressions per minute. The person conducting the compressions will perform them without interruption and will use the following mnemonic: "1-1000, 2-1000, 3-1000, 4-1000, 5-1000; 1-1000, 2-1000, 3-1000, 4-1000, 5-1000; etc." The first-aider performing the compressions will compress on 1, 2, 3, 4, 5. The first-aider performing the artificial ventilations must provide one breath after the word "five." Again, there must be no pause in the rhythm of the compressions. An interruption may cause the blood pressure to drop. From this discussion comes the ratio of five compressions and one ventilation.

In the situation where there is one first-aider performing CPR and another first-aider becomes available and identifies himself as being properly trained in CPR, the second first-aider ventilates once as soon as possible between any two compressions. When this occurs, the first-aider doing the compressions changes to the proper rate (60 compressions per minute) and mnemonic (1-1000, 2-1000, etc.) for two first-aider CPR.

Every three to five minutes the two first-aiders should stop the procedure for no more than five seconds to determine spontaneous return of respiration and circulation. In addition, the person performing the ventilations can check for effectiveness of the chest compressions by checking the carotid pulse. The first-aider is feeling for a pulsation with each chest compression and is performing this between ventilations.

When a switch of positions is necessary, it can be achieved with minimum interruption of the 5 to 1 cycle. The first-aider performing the compressions will change the mnemonic from "1-1000, 2-1000, 3-1000, 4-1000, 5-1000" to "WE, WILL, SWITCH, NEXT, BREATH." The person performing the ventilation will ventilate after the word "BREATH," move to the victim's side, and locate the landmark. In the meantime the first-aider giving the compressions continues giving two more compressions after the word "BREATH." The first-aider who has moved to the side of the victim will use the correct hand and take over the compressions on "3-1000." No compressions are missed. The other first-aider proceeds to the head, opens the airway, and gives one ventilation after "5-1000."

INFANT CPR

The procedure of CPR for infants and children is basically the same as the techniques previously discussed for adults with some exceptions. For purposes of emphasizing the correct procedure the differences will be noted in the discussion of the following steps for Infant CPR:

Respiratory and Cardiopulmonary Resuscitation (CPR)

FIGURE 8.4   INFANT CPR AT A GLANCE

Procedure	Suggested time for performance
Establish unresponsiveness	4–8 seconds
Open the airway	2 seconds
Establish breathlessness	3–4 seconds
Give four (4) ventilations	3–5 seconds
Establish pulselessness	5–8 seconds
Five (5) compressions and one (1) ventilation cycle	3–4 seconds per cycle

1   *Establish unresponsiveness.* With a small child or infant, the first-aider should either shout at the baby while shaking the shoulder or flicking the bottom of the infant's foot.
2   *Open the airway.* Open the airway by extension of or a slight backward tilting of the head. Overextending the head can result in collapse of the windpipe and obstruction of the breathing passage.
3   *Establish breathlessness.* After the airway has been opened, the first-aider should determine the presence or absence of breathing by putting an ear over the mouth of the child to feel and hear breathing and look towards the chest for movement.
4   *Give four (4) ventilations.* If the infant is not breathing, the first-aider should cover the mouth and nose of the infant with his mouth and use small puffs of air. The amount of air used is similar to puffing up the cheeks in the mouth.
5   *Establish pulselessness.* Normally with an adult it is suggested that the carotid artery be checked in order to establish pulselessness. The carotid arteries in the neck of an infant are small and may be difficult to locate. Therefore, the first-aider should check the pulse of an infant over the precordium (apical or aortic heartbeat) by gently placing the index and middle fingers on this area which is slightly left of the sternum and below the nipple line. The head tilt should be maintained during the pulse check.

   If a pulse is found, but the infant is not breathing, the first-aider should provide artificial ventilations (mouth-to-mouth) at the rate of 20 to 25 ventilations per minute or an average of one ventilation every three seconds. The precordium area should be checked every minute or so to see if a pulse can be determined. The pulse check should be accomplished without discontinuing the artificial ventilations.

   If no pulse was determined on the initial check or with the pulse check after starting artificial ventilations, the first-aider should continue to the next step.
6   *Locate midsternum, position tips of index and middle fingers over midsternum, and compress sternum five (5) times.* In preparing for the compressions on an infant, it is important for the first-aider to provide support

for the back of the infant. This can be done either by lowering the infant's head with proper hand support over the edge of a table and placing the hand closest to the infant's head under the back for support, allowing the head to fall back naturally, or by holding the infant on his arm, supporting the head of the infant in the palm, and providing support to the back with the forearm.

The proper area by which the first-aider should place the tips of the index and middle fingers is found by determining an invisible line between the nipples and placing one finger just above the line and the other finger just below the line. Both fingers must be placed together and on the sternum.

Five (5) compressions should be given with the finger tips in a downward direction so the chest is compressed one half to three quarters of an inch (13 to 19 mm). The compression rate should be approximately 100 compressions per minute. A puff of air should be delivered as quickly as possible after each five (5) compressions. As much as possible, the compressions should be smooth and regular even between the fifth compression of a cycle and the first compression of the next cycle.

7   Give one (1) ventilation. The one ventilation should be given immediately after the fifth compression. The first-aider must not attempt to ventilate and compress the chest at the same time because of the possibility of the lungs rupturing. The mouth of the first-aider should be close to the mouth of the infant in order to provide quick and proper ventilation.

8   Repeat steps 6 and 7 uninterrupted. The first-aider should continue with five (5) compressions followed by one ventilation until breathing and circulation is restored or someone else can take over. A pulse check taking no longer than five (5) seconds should be made approximately every minute. Artificial ventilations and compressions should be discontinued during these five (5) seconds.

FOREIGN BODY AIRWAY OBSTRUCTION

In a recent year, foreign body obstruction of the airway resulted in 2,900 persons dying in the United States.[5] Airway obstruction can result in respiratory and/or cardiopulmonary arrest.

One of the main causes of foreign body airway obstruction is food stuck in the trachea. Typically a person who chokes on food is wearing loose fitting dentures, drinking alcohol, or attempting to swallow large solid food. However, many other substances can cause airway obstruction including paper wads, balloons, small toys, and coins. These airway obstructions usually occur while the person is conscious. The victim can suddenly lose consciousness. For a person who is found unconscious, the most frequent cause of airway obstruction is that of the tongue falling

[5] National Safety Council, *Accident Facts*. Chicago: The Council, 1977, p. 7.

back into the upper airway. Also, vomiting of stomach contents into the upper airway can happen during a pulmonary or cardiopulmonary arrest or even during resuscitation attempts. Blood clots obstructing the upper airway can result from injuries to the head and neck area.

Prevention

Preventive care is the key to avoiding an airway obstruction. In order to avoid an airway obstruction one should

1. Keep small foreign objects from the reach of young children.
2. Try to keep young children from running while they have any type of foreign object in their mouths.
3. Cut food into small pieces.
4. Chew all food very thoroughly and slowly, particularly if one wears dentures.
5. Minimize talking and particularly laughing when chewing.
6. Restrict alcohol intake both before and during meals.

Symptoms

One will find that a foreign body in the airway can result in either a partial or complete airway obstruction. The key to successful first aid of an airway obstruction is early identification and recognition of its symptoms.

Partial Airway Obstruction When a victim has a partial airway obstruction, a good air exchange may exist.

1. With a good air exchange, the victim will usually be able to cough forcefully. However, a wheezing noise may sometimes be heard between coughs. When a good air exchange situation exists, the victim should continue to cough, and no attempt should be made to interfere with his attempt to get rid of the foreign object.
2. With a poor air exchange, a victim normally has a weak ineffective cough. Sometimes while the victim is inhaling, high-pitched sounds such as a crowing-like noise occurs. If the partial airway obstruction continues, there will probably be more respiratory difficulty and possible cyanosis. If these symptoms occur, the first aid for the partial airway obstruction should be managed as the first aid for a complete airway obstruction.

Complete Airway Obstruction This condition can occur to a conscious person from either eating food or from some other foreign object. The victim is unable to respond verbally or by coughing when asked, "Can you speak?" The victim may clutch his neck with his hand. Exaggerated

Foreign Body Airway Obstruction [123]

efforts to breathe might be evident, and air movement from the victim will not be detectable. Within a short time, the oxygen in the lungs will probably be exhausted because of the lack of air to the lungs. Unconsciousness will occur soon and death will follow.

Protection for Standing or Sitting Conscious Victim—Complete Airway Obstruction

It is important to remember the prompt and proper action that must be taken, preferably, while the victim is still conscious. Once the symptoms of a complete airway obstruction are recognized, the first-aider should

1. *Ask the victim if he can speak.* If the victim is unable to speak, an airway obstruction is a clear indication.
2. *Give the victim four (4) back blows.* The first-aider should stand behind the victim and slightly to one side, bend the victim forward, place one hand on the victim's chest for support, and deliver four (4) sharp, rapid, and forceful blows to the spine between the shoulder blades. If the airway is still obstructed, the first-aider should go to the next step. He should talk to the victim while working with him.
3. *Give the victim four (4) abdominal thrusts.* The first-aider stands behind the victim with his arms wrapped around the victim's waist. The first-aider places the thumb side of one fist between the xiphoid and the (umbilicus) navel, and presses the fist into the victim's abdomen with quick upward thrusts.
4. *Repeat steps 2 and 3 until effective or victim loses consciousness.* If steps 2 and 3 are ineffective, repeat the maneuvers of four back blows and four abdominal thrusts in rapid sequence until the airway is cleared.

Protection for Victim Who Loses Consciousness—Complete Airway Obstruction

If the victim loses consciousness while the first-aider is trying to provide protection (and the obstruction is still present), he should

1. Place the victim on the ground or floor and *roll the victim onto his side towards the first-aider,* supporting the victim's neck, and using the thigh for support of the abdomen area.
2. *Give four (4) back blows.* The first-aider gives four (4) forceful and rapidly delivered blows with the heel of one hand to the spine between the shoulder blades.
3. *Check for foreign body.* After giving the four (4) back blows, the first-aider should check to see if the object was successfully dislodged. The victim should be rolled on his back, maintaining the head to the side and using

[124]   Respiratory and Cardiopulmonary Resuscitation (CPR)

one or more of the following techniques for manual removal of a foreign object in the airway:
  a. *Cross Finger Technique.* In this technique the first-aider crosses his thumb under the index finger and slips them under the victim's lips in the upper corner of the mouth. The first-aider should brace his thumb against the lower teeth and the index finger against the upper teeth, push the thumb and finger in opposite directions to separate the jaws, and sweep out the mouth with the index finger of the opposite hand.
  b. *Tongue-Jaw Lift.* With this technique, the first-aider lifts both the tongue and lower jaw between the thumb (inside the mouth) and the fingers (outside the mouth on the jaw). The foreign body may become visible when lifting up the tongue and jaw. The index finger from the opposite hand should be used to check the mouth for a foreign object. The first-aider should use a hooking action to dislodge the object and take it gently out of the mouth. He should try not to force the object any deeper into the air passage.
4. *Open the airway and attempt to ventilate four (4) times.* Once the airway has been checked and a foreign body is not visible, the first-aider should use the head tilt while opening the airway and making attempts to ventilate. If the chest fails to rise, he will continue to the next step.
5. *Give four (4) abdominal thrusts.* The head of the victim should be turned to one side. The first-aider should straddle the victim's hips or one leg and place the heel of one hand between the umbilicus (navel) and xiphoid. The second hand is placed on top of the first hand, and the first-aider presses into the abdomen with quick upward thrusts. He should not press to either side. Up to four (4) abdominal thrusts should be performed.
6. *Check for foreign body.* With his head still turned to the side, the victim's mouth should be checked for a foreign object as described in step 3.
7. *Open the airway and attempt to ventilate four (4) times.* The first-aider repositions the head, using the head tilt, and attempts to ventilate.
8. *Repeat steps 1 through 7.* If after attempting to ventilate, the airway is still obstructed, repeat the steps described in items 1 through 7 in rapid succession up to four (4) times. If the airway continues to be obstructed after four (4) cycles, reposition the head with maximum head tilt and blow full, but slow, forceful ventilations into the mouth. It is hoped that this air will be forced around the foreign object and provide air to the lungs.
9. *If successful in clearing the airway, perform CPR, if necessary.*

Protection for Unconscious Victim—Complete
Airway Obstruction

If the first-aider while performing CPR to an unconscious person realizes that the victim has an airway obstruction, he should do the following. (The steps start out the same as performing CPR, and details for various steps are discussed in previous sections of this chapter.)

Foreign Body Airway Obstruction [125]

1. *Establish unresponsiveness.*
2. *Open the airway and establish breathlessness.*
3. *Attempt to ventilate.* The first-aider should try to ventilate four (4) times. If at any time the first-aider discovers an airway obstruction, he should continue to one of the manual methods of removal of foreign objects.
4. *Reposition the head and reattempt ventilation.* Many times the initial failure to inflate the lungs by the first-aider is a result of improper head tilt. The repositioning of the head may raise the tongue away from the air passage and allow the victim to breathe on his own. If airway obstruction is still present, the first-aider should continue on to the next steps.
5. *Give four (4) back blows.*
6. *Check for foreign body.*
7. *Open the airway and attempt to ventilate four (4) times.*
8. *Give four (4) abdominal thrusts.*
9. *Check for foreign body.*
10. *Open the airway and attempt to ventilate four (4) times.*
11. *Repeat steps 5 through 10.* Repeat these steps in rapid sequence. If unsuccessful after four cycles of the aforementioned steps, reposition the head with maximum head tilt and blow forcefully into the mouth.
12. *If successful in clearing the airway, continue with CPR, if necessary.* The first-aider should give four (4) ventilations, check for pulse and if there is no pulse, continue with external cardiac compression and the proper CPR procedures.

Protection for Infants and Small Children—Airway Obstruction

The first aid procedure and techniques for airway obstruction in infants and small children up to forty pounds is different than that just described. With infants and young children up to forty pounds, the first-aider should

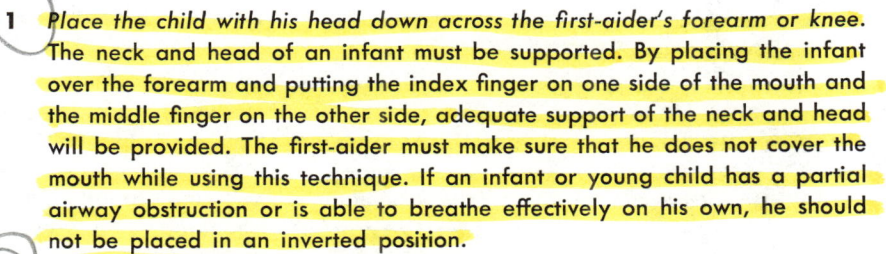

1. *Place the child with his head down across the first-aider's forearm or knee.* The neck and head of an infant must be supported. By placing the infant over the forearm and putting the index finger on one side of the mouth and the middle finger on the other side, adequate support of the neck and head will be provided. The first-aider must make sure that he does not cover the mouth while using this technique. If an infant or young child has a partial airway obstruction or is able to breathe effectively on his own, he should not be placed in an inverted position.
2. *Give four (4) gentle sharp blows between the shoulder blades.*
3. *Provide pressure upwards along the lower portion of the child's back.* This technique can be used if the back blows are ineffective. The pressure is applied on the back in the same position as the abdominal thrust is applied on an adult.
4. *If successful in clearing the airway, continue with Infant CPR, if necessary.*

[126] Respiratory and Cardiopulmonary Resuscitation (CPR)

The Chest Thrust—Alternative Technique to the Abdominal Thrust

When the victim of an airway obstruction is markedly obese or in advanced stages of pregnancy, the chest thrust method of relieving an airway obstruction might be considered. The first-aider should consider the following sequence if the victim is standing or sitting. He should

1. Ask the victim to speak if conscious.
2. Give the victim four (4) back blows.
3. Give the victim four (4) chest thrusts. While standing behind the victim, the first-aider will place his arms under the victim's arms and encompass the victim's chest. One of the first-aider's fists will be placed thumb side against the lower part of the sternum. The other hand is placed over the fist and quick backward thrusts should be applied in rapid succession.
4. Repeat steps 2 and 3 until effective or victim loses consciousness.

If the pregnant or obese victim is lying on the ground or floor, the first-aider should

1. Place victim on side with face toward the first-aider.
2. Give four (4) back blows.
3. Check for foreign body. If the person is conscious, the first-aider should consider going to step 5.
4. Open the airway and attempt to ventilate four (4) times. Again, if the victim is conscious, the first-aider must go to step 5.
5. Give four (4) chest thrusts. The first-aider should turn the victim's head to one side and straddle the hips or kneel close to one side of the victim's body. The first-aider should place the heels of his hands on the sides of the victim's chest at the level of the nipples. The thumbs of the first-aider should rest on either side of the sternum, and the fingers should curl around the rib cage. While being in a perpendicular position to the chest, he should exert a rapid downward and inward thrust with a squeezing action, thereby compressing the chest.

GASTRIC DISTENTION

In many cases distention of the stomach results from too much air being blown into the mouth or the airway being obstructed. The American National Red Cross has identified five possible effects of stomach distention:

1. The distended stomach elevates the diaphragm, which compresses both lower lungs and reduces the effectiveness of artificial respiration.
2. The elevated diaphragm may also distort the position of the heart and great vessels and impair venous return.

Chest-Pressure Arm-Lift Artificial Ventilation Method [127]

3. The enlarged stomach compresses the abdominal organs and reduces venous return and ultimately cardiac output.
4. The distended stomach may promote reflexes that are harmful to the circulation.
5. The distended stomach is prone to sudden regurgitation, which carries liquid gastric contents into the pharynx, which in turn is followed frequently by aspiration into the trachea and lungs.[6]

Protection

For the unconscious person, gastric distention probably can be alleviated. The first-aider should

1. Stop CPR for a very short period of time.
2. Turn the victim on his side or just turn his head to the side.
3. Apply moderate pressure with the hand over the upper abdomen of the victim. The upper abdomen is located between the rib cage and navel.

CHEST-PRESSURE ARM-LIFT ARTIFICIAL VENTILATION METHOD

This is one of the older manual methods. It was first developed by Silvester, an Englishman, in the 1850s. It is only recommended when mouth-to-mouth, mouth-to-nose, or mouth-to-stoma resuscitation cannot be used. This occurs when severe facial injuries on the victim result in one of the preferred methods being unacceptable.

The steps in the chest-pressure arm-lift method are as follows:

1. The victim is placed on his back. The mouth should be examined and any foreign matter or object removed. If pillows, blankets, or other materials are readily available, they should be placed beneath the shoulders to raise them and to permit the head to fall sharply backward. A special effort should be made to cause the chin to jut forward and upward to help keep the breathing passage open.
2. The rescuer then assumes the kneeling position on one or both knees and then alternates his knees to keep them from becoming too uncomfortable. The rescuer grasps the victim's wrists and crosses them or places them side-by-side over the victim's chest in the region of the diaphragm or lower rib-cage. It is important that the victim's wrists not be positioned too high on the chest or down on the stomach or abdomen. If a second rescuer is available he can concentrate on the victim's chin and keep it properly positioned. The rescuer rocks forward keeping his arms straight, permitting the weight of his body to force the air from the victim's lungs.

[6] American National Red Cross, *Cardiopulmonary Resuscitation*. Washington, D.C.: American National Red Cross, 1974, p. 37.

[128] Respiratory and Cardiopulmonary Resuscitation (CPR)

3 The rescuer releases the pressure on the victim's chest and then moves the victim's arms upward and outward in the widest possible movement. This enables the chest to expand and causes the lungs to be filled with air. Then the victim's arms are moved back to his chest and a new cycle is begun.

If used, this method should be applied at the rate of 14 to 16 times per minute for the adult and some 18 to 20 times per minute for children.

ACTIVITIES

1 Take a CPR course from a local Heart Association or American National Red Cross. Develop proficiency in unwitnessed CPR, infant CPR, and helping a person with an airway obstruction.
2 Visit a local hospital and determine the equipment used in the medical treatment of respiratory and/or cardiac arrest.
3 Compare and contrast the techniques used in adult CPR and infant CPR. Prepare the findings for a presentation to a peer group.
4 Become an instructor in Basic Life Support—CPR through the American National Red Cross or state Heart Association. Teach two to three classes of CPR each year to the general public.
5 Organize and give a presentation to the class on the merits of different methods of artificial ventilation.

QUESTIONS TO ANSWER

1 What are the symptoms of respiratory arrest?
2 What are the symptoms of cardiac arrest?
3 What parts of the body are the first to be affected by the lack of oxygen?
4 What is the difference between clinical death and biological death?
5 Describe the breathing system. Describe the cardiovascular system. Identify how they are interrelated.
6 Define the A-B-C steps of CPR.
7 Describe when CPR should begin and be terminated.
8 How much pressure should be applied in performing the compressions to the sternum of an adult?
9 Describe the different symptoms of a partial airway obstruction and a complete airway obstruction.
10 Is the airway obstruction technique different for an infant than an adult? If so, describe the differences.

SELECTED REFERENCES

AMERICAN HEART ASSOCIATION, *CPR in Basic Life Support for Unwitnessed Cardiac Arrest*. Dallas, Texas: American Heart Association, 1977.

AMERICAN HEART ASSOCIATION, *Heart Attack*. Dallas, Texas: American Heart Association, 1975.

AMERICAN NATIONAL RED CROSS, *Cardiopulmonary Resuscitation*. Washington, D.C.: American National Red Cross, 1974.

AMERICAN NATIONAL RED CROSS, *CPR Workbook—Modular System*. Washington, D.C.: American National Red Cross, 1975.

AMERICAN NATIONAL RED CROSS, *First Aid for Foreign Body Obstruction of the Airway*. Washington, D.C.: American National Red Cross, 1976.

AMERICAN NATIONAL RED CROSS, *Instructor's Manual—Cardiopulmonary Resuscitation Basic Life Support*. Washington, D.C.: American National Red Cross, 1974.

"CARDIAC EMERGENCIES," *Emergency Medicine*, March, 1974, pp. 48–73.

HUSZAR, ROBERT J., *Emergency Cardiac Care*. Bowie, Md.: Robert J. Brady, 1974.

JUDE, JAMES R., *Closed Chest Cardiac Resuscitation: Methods—Indications–Limitations*. New York: American Heart Association, 1966.

"STANDARDS FOR CARDIOPULMONARY RESUSCITATION (CPR) AND EMERGENCY CARDIAC CARE," Supplement to *Journal of the American Medical Association*, Vol. 227, No. 7 (February 18, 1974), pp. 833–868.

9. TEMPERATURE PROBLEMS

Any time the human body is exposed to extremes in temperature, there can be damage or injury to the skin, tissues, muscles, bones, and vital organs. The extremes in temperature can be either excessive heat or cold. The purpose of this chapter is to discuss the major injuries that are attributed to temperature problems and to describe how first-aid rescuers can protect victims until medical help is obtained.

BURNS

Accidental deaths from fires and burns took between 6,000 and 10,000 lives in a recent year. Most of these deaths could have been prevented if smoke detectors were installed in all homes. Fires and burns continue to be major safety problems for people of all ages but especially so for the child under age 4 and the older segment of our population, age 65 and over. Many burn victims do not lose their lives but suffer great pain, are disfigured and scarred, and suffer emotionally as well as physically. Severe burns require much time to heal, and hospital care can be very costly. Thermal burns are usually classified as first-degree, second-degree, third-degree, and, by some, fourth-degree.[1] The degree indicates the intensity and severity of the burns.

In many cases it is impossible to determine the extent or severity of a burn injury through a cursory visual examination. The seriousness of a burn may only become apparent after several hours or days. For example,

---

[1] John Henderson, *Emergency Medical Guide*, 4th ed. New York: McGraw-Hill, 1978.

a third-degree burn caused by a leg coming in contact with a hot motorcycle exhaust pipe may initially resemble a first-degree burn. Later, blisters form around the outer periphery of the burned area, swelling occurs, and after a few days the skin may start to slough off in the central area of the burn. Burns caused by microwave radiation are particularly difficult to ascertain because subsurface tissue damage may be quite extensive even though the skin surface shows little initial change.

Pain is not a particularly good initial indicator of the seriousness of burn injuries because the nerves may be burned away and pain be in little evidence. The psychological state of the burn victim may further mask the true gravity of the burn injury. Great pain may be present even when the area of the burn and depth of tissue damage is rather negligible. All burns should be considered possible sources of infection. Regardless of the apparent seriousness of a burn, the first-aider should be particularly careful to protect against contamination of the wound.

First-Degree Burns

First-degree burns are characterized by an intense reddening of the skin, usually covering a large area, such as in the case of sunburn. A common cause of first-degree burn is steam from boiling water. The pain from a first-degree burn may range from moderate to very painful, but as a rule it will heal with little assistance and without a scar.

Sunburn can be serious. It is important that the first exposures to the sun in the spring and summer be moderate and that they not exceed 30 minutes. For persons with light complexions, the exposure should be about half of that duration. It is recommended that a person avoid the noonday sun and that the exposure be in the morning or late afternoon when the rays are not so intense.

Many persons are victims of severe sunburn because they underestimate the sun's power, particularly on semicloudy days. Reflecting surfaces such as water or snow also intensify the effect of the sun. Too much exposure to the sun can produce a dangerous result and lead to the formation of precancerous keratotic lesions of the skin.

Numerous suggestions have been made for the protection of the first-degree burn—e.g., the use of white petrolatum or any of several good burn ointments, then covering with a sterile dressing. A more recent protection for the first-degree burn is the use of cold water. This method is recommended by Dr. Alex G. Shulman.[2] It consists of placing the burned part in cold water, 70°F or colder, and leaving the burned part in the cold water until it can be removed without feeling pain. This is an excellent method, especially for children, because it checks the pain quickly.

[2] Alex G. Shulman, "Burned, Try Cold Water." *Family Safety*. Chicago: National Safety Council, Summer, 1963.

[132]   Temperature Problems

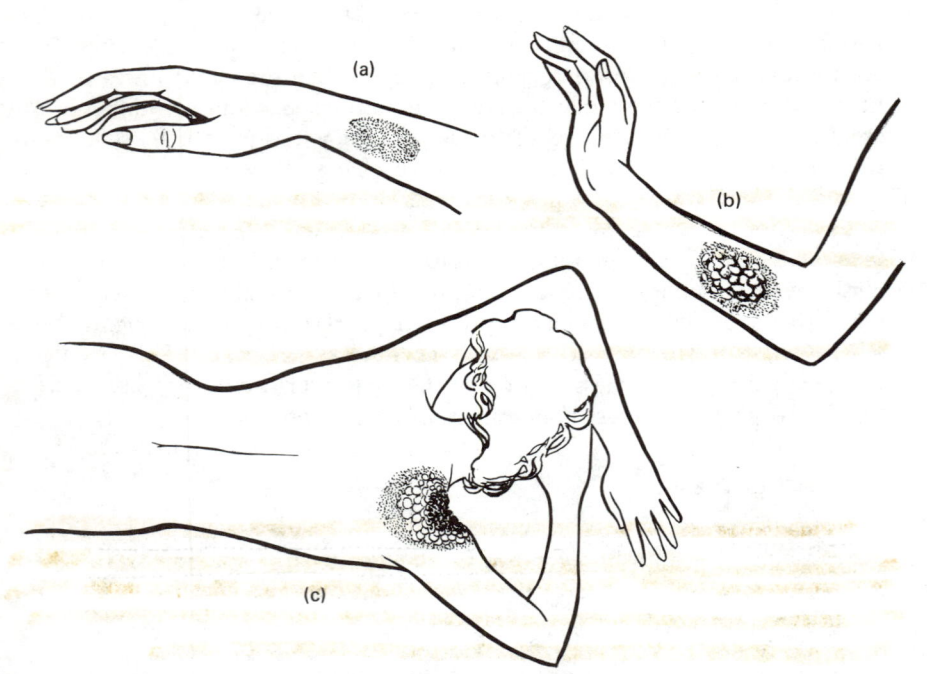

FIGURE 9.1 Degrees of burns: (a) first degree, such as from sunburn or steam—reddening of skin; (b) second degree—formation of blisters; (c) third degree—damage to underlying tissues.

Second-Degree Burns

Second-degree burns are characterized by the formation of blisters. The heat has penetrated more deeply into the skin and has caused body fluids to leak and to collect beneath the skin and to rise as a blister. These burns present a greater problem because the blister must be protected to prevent a skin rupture and to keep infectious organisms from entering the body. The second-degree burn normally will not result in a scar formation. If second-degree burns are intense, such as in severe sunburn, blisters may arise at a later time and cover a large area.

To protect the second-degree burn it is suggested that the first-aider cleanse the area of the burn by washing carefully, preferably with sterile soap. If the burn is in an area where it is subject to rupture, it should be covered with a sterile dressing. It is suggested that the blister not be opened. The cold water method described previously is also useful in the protection of second-degree burns. This method as outlined by Dr. Schulman is very effective and is an excellent protective measure for the first-aider to use until medical help is obtained.

Third-Degree Burns

Third-degree burns penetrate through the entire thickness of the skin and cause a complete destruction of the skin tissues. A third-degree burn is the most serious type burn. It leaves the terrible scar with its emotional impact. The scar can be removed and corrected only by a skilled surgeon. This type of burn not only destroys the outer covering of the skin but also destroys tendons, bones, and muscles and other underlying tissues in its path. Great care should be exercised in the home, at play, and in all types of industry to prevent third-degree burns.

First-aid rescuers can help the victim of a third-degree burn by giving some protection against infection and shock by getting him to a hospital. This is the limit to which the first-aider should go in working with the third-degree burn victim. All such victims belong in the hospital under expert care.

A common mistake made by the lay person (not by the first-aider, it is hoped), is to apply some home remedy such as butter, oleo, lard, cream, salad dressing, or mayonnaise on the burned area. These home remedies create problems by obscuring the appearance of the burned area and must be removed by medical personnel before they can access the wound. An even greater danger is that the substance will be a source of infectious organisms which will contaminate the burned area and lead to serious problems.

It is recommended that the burned area be covered with a dry burn dressing several layers thick if possible. In the home this could be a clean sheet or tablecloth; it should be unfolded and its unexposed or inner part placed over the burn. The use of aluminum foil or a cello-wrap over the burned area also can prevent contaminants from entering the wound. An unused plastic bag of the type used by dry cleaning establishments also may serve to cover the wound.[3] These would not be sterile but would be helpful. Nothing should be placed on the burned area other than one of these dry burn dressings. The victim should be protected against chilling.

A badly burned person is a shock case. Shock can mean loss of life. Drinking salt and soda in water will help to control shock. Start salt and soda at the earliest possible moment.

The U.S. Public Health Service suggests the following for the protection of severe burns:

A—Give salt and soda in water to drink.

In 1 quart of cool water, dissolve 1 level teaspoon of table salt and one-half teaspoon of baking soda.

---

[3] American National Red Cross, *Standard First Aid and Personal Safety*. New York: Doubleday, 1973.

[134]   Temperature Problems

If the burned person is conscious, have him drink this solution and nothing else, except on doctor's orders. Keep giving him this solution. He may need as much as 10 quarts in 24 hours.

Encourage him to drink just as much as he can, so long as he does not vomit. He will be thirsty, and he will want to drink. But do not give him anything else except the salt and soda solution. If vomiting begins, get him to a hospital at once.

Always be sure there is exactly 1 teaspoon of salt and one-half teaspoon of soda to a quart of cool water. Too much salt may upset the stomach; to little will not do the job.

B—Protect the burn

Leave bad burns for the doctor to treat, but try to keep burns from being contaminated. Cover burns to keep them from getting dirty or infected.

C—Keep the person comfortable

Do not move the burned person unless it is absolutely necessary. Have him lie flat. Make him as comfortable as you can. Do not let him get chilled.[4]

The first-aider should not pull or tear any debris from the third-degree burn area. Charred clothing or similar matter should be carefully cut away with sharp scissors, taking care not to touch the wound.

Fourth-Degree Burns

Henderson [5] describes the term *fourth-degree burn* as that burn which affects the tissues underlying the layers of the skin, such as a bone, tendon, muscle, or blood vessel. An attempt to distinguish between third- and fourth-degree burns from the standpoint of protection for the first-aider is not made. The first-aider should protect against shock and infection and make every effort to obtain medical assistance immediately.

Position of Burn Victim

Normally a flat position is best for the burned victim, depending upon the location of the burns. It is helpful to elevate the feet and also to elevate the burned part above the body and keep it in this position.

---

[4] U.S. Public Health Service, "ABC's of Salt and Soda for Shock in Burns," Publication No. 43. Washington, D.C.: U.S. Government Printing Office, 1950.

[5] Henderson, op. cit.

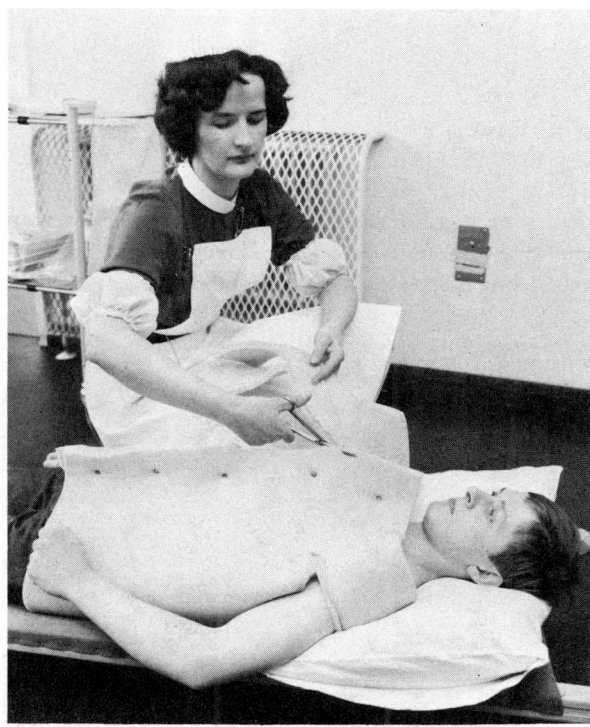

FIGURE 9.2 Use of polyurethane foam in the treatment of burns. (Roehampton Medical Supply Company Ltd. *Nursing Mirror* photographs)

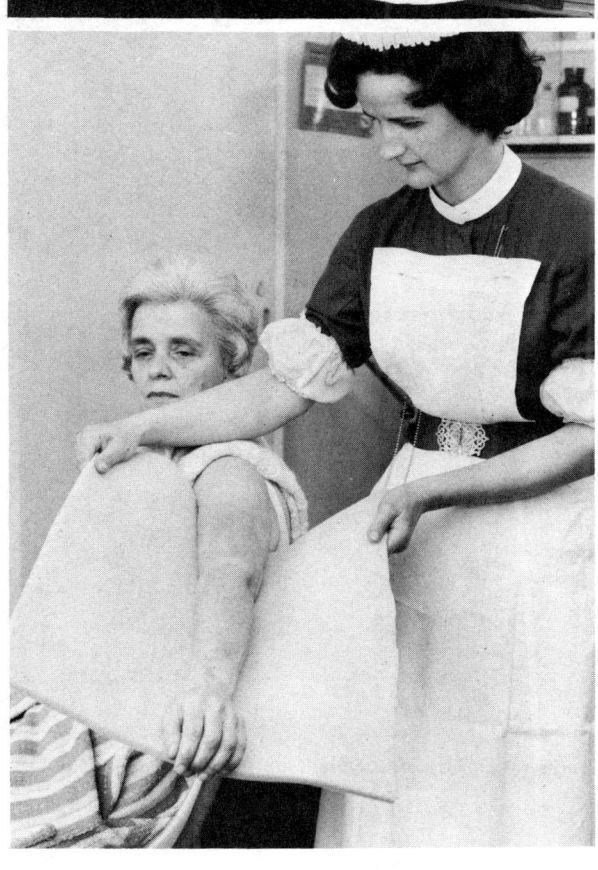

[136] Temperature Problems

CHEMICAL BURNS

If strong acids or alkalis such as battery fluid, drain cleaners, oven cleaners, paint removers, and a host of industrial chemicals come in contact with the body, chemical burns may result. These substances are very

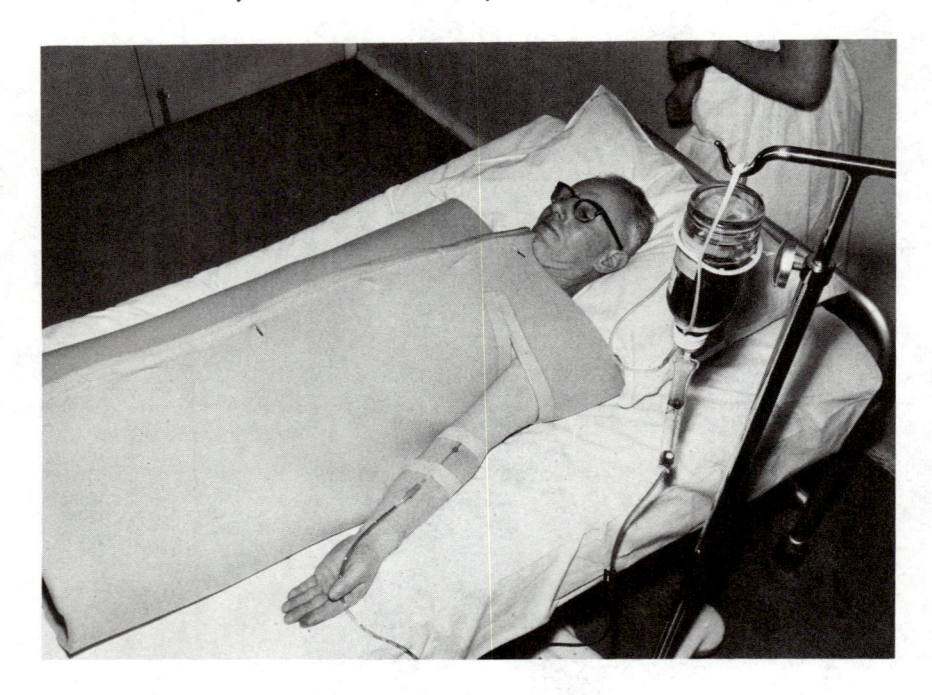

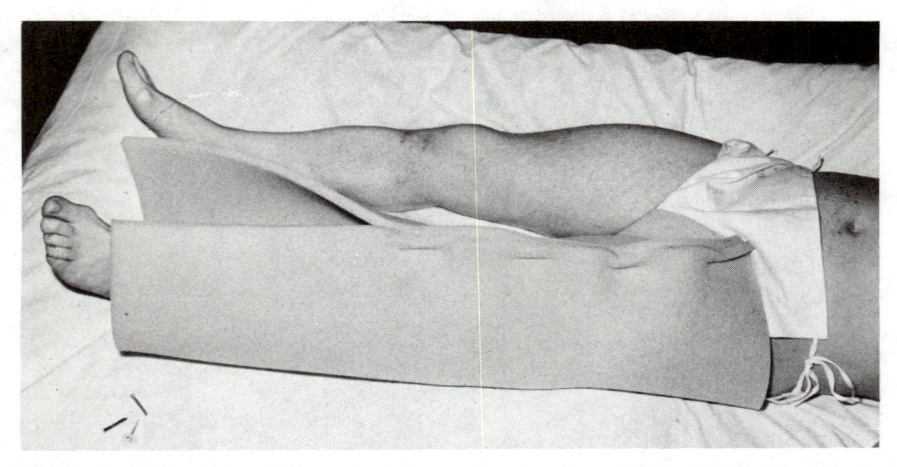

FIGURE 9.3 Protection of burns by the use of polyurethane foam. (Roehampton Medical Supply Company Ltd.)

Chemical Burns [137]

caustic and fast-acting. The first-aider should act quickly to protect the victim.

It is not suggested or recommended that the rescuer attempt to neutralize the effects of the poisonous substance. However, it is suggested that the part of the body that has been exposed to the chemical be flooded with water. For example, if the eyes are exposed, as when an automobile battery explodes while a car is being jump-started, the process of irrigation of the eyes should be started immediately. The head and eye or eyes can be placed beneath a tap of running water, or water can be poured from a container into the eyes. It is preferable to use water, but if it is not avail-

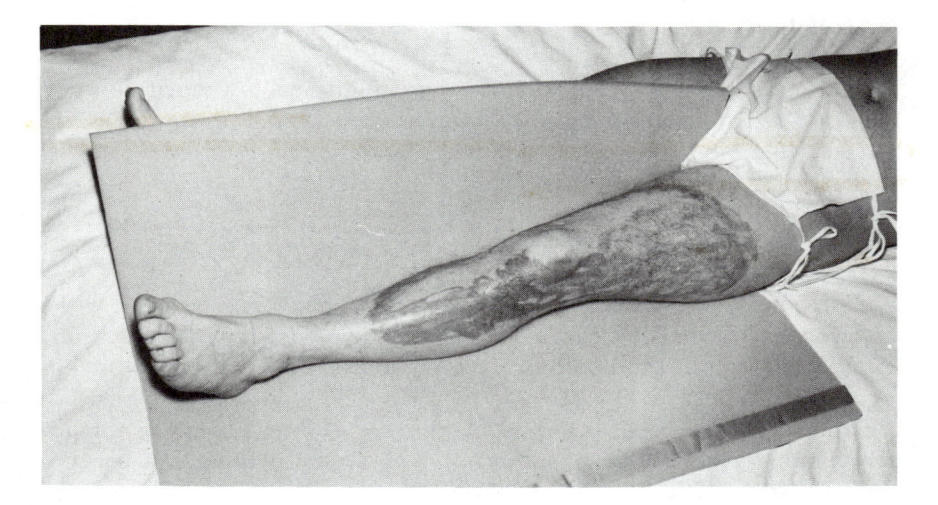

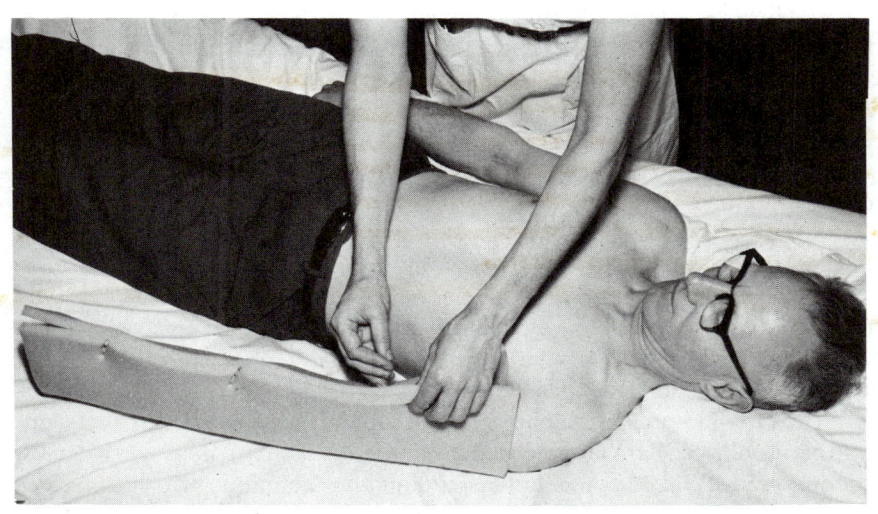

FIGURE 9.3 (Continued)

[138] Temperature Problems

able, fruit juice, soda pop, milk, or a similar fluid should be poured over the burned eyes immediately to dilute the caustic substance. Irrigation of the eyes should be continued while the person is transported to medical help. If the clothes have been saturated with the acid or alkali, the clothes should be removed and the burned area flooded. Many industries have special showers for such cases. After the first-aider gives protective care, the victim should be seen and treated by a physician. There are specific antidotes for specific acid and alkali burns that the first-aider may want to investigate. As such action constitutes treatment, a medical person needs to be consulted.

MAJOR HEAT PROBLEMS

The major heat problems involve both high and low environmental temperatures and man's struggle to adapt to them. Man is a warm-blooded animal, which implies that his body temperature should remain constant regardless of his surroundings.

Acclimatization

Individuals vary in their adaptability to bodily stress caused by the variations in temperature and climate from the norms in which they feel comfortable. When this bodily stress is combined with the severe psychological stress of suddenly being lost in a hostile environment (blizzard, capsizing, marooning) or being unable to cope with an adventure (mountain climbing, backpacking), survival is both a physiological and psychological matter. Cases of persons dying of exposure in temperatures of 60°F when well clothed and equipped are in direct contrast to the remarkable feats of those surviving many months in subzero temperatures.

The body can and will adapt to great changes in temperature whether it be hot or cold; however, it does require time and there are limitations. If a person realizes this, does not panic, and takes appropriate measures to control to the extent possible the stresses placed upon him (prevention of loss of body heat in cold temperatures and avoidance of unnecessary fluid loss and exposure to the sun in hot temperatures) then the body is given time to adapt and survive.

Perhaps the most important variable in survival is a person's desire to live. If a person gives up, he probably will die. However, if he wishes to live, he probably will survive provided he does not make mistakes that sap the body of its necessary heat and fluids.

A thorough study of acclimatization and survival is beyond the scope of this book. It can be mastered best by carefully studying situations encountered by others and understanding the techniques they employed to endure and survive their circumstances.

Major Heat Problems [139]

FIGURE 9.4 WIND-CHILL CHART

Estimated Wind Speeds MPH	\multicolumn{11}{c}{ACTUAL THERMOMETER READING}
	50	40	30	20	10	0	—10	—20	—30	—40	—50	—60
	\multicolumn{12}{c}{EQUIVALENT TEMPERATURE °F.}
Calm	50	40	30	20	10	0	—10	—20	—30	—40	—50	—60
5	48	37	27	16	6	—5	—15	—26	—36	—47	—57	—68
10	40	28	16	4	—9	—21	—33	—46	—58	—70	—83	—95
15	36	22	9	—5	—18	—36	—45	—58	—72	—85	—99	—112
20	32	18	4	—10	—25	—39	—53	—67	—82	—96	—110	—124
25	50	16	0	—15	—29	—44	—59	—74	—88	—104	—118	—133
30	28	13	—2	—18	—33	—48	—63	—79	—94	—109	—125	—140
35	27	11	—4	—20	—35	—49	—67	—82	—98	—113	—129	—145
40	26	10	—6	—21	—37	—53	—69	—85	—100	—116	—132	—148

Wind speeds greater than 40 mph have little additional effect	LITTLE DAMAGE FOR PROPERLY CLOTHED PERSON	INCREASING DANGER	GREAT DANGER
		DANGER FROM FREEZING OF EXPOSED FLESH	

TO USE THE CHART, find the estimated or actual wind speed in the left-hand column and the actual temperature in degrees F. in the top row. The equivalent temperature is found where these two intersect. For example, with a wind speed of 10 mph and a temperature of —10°F. This lies within the zone of increasing danger of frostbite, and protective measures should be taken.

Hypothermia

Hypothermia is the lowering of body temperature through exposure to cold air or water, or a combination of low temperature and wind. It can be a great danger to outdoorsmen, snowmobilers, and motorcyclists because it affects judgment and reaction time. It is best prevented by selecting proper clothing and preplanning to provide warmth or to include muscular activity that increases circulation and body heat.

Wind chill causes the effect of a given air temperature to be greatly increased in its ability to take heat from the body. Many newspapers and radio stations report wind chill temperatures as well as still air temperatures in local weather reports and forecasts.

Shivering is the way the body informs a person that he should get out of the cold or start moving in order to generate heat. If unheeded, numbness is often the prelude to frostbite.

Temperature Problems

Frostbite

Frostbite means that the tissues are frozen. Ice crystals form between the cells of the body. As these crystals of ice get larger, they draw water from the body cells and thus cause injury to the cells. The tissues of the body most susceptible to freezing are the skin, blood vessels, nerves, and muscles. The combination of a freezing temperature and a cold blowing wind sets the stage for frozen body tissues. The external parts of the body commonly affected are the ears, fingers, toes, and face. These parts need good protection from the cold.

Goose down and other types of down provide exceedingly good protection against cold. Its extremely light weight and the small space necessary to store it are its advantages over other types of cold weather clothing. However, it is somewhat expensive to purchase. Woolen clothing, with its many air spaces and ability to provide warmth when wet, also is quite good for cold weather warmth and protection against exposure and frostbite. Some of the newer synthetic materials provide some warmth at lower cost than down or wool. Insulated boots have proven to be very comforting to the person who works in or enjoys the outdoors during the winter season.

The use of alcohol, smoking, excessive perspiration, fatigue, advanced age, and exertion are contributing factors to frostbite. The first signs of trouble are the blanched skin, which turns gray in color, discomfort, and the loss of pain in the frozen part. The part becomes numb and the skin turns from white to glossy. To protect against frostbite, the rescuer should heed the following advice.[6]

1. Cover the frozen part and wrap the victim in a blanket or extra clothing.
2. Take the victim indoors (preferably a 70° to 80°F room) as soon as possible.
3. Give the victim warm fluids (water, coffee, tea, or broth) to drink if he is conscious and not vomiting.
4. Rewarm the frozen part by immersing it in water that is 102° to 105°F. If available, a thermometer should be used to check the temperature of the water. NOTE: If the affected part has been thawed and refrozen, it should be warmed at room temperature.
5. If warm water is not available or practical to use, gently wrap the affected part in a sheet and warm blankets.
6. Never rub or roughly handle the frozen part. Boots and gloves should be cut off, and if frozen they should be soaked and then cut.
7. Never use a heat lamp or hot water bottle on the affected area.
8. Never allow the victim's frozen part near a fire or hot stove.

---

[6] American National Red Cross, *Standard First Aid and Personal Safety*. New York: Doubleday, 1973, pp. 162–163.

9. Never break the blisters.
10. Never let the victim walk if his feet have been frozen.
11. Discontinue warming the victim as soon as the affected part becomes flushed, since severe swelling develops very rapidly after thawing.
12. Once it is warmed, have the victim exercise the affected area and also elevate it.
13. If fingers and toes are part of the affected area, place dry sterile gauze between them to keep them separated.
14. Never apply tight dressings or any other dressings than those mentioned previously.
15. Obtain medical assistance as soon as possible.

Frostbite is not a problem in all areas of the United States; it is rarely experienced in some areas, but it is a major problem in others. Where frostbite occurs it is important that people learn the first-aid protection.

Heatstroke; Sunstroke

This condition is also referred to as red heat because the skin becomes red. Sunstroke is caused by too much exposure to the direct rays of the sun, whereas heatstroke is due to continuous exposure to heat, outdoors or indoors. The condition is much more prevalent in the male than in the female. Heatstroke and sunstroke have similar symptoms, and the emergency care and first-aid protection for them is the same. They will be treated as the same in this text.

The danger from sunstroke and heatstroke is significant and the persons most likely to be affected are the elderly, the overweight, those unduly tired, and those who overindulge in the use of alcohol. If an individual recovers from a sunstroke or heatstroke, there is evidence that he may be more likely to have a second such occurrence. Some authorities feel that the heat-regulating part of the brain is affected, and this is the explanation for the second or third occurrence being more likely.

To guard against sunstroke or heatstroke, the body should be protected from continuous extreme hot temperatures and from the direct rays of the sun. The body should be covered, especially the head. Rests should be taken frequently, and the individual should drink sufficient water. It is also important to take sufficient salt.

Indications of sunstroke and heatstroke are red, dry, hot skin, cessation of perspiration, headache, rapid and strong pulse, nausea, and dizziness. The victim will be semiconscious or in severe cases unconscious, and his temperature may be as high as 110°F, sometimes higher. The condition is extremely dangerous, and the death rate from sunstroke is high.

To protect the sunstroke or heatstroke victim, action should be taken immediately to lower his body temperature. The first-aider should

[142] Temperature Problems

1. Immerse the victim in cool water if available or
2. Immediately move the person to shade or a cool place, loosen or remove his clothing, and cool with wet towels while fanning air over him.
3. Summon medical aid as soon as possible.
4. Continue to cool the victim to normal body temperature and monitor his temperature with a thermometer.
5. Give water to the victim only if conscious. If unconscious, an enema may be given to provide needed fluids.

Muscle Cramp; Heat Cramp

This is a condition associated with fatigue, hard work, high temperature, the drinking of large amounts of water, and the loss of body salt and water through much sweating. It seems to be triggered by an upset of the electrolytic balance of the body. It should be noted that too much salt can have severe consequences.

The condition is quite common in athletes, but also can be found in some industrial workers as well as military personnel during basic training.

Indications of heat cramps or muscle cramps, especially in the legs and sometimes in the abdomen, are exhaustion, weakness, dizziness, faintness, prostration, and nausea. The victim is pale and perspiring, stuporous and sometimes in a coma; the pulse is strong but fast, with the body temperature normal. The victim will probably be very thirsty.

To protect against heat cramps

1. Condition yourself gradually to play or work.
2. Guarantee that the water supply is adequate and the salt intake sufficient.
3. Get sufficient rest.
4. Have rest periods during practice or work sessions.
5. If injury occurs use firm pressure and warm applications.
6. Give salt water solution as is recommended—one-half teaspoon to a pint of water.

The following are some excellent hot weather suggestions for the family, athletic coach, and the working person:

When preseason football practice is conducted in very warm and highly humid weather, warns the AMA Committee on the Medical Aspects of Sports and National Federation of State High School Athletic Associations, players may be subject to heat fatigue, heat exhaustion and heat stroke.

Heat fatigue—brought about by sweating which drains the body's salt and water—dulls the athlete's alertness, making him vulnerable to injury. Heat exhaustion and heat stroke can cause death.

Heat exhaustion is brought on by excessive depletion of the body's salt and water and is marked by profuse sweating and weakness.

Major Heat Problems   [143]

Heat stroke occurs when the sweating mechanisim breaks down and the body overheats. Symptoms are collapse, dry warm skin, and rising body temperature.

Heat illnesses are preventable only by careful control of the athelete's conditioning program. Basic, of course, is to require each boy to get a thorough medical examination before allowing him to participate in practice.

When practice begins, it's essential that players be acclimated gradually to hot-weather activity. Equally important is the need for the boys to increase their salt and water intake.

As the athlete becomes accustomed to hot-weather activity, he perspires more freely, dissipating body heat and excreting less salt. With gradual training, such acclimation can be expected to take place over a period of a week.

The old idea that water should be withheld from athletes during workouts has no scientific foundation. In fact, such a restriction can lead to heat illness. During exercise in the heat, players should be allowed to replace at least hourly the water lost by perspiration.

Salt also needs to be replaced, particularly during the adjustment period. Extra salting of the athlete's food within the bounds of taste is one way. Adding salt to water—one teaspoonful to six quarts—for drinking during workouts is another. Salt tablets can irritate the stomach.

Even after acclimation, periods of strenuous exercise should be alternated with periods of rest during hot weather. It also is important for the coach and his assistants to observe their athletes carefully for signs of heat illness such as inattention, unusual fatigue, or stupor. Symptoms may include headache, nausea, hallucinations, and/or weak and rapid pulse. If heat illness is suspected, the athlete should be given immediate attention.

Delay in treating a victim of heat stroke could be fatal. He must be cooled by the most expedient means. Immersion in cool water is the best method. Medical care must be obtained at once.

An athlete suffering from heat exhaustion should be placed in the shade with his head level or lower than his body and given sips of diluted salt water if conscious. Medical care must be obtained immediately.

The following suggestions are offered to help coaches prevent heat illness during hot-weather athletic activity:

[144]   Temperature Problems

Advise candidates to conduct their personal summer conditioning program out-of-doors.

Require a medical history and checkup prior to the beginning of practice.

Schedule workouts during the cooler morning and early evening hours.

Acclimate athletes to hot-weather activity by carefully graduated practice schedules.

Provide for rest periods of at least 15 minutes during workouts of an hour or more.

Furnish water and salt generously.

Supply lightweight clothing that is white—to reflect the heat—brief, loose, and comfortable.

Watch athletes carefully for signs of trouble, particularly interior linemen and the determined athlete who may not report discomfort.

Remember that temperature and humidity, not the sun, are the crucial factors.

Know what to do in case of an emergency, including first aid.

Outlaw use of rubberized apparel or any air-tight garment used for weight reducing.[7]

The following are some hot-weather suggestions for keeping fit. A person should

1. Drink plenty of cool water—not ice cold water, and never gulp it down.
2. Eat moderately of simple food, and do not confine eating to uncooked food.
3. Exercise every day.
4. Guarantee adequate daily intake of salt. The more a person perspires, the more salt he should use.
5. Avoid alcoholic drinks. Alcohol does not cool.
6. Get sufficient rest and sleep to meet daily needs.
7. Take baths as needed. Preferably they should be at body temperature.

[7] American Medical Association, "Tips for Home and Family." *Today's Health*, August, 1968, pp. 69–70. (*Today's Health*, published by the American Medical Association. Used by permission.)

8   Keep busy; one should not watch the thermometer and worry about the temperature.
9   If working outside in hot weather, mowing the yard or gardening, work during the cooler parts of the day.
10 Keep body weight under reasonable control.

BODY TEMPERATURE

Normally, the body temperature is 98.6°F when taken by mouth. If taken in the armpit, it will be about one degree lower, and if taken through the anus (rectal temperature), one degree higher. Take the temperature of an unconscious victim some way other than orally.

The thermometer (oral or rectal) should be washed and rinsed carefully in cool water, shaken down to 95°F, placed in the mouth or anus and left in place for one or more minutes. It is well to use petrolatum on the anal thermometer and in the anus to guard against breakage. If the temperature is taken at the armpit, the arm should be kept as close to the body as possible.

It is possible that the normal temperature can vary as much as one degree in the perfectly well person. The temperature also varies somewhat during the day. Usually 100° or more is considered as fever. Fever is a

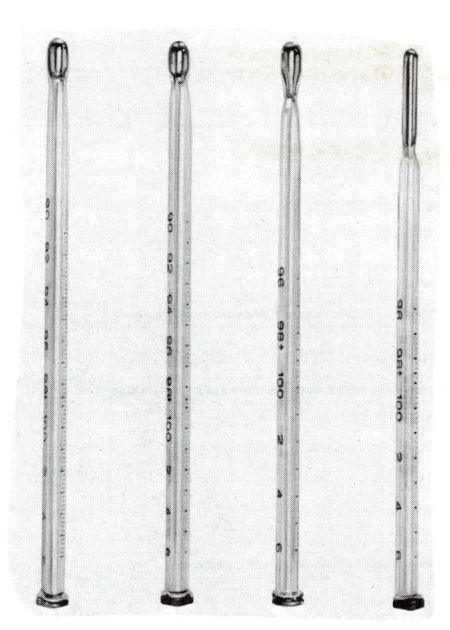

FIGURE 9.5   Various types of fever thermometers. (Becton, Dickinson and Company)

[146] Temperature Problems

protective reaction which assists the body in overcoming infection. If the fever persists for more than a day, this can indicate that the body cannot solve its own problems and that medical help is needed. A persistent low fever can also be an indication of other problems, and medical assistance should be sought.

It is not advisable for parents to give their children fever-reducing medication unless their physician so indicates. If the fever persists or reaches a dangerous level, the physician is needed. He should be called or the victim taken to the physician or hospital. Unfortunately, there is far too much publicity and commercial advertising praising the merits of fever-reducing patent medicines.

General Note: You will read from scale markings and numbers. Do not touch bulb end of the thermometer.

Scale markings or graduations

Numbers

1. Hold the thermometer *in right hand, at the end away from the bulb*, between your thumb and index finger.

   Note: Do not touch the bulb end. Accidentally squeezing the bulb with your fingers would raise a reading.

2. Turn the thermometer between your thumb and index finger *until you see the numbers on the bottom and the scale markings on top*.

   Note: Follow the picture to be sure position is correct—instrument in right hand, *numbers on bottom, scale on top*.

3. Hold the thermometer slightly below eye level and turn it *slowly until you see a wide, shining mercury band between the scale and the numbers*.

4. Read the temperature registered at the end of the mercury band.

   A. Fahrenheit scales are marked in *two tenths* of a degree:

   One degree
   Two tenths of a degree (0.2°)

   a. This Fahrenheit scale reads 100.2°F, *not* 101.2°F.

   b. This Fahrenheit scale reads 101.2°F, *not* 100.2°F.

   B. Centigrade scales are marked in *one tenth* of a degree:

   One degree
   One tenth of a degree (0.1°)

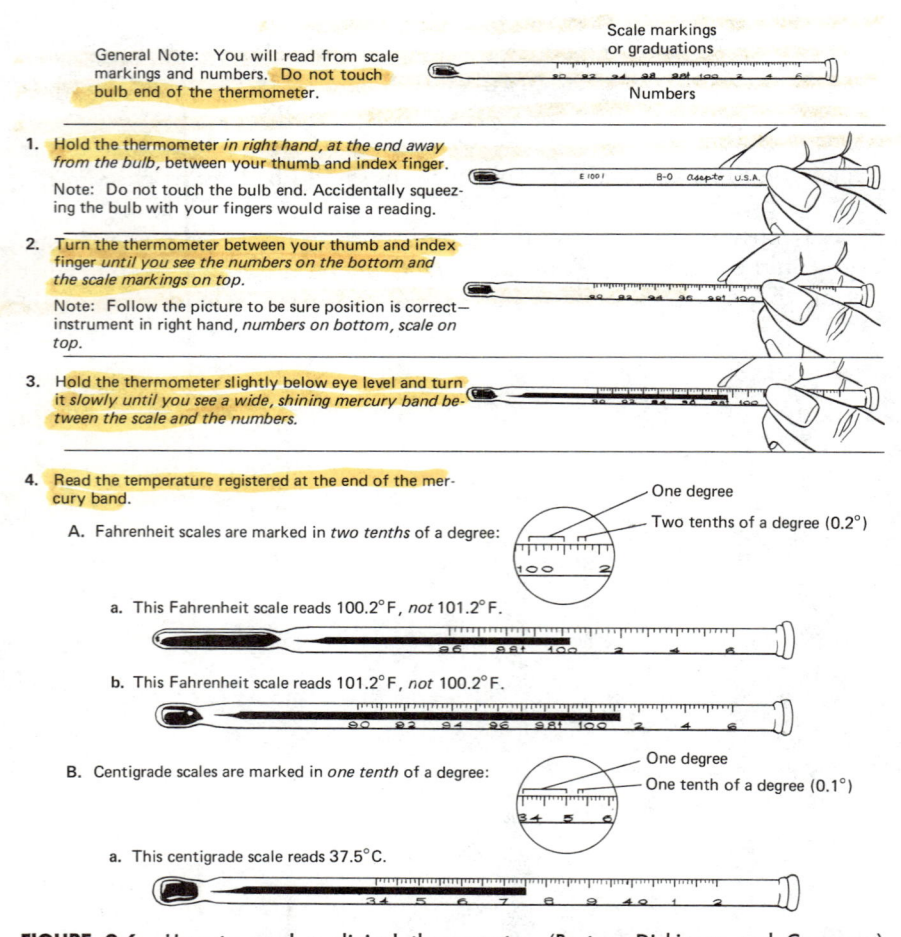

   a. This centigrade scale reads 37.5°C.

FIGURE 9.6 How to read a clinical thermometer. (Becton, Dickinson and Company)

ACTIVITIES

1 Consult the local health authorities and determine the common temperature problems of the area. Develop a paper for class presentation on the protection for the temperature problems.
2 Prepare charts, including drawings, to show the difference between heatstroke, heat exhaustion, and heat cramp.
3 Research the topic and explain in detail to the class the difference between the protection and treatment for burns.
4 Consult *Accident Facts,* published by the National Safety Council, for the past five years and review the statistics concerning the trend in fires, burns, and persons affected.
5 What are some of the conditions that a low body temperature may indicate? What does a high temperature mean? Develop a chart depicting the relationship between the conditions and the temperatures.

QUESTIONS TO ANSWER

1 What are the differences between sunstroke and heat exhaustion?
2 What is the correct use of a thermometer? How is the temperature taken orally, rectally, and at the armpit? How are the readings interpreted?
3 What are the most important dangers resulting from severe burns?
4 What is meant by the problem "muscle cramp"? What can be done to prevent or help to eliminate such cramping in the muscles?
5 What are the protective steps that help the frostbite victim?
6 In what position should a person be placed if he has severe burn, sunstroke, frostbite, or heat exhaustion?
7 What protection should be given the victim of a sunstroke until or before the physician arrives?
8 What protection should be given the first-degree burn, second-degree, and third-degree?
9 What is meant by the "cold water" method of protecting burns? What does this method accomplish?
10 What are the "don'ts" regarding the protection of burns?

SELECTED REFERENCES

AMERICAN MEDICAL ASSOCIATION, "Tips for Your Home and Family," *Today's Health,* August, 1968, pp. 69–70.

AMERICAN NATIONAL RED CROSS, *Red Cross First Aid Module: First Aid for Burns*. Washington, D.C.: The American National Red Cross, 1977.

AMERICAN NATIONAL RED CROSS, *Standard First Aid and Personal Safety*. New York: Doubleday, 1973.

COLE, WARREN H., and PUESTOW, CHARLES B., *First Aid: Diagnosis and Management*, 6th ed. New York: Appleton-Century-Crofts, 1965.

GREEN, MARTIN I., *A Sigh of Relief*. Toronto, Canada: Bantam Books, 1977.

HAFEN, BRENT Q., and KARREN, KEITH J., *First Aid and Emergency Care Workbook*. Denver, Colo: Morton Publishing Co., 1977.

HAFEN, BRENT Q., and PETERSON, BRENDA, *First Aid For Health Emergencies*. St. Paul, Minn.: West Publishing Co., 1977.

HENDERSON, JOHN, *Emergency Medical Guide*, 4th ed. New York: McGraw-Hill, 1978.

MCKEE, ALEXANDER, *Death Raft*. New York: Warner Books, 1975.

ROBERTSON, JAMES C., *Introduction To Fire Prevention*. Beverly Hills, Calif.: Glencoe Press, 1975.

U.S. AIR FORCE, *Search and Rescue Survival*. Washington, D.C.: U.S. Government Printing Office, 1969.

10. POISONS

Poisoning is caused by a wide range of substances such as chemicals, bacteria, and plants when they enter the body in various ways. Oral or ingested poisoning is the most common mode of entry into the body. This can occur from numerous types of household products, garden, garage, and agricultural supplies, drug and medicinal substances, food poisoning, and from ingesting plants or parts of some plants. A second mode of entry is by inhalation of poisonous vapors or fumes. Gases, such as carbon monoxide or carbon tetrachloride, enter the respiratory system and cause damage or death. Absorption is the third way a poison can enter the body. Absorption directly into the skin can result from insecticides or plant sprays when there is prolonged contact with the skin. This can occur in factories where chemicals are commonly used for industrial purposes, and it can be chronic in nature, as lead poisoning. Poison ivy, oak, and sumac, which irritate the skin, are fully covered in Chapter 14. The fourth and last mode of entry is injection by insect stings and snakebites. This subject is discussed in Chapter 13.

PREVENTION

Nearly all cases of poisoning could be prevented. This is why it is such a tragic accident. Usually poisoning is a result of carelessness or a lack of awareness of the potential danger of many common substances in the house, garage, or storage area. It is the responsibility of parents and other adults to prevent the needless cases of accidental poisoning in children. The period of 18 months to 2 years of age is the most vulnerable and hazardous, as children are beginning to investigate their surroundings

[150] Poisons

during this growth period. It seems to be a natural tendency for them to put everything into their mouths. Children at this age have poor discrimination and no sense of danger.

Having a knowledge and awareness of potentially dangerous substances could greatly reduce the occurrence of accidental poisonings. Also, taking heed and utilizing the following preventive measures will greatly lessen the possibility of poisoning:

1. Shake all liquid medicine thoroughly before measuring.
2. Store all poisonous substances away from food.
3. Be extremely careful with colored or flavored medicine which children may relate to candy. Never encourage children to take medicine by referring to it as candy.
4. Never take medicine in the presence of children.
5. Eliminate all unnecessary poisonous substances from your home.
6. Keep all necessary poisonous substances out of sight and out of reach of children, preferably locked in a cabinet or closet.
7. Keep all poisons in their original containers and properly and clearly labeled. Transparent tape will help protect the label. Using the Mr. Yuk labeling may help with young children.
8. Read all labels carefully and follow directions when using any poisonous substance. Never take medicine in the dark.
9. Date all medications and drug supplies when they are bought. Never allow medicines to accumulate. Discard old preparations.
10. When discarding hazardous substances, flush the material down the toilet and dispose of the containers where they cannot be found by children or pets.
11. Carefully follow the physician's directions when taking or giving prescription drugs.
12. Read carefully and follow exactly all directions for insecticides, plant sprays, and other fumigants.
13. Never offer to or accept from others medications for seemingly similar symptoms.
14. Never take two or more drugs (including alcohol), prescription or over-the-counter, without the knowledge and consent of a physician.

POISON CONTROL CENTERS

The first Poison Control Center was established in November 1953 in Chicago. Some 20 hospitals, four health departments, five medical colleges, The American Public Health Association, the American Academy of Pediatrics, and other associations worked together in this first project.[1]

---

[1] Henry L. Verhulst and John Crotty, "Poison Control Activities in the United States." *The Journal of School Health*, Vol. 37, No. 2 (February, 1967), p. 50.

Soon Poison Control Centers were being organized all over the United States, usually on a voluntary basis. The purpose of the Poison Control Center is to give 24-hour emergency service, improve first aid for poisoning, and make the emergency care easily available to the population. The Poison Control Center personnel can readily obtain and give the chemical composition of commercial products, and they can give antidotes for poisoning.

The centers are usually associated with a large hospital or medical school. Directories and card files are kept up-to-date on the commercial name and ingredients of new products that manufacturers develop and put on the market. The information center is a valuable reference for physicians as well as individuals who must decide the course of action to take in case of poisoning. The telephone numbers of the family physician and the nearest Poison Control Center should be near each phone.

NONCORROSIVE POISONING

Speed is most important in giving emergency care to a victim of poisoning. The longer a poison remains in the stomach, the greater the absorption and the less chance of recovery. Immediate removal of the poison is essential in most situations; however, this is only possible when the victim is conscious.

Conscious Victim

When poisoning is first suspected, a rescuer should try to find out what type of substance caused the condition, try to determine the time elapsed since ingestion, and try to determine the amount ingested. He should look for the container, and the label should advise if vomiting is to be induced. However, the first-aider must be careful about the labels on products listing first aid for poisoning; many such instructions are incorrect regarding antidote. It would be better that he follow the directions of the Poison Control Center or physician. If possible, help should be enlisted. One person can seek medical help while the other gives first-aid protection.

If it is positive that the poison was noncorrosive, the poison should be diluted immediately with a glass of water or milk if the person is conscious and not having convulsions. Second, an emetic should be given to induce vomiting to remove the poison from the stomach. An emetic should be given only upon the advice of the Poison Control Center or physician. The best emetic is syrup of ipecac which is available at drugstores and should be kept on hand in case of an emergency. The recommended dosage is one tablespoon for children and two tablespoons for adults. If syrup of ipecac does not bring results, the back of the throat should be stimulated with a finger or the blunt end of a spoon to induce vomiting.

[152]   Poisons

If medical help is not obtainable, vomiting should be induced as just described only (1) when an overdose of drugs or medicines has been taken, or (2) when it is certain that the poisoning was not a strong acid, alkali, or petroleum product.

When inducing vomiting in a child, special care must be taken so that the victim will not aspirate vomitus into the lungs. One method to help keep vomitus from being inhaled is to wrap a large towel around the child's body to restrict movement of the extremities and place the child across the lap, head down.

All evidence of the poison should be saved for medical examination. This includes the original container, the vomitus material, and soiled clothing. A plastic bag could be used to secure these materials.

If medical assistance is still not available and the victim cannot be moved immediately to a hospital or emergency room, the antidote for the poison should be given only upon the advice of the nearest Poison Control Center or physician.

After the poison has been removed from the stomach and an advised antidote has been administered to counteract the effects of the poison, the victim should be kept as warm and comfortable as possible to reduce the chance of shock. When there is a problem with breathing, artificial respiration should be given until a medical person is available. If medical assistance cannot be obtained, the victim should be taken to the nearest hospital.

Use of Activated Charcoal and Epsom Salts   The two ingredients—activated charcoal and epsom salts—can be used for incidents of poisoning by mouth. However, it is important to note that each substance should be used only upon the advice and direction of the Poison Control Center or physician. Under no circumstances should a first-aider use such items without proper medical instructions.

Activated charcoal is used for deactivating or absorbing poisons that are in the stomach. It should be taken by mouth after syrup of ipecac is given because it tends to prevent vomiting. When activated charcoal is advised by the Poison Control Center or physician, the probable dosage will be one to two tablespoonful mixed thoroughly in a 12 ounce glass of water.

Epsom salts function as a laxative. Again, the first-aider should get medical advice before administering it. The normal recommendation is one tablespoon of epsom salts blended in a glass of sweet liquid, e.g., sweetened orange juice, for adults and a smaller dosage for children.

Unconscious Victim

In any case that the victim is unconscious, no liquids or other matter should be given orally, and no attempt should be made to induce vomiting because vomitus material might get into the lungs. An open airway must be maintained, and when necessary, artificial respiration and cardiopulmonary resuscitation should be administered. The suspected poison container should be kept, and if the victim has vomited, a sample of the vomited material should be put into a plastic bag. If he can be awakened, the emergency care procedure for poisoning should be followed. However, if the victim cannot be awakened, medical aid must be sought immediately. Meanwhile, cardiopulmonary resuscitation should be administered if there is depressed breathing or the skin has a bluish color. The victim should be kept warm to counteract shock until medical aid is available.

Victim Having Convulsions

A person who has taken a substance such as strychnine or an overdose of digitalis may start having convulsions. It is important that the first-aider get medical help as quickly as possible and call an ambulance and/or emergency squad. No attempt should be made to restrain the victim; however, he should be protected from injuring himself on surrounding objects.

The first-aider should watch for possible airway obstruction and loosen tight clothing around the neck. If necessary artificial respiration or CPR should be given.

If the victim is vomiting, it is necessary that the vomitus matter drain from the person's mouth. Placing the person on his side will help in achieving this goal. In no case should the victim be given liquids or be caused to vomit.

CORROSIVE POISONING

Corrosive poisons destroy body tissues. The esophagus leading to the stomach and the stomach walls are immediately weakened by the burning action of corrosives. Usually there are burns about the lips, tongue, and mouth if a corrosive substance has been ingested. Following ingestion of the substance there is burning pain, often severe, in the mouth and throat and a cramplike or burning pain in the stomach. If the poison was swallowed some time before discovery, there may be mental confusion and shock. A corrosive poisoning victim should not be induced to vomit, nor should a tube be inserted into the esophagus, because these actions may cause a break or rupture of the esophagus or stomach wall. There are two types of corrosive poisons, acids and alkalis, which are very dangerous substances if ingested.

Poisons

FIGURE 10.1 POISONS THAT BURN OR STAIN THE MOUTH

Strong Acids

Acid	Source	Discoloration	First Aid
Acetic (concentrated)	"Essence of Vinegar" (flavoring agent): glacial acetic acid (industrial)	Grayish-white	**DON'T MAKE VICTIM VOMIT** 1 Give glass of water or milk
Hydrocloric (muriatic)	Metal cleaners, soldering solutions	Gray	
Nitric	Industrial plants	Yellow	2 Rush to hospital or medical facility
Sulfuric (oil of vitrol)	Battery acid, industrial plants	First white, then black	**Note:** External injuries (eyes, skin): flood with large amounts of water.

Strong Alkalis

Alkali	Source	Discoloration	First Aid
Ammonia	Household cleaners, certain medications	Lips dry, cracked; tongue raw	**DON'T MAKE VICTIM VOMIT** **DON'T DILUTE**
Lime, quicklime, burnt lime, unslaked lime	Building trades, chemical industry, agriculture		
Lye, caustic potash, caustic soda	Drain openers, paint removers	Whitish, later becoming brown	Rush to hospital or medical facility
Washing soda	Household cleaners, laundry		**Note:** External injuries (eyes, skin): flood with large amounts of water.

Acids

Acids are chemical substances that have a sour taste, are soluble in water, and redden litmus paper. The most common acids are

1. Sulphuric acid—found in automobile batteries, metal cleaners and polishes.
2. Hydrochloric acid—an ingredient in metal cleaners and polishes.
3. Nitric acid—found in cleaning solutions.
4. Acetic acid—an ingredient in permanent wave neutralizers.
5. Oxalic acid—cleaning solutions, furniture and floor polishes and waxes, bleach.
6. Phosphoric acid—metal cleaners and polishes.
7. Carbolic acid or phenols—antiseptics, disinfectants, and preservatives.

Symptoms Symptoms of acid poisoning are severe burning pain in the mouth, throat, and stomach. It may be followed by vomiting and diarrhea with blood and finally collapse.

Protection The rescuer immediately should call for and get the victim to medical help. Then, he should attempt to relieve the victim by quickly diluting the stomach contents with water, but not too much or it might induce vomiting. No attempt should be made to use a neutralizing agent such as milk of magnesia, lime, chalk and water, or baking soda. The first-aider is not to give olive oil, vegetable oils, or any other oils. They have no value for emergency care of poisoning and may cause damage if aspirated into the lungs.

It is important to keep the victim warm and quiet because the pain is usually severe and the danger of shock is immense. If the victim has trouble breathing, artificial respiration or CPR should be administered. However, it is imperative that all poison victims receive medical attention regardless of the extent of the poisoning and the amount of emergency care received.

Alkalis

An alkali is a chemical substance that dissolves in water and produces a solution that has soapy characteristics. Some of the common alkalis are

1. Caustic soda and lye (sodium hydroxide)—used in soapmaking.
2. Potash (potassium hydroxide)—found in drain cleaners.
3. Lime (calcium hydroxide)—unslaked lime or quicklime used in building construction.
4. Ammonia (ammonium hydroxide)—found in strong ammonia water for household and industrial uses.

[156] Poisons

Symptoms The symptoms of alkali poisoning are similar to those of acid poisoning—burning in the mouth, throat, and abdomen followed by vomiting, diarrhea, and finally collapse.

Protection Medical help should be summoned immediately. However, emergency care must be given until the medical assistance is available. In recent years, the scientific community has questioned the value of diluting strong alkalis when they have been swallowed. Taking time to dilute may not be valuable since strong caustics do most of their damage 30 to 60 seconds after ingestion. Giving water or milk to dilute the strong alkali may cause the person to vomit resulting in further damage to body tissue. Therefore, the most important first-aid technique is to get the person to medical help.

Corrosive acids and alkalies can also be dangerous if they come in contact with the skin or eyes. Any corrosive substance in contact with the skin should be drenched with water for several minutes. After rinsing, the skin should be thoroughly cleansed with soap and water. Eyes contaminated with a corrosive should be flushed with cold water for 15 minutes. As always, a doctor should be consulted.

PETROLEUM PRODUCTS AND DISTILLATE POISONING

The products in this group include kerosene, gasoline, benzine, naphtha, lighter fluid, mineral spirits, paint thinner, and furniture polish. These substances are irritants that cause inflammation of the tissues with which they come in contact. Certain petroleum substances contain materials that are toxic when the poison enters the circulatory system.

Symptoms Upon ingestion the victim will choke, gasp, and cough. Weakness will develop followed by dizziness and slow and shallow respiration. There may be vomiting and coughing of bloody sputum. Finally, there will be unconsciousness and convulsions.

Protection Prompt medical care is necessary. Vomiting should not be induced except on advice from the Poison Control Center or physician. Vomiting can be very dangerous because the person may get vomitus into his lungs. Aspiration of the substance of fumes into the lungs can cause chemical pneumonia. If the victim does vomit, his head should be kept down so there will be less possibility of inhalation of the substance. Hospitalization is necessary as soon as possible where expert care and treatment can be given. Serious infection of the lungs, pneumonia, or congestive heart failure may occur even under medical treatment.

OTHER CASES OF DRUG AND CHEMICAL POISONING

Around the home, at school, or at industrial plants there are many opportunities for individuals to become poison victims. In addition to those already presented, the following discussion identifies a number of special cases of drug and chemical poisoning and their particular symptoms. *The first aid for each would be the same as described under non-corrosive poisoning.* The specific first aid would depend on whether or not the person was conscious, unconscious, or having convulsions.

Depressant Drugs, Sedatives, and Barbiturates

This group of drugs includes numerous trade and brand names of different chemical compositions. Chloral hydrate, phenobarbital, sulfonethylmethane, and thiopental are included in the depressant drugs.

It is important to stress the effect of alcohol and barbiturates or any depressant. Both alcohol and barbiturates are depressants of the central nervous system, and if both are taken into the system the effects are compounded, often resulting in accidental poisoning.

Symptoms The first symptoms of poisoning are drowsiness, headache, mental confusion, and incoordination; as the poison is absorbed breathing will become noticeably shallow, hallucinations may occur, and the victim will fall into a sleep which will deepen into a coma and death will result. On occasion there may be vomiting and diarrhea.

Narcotics

In the narcotic group of depressants are included codeine, opium, morphine, paregoric, heroin, and many others. These are drugs utilized to relieve pain, coughing, and vomiting. They must be prescribed by a physician, as continued use of them can lead to dependence, or addiction.

Symptoms Soon after ingestion the person will become mentally stimulated, but this stimulation is quickly followed by drowsiness. As the absorption of the narcotic continues, the victim will experience headache, slow shallow breathing, and finally unconsciousness and coma. The pupils become pinpoint in size.

Salicylates

This substance, salicylate, is an ingredient in aspirin and is found in almost all analgesic preparations. Oil of wintergreen, an ingredient in many skin ointments, is also high in salicylate content.

[158]   Poisons

Symptoms   There is a wide range of variance in the symptoms of salicylate poisoning because it depends on a person's age and the amount swallowed. Onset of the symptoms may be delayed for 12 to 24 hours. Rapid and deep breathing are the first signs that poisoning may have occurred. Problems in breathing are followed by irritability, dizziness, hearing loss, fever, and sweating. There may be nausea and vomiting at this point. In the final stages there will be delirium, convulsions, coma, and respiratory failure.

Atropine and Belladonna

Atropine and belladonna are ingredients in medicines used for medical treatment of gastrointestinal diseases, colds, hay fever, and asthma. Drugs containing the two substances are used extensively.

Symptoms   The first symptoms are dryness and burning of the throat and mouth, with blurring and double vision. The pupils are widely dilated and not responsive to changes in light. The skin is red, hot, and dry and there may be a rash. The pulse is weak and rapid, and hallucinations may occur. Rapidly rising temperature may sometimes reach 108°F. Circulatory collapse and death result from these effects on the autonomic nervous system.

Cardiovascular Drugs

The most common component of drugs used in the medical treatment of cardiac disease is digitalis. It is highly dangerous if an overdose is taken. Precaution must be practiced by heart patients to keep digitalis-containing drugs out of the reach of children.

Symptoms   Absorption of the drug results in headache and pain in the chest and stomach. Vomiting, a slow and irregular pulse, delirium, convulsions, and finally heart failure are also present.

Iron

The type of iron that usually results in poisoning is in the medical compound to relieve anemia. Adults should be extremely careful to keep medications out of the reach of children. Iron tonics and pills are sold under numerous brand names.

Symptoms   Symptoms of iron poisoning are nausea, pallor, restlessness, vomiting, bloody diarrhea, and shock. The person will lapse into coma within one-half to one hour.

Other Cases of Drug and Chemical Poisoning [159]

Iodine

Iodine is chiefly used as an antiseptic. If poisoning of this type is suspected, look for brown stains about the lips and mouth. Also, there may be a metallic taste in the mouth.

Symptoms The first symptom is a burning pain in the mouth, throat, and stomach followed by nausea, severe vomiting, shock, fever, delirium, coma, and death.

Boric Acid and Borates

These substances are used as antiseptics, for food preservation, cleaning agents, mouthwashes, and dentifrices. Over 50 percent of the infants poisoned by boric acid die from it. Individuals need to get in the habit of reading labels on proprietary drugs and household cleaners. The best preventive measure is to discontinue use of these substances and use less dangerous ones.

Symptoms Symptoms are vomiting, diarrhea, convulsions, and coma. Death is usually imminent.

Camphor

This is basically an ingredient in moth preventives and camphorated oil. One teaspoon of camphorated oil can be fatal to a small child.

Symptoms The symptoms of camphor poisoning are a burning in the throat and chest. In addition headache, thirst, nausea, vomiting, dizziness, unconsciousness, spasms, and convulsions are primary symptoms to be checked out.

Methyl or Wood Alcohol

Methyl alcohol is used in antifreeze, in paint remover, as a solvent in shellac and varnish, and as a window cleaner. It affects the optic nerve and may result in sudden blindness.

Symptoms Symptoms begin with headache, nausea, vomiting, dizziness, weak pulse, and dimming of vision. As the poison is absorbed, delirium and death from respiratory failure occur.

[160]   Poisons

Lead

Lead is used in type metal and insecticides but is found chiefly in lead paint. Chronic poisoning most commonly results from gradual ingestion. For example, many children chew it off walls, floors, or objects. One danger of this type of poisoning is the effect on the kidneys.

Symptoms Symptoms of this poisoning are vomiting, constipation, irritability, convulsions, metallic taste, dizziness, weakness, and abdominal pain. In more chronic cases there will be weight loss, lethargy, and pallor, and jaundice may develop.

Phosphorus

Phosphorus is an ingredient in rodent and insect poisons, fireworks, fertilizers, and matches. These substances are common in most homes and therefore constitute a hazard to the welfare of all family members. The presence of such products is a special hazard where small children are found.

Symptoms After ingesting the poison, within one to two hours, nausea, vomiting, and diarrhea may develop. There is a distinctive odor on the breath and excreta. After poisoning, death may occur within a week.

Strychnine

Strychnine is a component of many rodenticides. It is also used for several medicinal purposes.

Symptoms The poison affects the central nervous system. First there are restlessness and excitement of the muscles, followed by a stiffness of the face, neck, and knees, along with twitchings of the entire body muscles. As the effects of the poison progress, any sound or movement will elicit a spasm. Convulsions will continue until death occurs from respiratory failure.

Arsenic

Arsenic is used widely in insecticides, weed-killers, and paint. Some medicines also contain arsenic.

Symptoms There will be a metallic taste in the mouth and obvious odor on the breath. Burning pain in the throat and stomach are followed by thirst, nausea and vomiting, weakness, diarrhea, and death from circulatory failure.

Poisonous Gases [161]

Cyanide

Cyanide is a component in insecticides and rodenticides, fertilizers, metal cleaners, and is used in the refining industry. It is one of the most fatal and fast-acting of all poisons.

Symptoms Large doses are almost certain to be fatal. Death can occur within minutes. If a smaller amount is ingested, there will be nausea, vomiting, headache, convulsions, unconsciousness, and death from respiratory failure.

POISONOUS GASES

Some toxic vapors and fumes can be present without giving any warning of their presence. This is one reason why it is important to know the conditions that cause gas or fumes to escape. Gases may be the by-product of certain operations such as exhaust from internal-combustion engines or bacterial decomposition of substances. Poisonous fumes also are given off from substances that are themselves poisonous if taken internally.

Carbon Monoxide

A frequent cause of fatal poisoning in the United States is by carbon monoxide fumes from motor vehicles. It is unusually hazardous because the gas is colorless, odorless, and tasteless and gives no warning of its presence. It is formed when fuel burning takes place in a poorly ventilated area. Any flame or combustion device will probably emit some carbon monoxide. Carbon monoxide is present in the exhaust of internal-combustion engines and in manufactured utility gas sometimes used for heating and cooking. Natural gas is the type chiefly utilized by city gas supplies and utility companies. However, on occasion manufactured gas may be added to the natural gas. Through faulty equipment or carelessness, carbon monoxide fumes may escape, thus creating a dangerous condition.

Symptoms The symptoms of carbon monoxide poisoning are headache, irritability, shortness of breath, chest pain, dizziness, nausea, and fainting. The lips and skin may be bright red. If exposure is continued, mental deterioration, stupor, unconsciousness, and death will follow. The symptoms depend largely on the concentration of carbon monoxide in the air.

Protection for All Gas Poisoning The emergency care for all gas poisoning cases is the same. First, the victim should be removed immediately to a well-ventilated area, but not out-of-doors in cold weather, as this can be dangerous. A warm, well-ventilated area is necessary. Artificial respira-

[162] Poisons

tion or CPR should begin immediately if necessary. Medical aid should be summoned or the victim removed to a hospital as soon as possible. The victim should have oxygen inhalations to help replace the carbon monoxide in the blood cells. Be sure the victim is kept warm and quiet to combat shock, and that he is lying down.

Carbon Tetrachloride

Carbon tetrachloride is one of the most toxic household substances. It is used in cleaning agents, fire extinguishers, insecticides, and dry cleaning materials. This is highly dangerous taken orally or inhaled. The fumes are not easily recognized and a very small amount can be dangerous in a poorly ventilated area.

Symptoms The symptoms of poisoning usually are delayed until after the damage has occurred. Vapors cause irritation of the respiratory tract, eyes, nose, throat, and lungs. After inhaling, dizziness, headaches, nausea, coughing, and mental confusion will follow. The symptoms resemble a kind of intoxication similar to that of alcohol. The chief danger of this chemical is kidney failure, which is usually fatal.

Petroleum Distillates

There are several substances that cause poisoning if they are ingested or inhaled. One group of these is the petroleum distillates. Gasoline, benzine, and kerosene and other products can cause a kind of intoxication similar to that of alcohol if they are inhaled. Death from asphyxiation can result from intoxication by the fumes of petroleum distillates.

Symptoms Feeling of well-being and security, uncoordination, and mental disorder are the symptoms of petroleum gas poisoning. This is followed by unconsciousness and death.

Hydrogen Sulfide

Hydrogen sulfide is a colorless gas released spontaneously by the decomposition of sulfur compounds. It is most likely found in petroleum refineries, tanneries, and mines. It may be present as sewer gas, and is found in high concentrations where animal matter has burned or decayed. The gas in high concentrations may paralyze the sense of smell, and therefore its presence will not be recognized.

Symptoms The first symptom of hydrogen sulfide poisoning is the appearance of a halo around lights, followed by eye, nose, and throat irritation. There is observable breathing difficulty, and finally paralysis of respiration.

Methane or Marsh Gas

Methane is similar to hydrogen sulfide in that it is a product of decomposition of organic matter in marshes and mines and of dry distillation of organic substances. It may also be present as sewer gas. However, it differs in that it is completely odorless and gives no warning of its presence. It is a hydrocarbon and inflammable. A highly toxic gas, it can result in asphyxiation.

Ammonia

This is an industrial gas that is used in many ways. It is used as a refrigerant and as a fertilizer. Ammonium hydroxide is used as a cleaner and as an organic synthesis. It is extremely irritating and causes coughing and spasms of air passages. Ammonia fumes can cause death from asphyxiation.

Chemical Warfare Gases

This area consists chiefly of the nerve gases which are poisonous and lethal in a short period of time. They directly paralyze the nervous system and in just a few minutes death can occur. This area is related to civil defense, but mention is made of them here because they are poisonous gases.

FOOD POISONING

There are three major classifications for food poisoning. One of these is chemical poisoning, where the chemical is somehow ingested with food. Such chemicals are discussed in detail previously in this chapter. A second type of food poisoning, as discussed in Chapter 14, is ingesting foods that are by their nature poisonous. The third type of food poisoning is caused by bacteria that infest the food. Food poisoning caused by bacteria is discussed here.

Prevention

There are many measures and precautions that can be taken to lessen the possibility of bacterial food poisoning. These are as follows:

1. Hands and utensils should be clean while preparing food.
2. Anyone who has a sore, cut, or boil, or is coughing should not prepare food.
3. Canned vegetables should be boiled at least 10 to 15 minutes before tasting.

[164]   Poisons

4   Canned food that does not smell right or is exceptionally soft or cloudy should be discarded immediately.
5   Contents of a can that is bulging at the ends should never be used. This is caused by a gas and the food is spoiled.
6   Food should be kept hot until it is eaten, and the leftovers should be refrigerated immediately.
7   Only pasteurized milk or milk products should be used.

Botulism

The botulinus toxin is fatal. The bacterium, *Clostridium botulinum*, is responsible for contamination of the food. The organism is found around any farm and is present on all vegetables. The growth occurs in underprocessed, nonacid canned foods that are in an anaerobic state. The bacteria multiply profusely in the absence of oxygen. Soil is the habitat of the organism, which is why it is naturally found on all vegetables.

Symptoms   Symptoms will begin with weakness, headache, nausea, vomiting, and sometimes diarrhea and abdominal distress. Usually there are constipation and retention of food in the stomach. If untreated by medical help, death will occur in three to seven days. Between 12 and 24 hours muscle involvement occurs with double vision and difficulty in talking and swallowing. The central nervous system is also affected. Botulism results in cardiac or respiratory failure. Over 50 percent of those poisoned die.

Protection   The victim should be removed to a hospital immediately, where an antitoxin can be administered by the doctor. The effectiveness of the serum depends on how soon the patient receives it as well as the amount of poison ingested. The victim should be kept quiet and bedfast. There should be no muscular exertion whatever.

Salmonella

A second type of food poisoning is caused by the bacteria *Salmonella*. This type of poisoning often results in epidemics when many persons may eat the same food. Contamination of the food may be caused by a carrier of bacteria who does not properly wash before handling food. The carrier may be free of symptoms. The foods so contaminated will then transmit the disease. Refrigeration of contaminated food will not be sufficient because the bacteria lie dormant until they reach the digestive tract. The foods most often affected are fish, poultry, egg products, meat dishes, cheese and other dairy products. The feces of infected animals can also contaminate food.

Symptoms This type of food poisoning appears about eight hours after ingestion. The first signs are headache, chills, fever, muscular aches, vomiting, abdominal cramps, and diarrhea. The danger lies in the possibility of dehydration if vomiting and diarrhea are severe.

Protection The victim should be put to bed and given fluids such as hot tea after vomiting subsides. Rest and quiet are necessary. The duration of the attack is usually about two days. Medical assistance is necessary if the illness is severe.

Staphylococci

Staphylococcal bacteria are the main cause of food poisoning. These bacteria are found in open sores, pimples, boils, infected cuts, or scratches. Also, the staphylococci are found in the nose, in saliva, and on the skin. When the bacteria get on food, they multiply rapidly. Heat will destroy the bacteria and refrigeration will prevent the formation of the toxin.

This kind of food poisoning occurs most often during the picnic season. The bacteria multiply rapidly in moist food stored in a warm place. Within three to five hours a food can become a reservoir of toxin. The safest method is to keep food piping hot or under good refrigeration until it is eaten. Foods most responsible for this poisoning are meats, fish, poultry, milk and milk products (cream and cream-filled bakery goods), and eggs. Although epidemics result many times, the fatality rate is very low.

Symptoms The onset of poisoning is noticed by nausea, vomiting, prostration, diarrhea, and abdominal pain from three to six hours after ingestion. It may last for 24 hours and then subside. The symptoms are caused by the effect of the toxins on the body.

Protection Emergency care should consist of bed rest and nothing to eat or drink for several hours until vomiting has subsided. Then liquids should be given for one day before solids are started. Some antibiotics relieve the severity of the poisoning, so medical attention should be sought for the victim.

ACTIVITIES

1 Visit a local Poison Control Center. Discuss with the person in charge the various types of poisoning that occur in the home and the emergency care measures for each. Report the nature of the visit to the class.
2 Inspect your home or place of work and determine the substances that should be locked up or kept out of reach of children. Mark those that

[166] Poisons

should be thrown away or have been put in the wrong containers. Take the necessary steps to make your home or place of work a poison-free environment.
3 Have the community or class organize and implement a poison prevention program during National Poison Week, usually in March.
4 Write a paper on the hazards of using neutralizing agents with corrosive poisoning.
5 Develop a home emergency care kit. Include the antidotes to the poisons that are in your home.

QUESTIONS TO ANSWER

1 List six preventive measures that will greatly eliminate the possibility of poisoning.
2 What is the purpose and function of a Poison Control Center?
3 Name three emetics that can be given to induce vomiting.
4 List the three essential ingredients of the universal antidote.
5 Differentiate between the emergency care of corrosive acid and corrosive alkali poisoning.
6 What poisoning results in death to children more frequently than any other type?
7 Discuss the benefits and hazards for a person using digitalis.
8 What can result if a person vomits after ingesting a petroleum product such as kerosene?
9 Why shouldn't vomiting be induced if the symptoms of strychnine are visible?
10 Discuss the measures necessary for prevention of carbon monoxide poisoning.

SELECTED REFERENCES

AMERICAN ACADEMY OF ORTHOPAEDIC SURGEONS, COMMITTEE ON INJURIES, *Emergency Care and Transportation of the Sick and Injured.* Chicago: The Academy, 1971, pp. 166–170.
AMERICAN NATIONAL RED CROSS, *Advanced First Aid and Emergency Care.* New York: Doubleday, 1973, pp. 95–133.
AMERICAN NATIONAL RED CROSS, *First Aid for Poisoning.* Washington, D.C.: The American National Red Cross, 1977.
AMERICAN NATIONAL RED CROSS, *First Aid for Poisoning* (Poster). Washington, D.C.: The American National Red Cross, 1977.
ARENA, JAY M., "Poisoning—General Treatment and Prevention." *Journal of the American Medical Association,* Vol. 233, No. 8 (August 25), 1975, pp. 900–903.

DONE, ALAN K., "The Toxic Emergency," *Emergency Medicine*, May, 1974, pp. 252–258.

DREISBACH, ROBERT H., *Handbook of Poisoning*, 5th ed. Los Altos, Calif.: Lange Medical Publications, 1966.

ERVEN, LAWRENCE W., *First Aid and Emergency Rescue*. Beverly Hills, Calif.: Glencoe Press, 1970, pp. 183–200.

GREEN, MARTIN I., *A Sigh of Relief*. New York: Bantam Books, 1977, pp. 180–183.

SELIGER, SUSAN, "Antidotes May Worsen Poisons' Damage." *The National Observer*, October 23, 1976, pp. 1, 11–12.

11. BONE, JOINT, AND MUSCLE INJURIES

Injuries to the skeleton, bones, ligaments, and tendons are common. Because these injuries are so frequent, the potential long-term disabling effects and the acute concerns presented by these types of injuries may often be overlooked by the first-aider. These injuries can cause muscle, nerve, and blood vessel damage. Fractures of the long bones as well as many of the other portions of the skeletal structure can result in complications causing the loss of the limb or even prove fatal to the victim. Skeletal injuries result from a variety of physical activities, work experiences, and motor-vehicle crashes. The contact-sport participant, the worker who climbs and works in the air, and the miner who labors deep beneath the ground frequently encounter such injuries. Nothing can match the automobile's ability to shatter skeletal parts. This, of course, is due to the impact of the body against the car's interior during collision.

In a recent year, the National Safety Council reported approximately 11 million disabling accidents for the United States. Some 2 million of these accidents were motor-vehicle related. Although there was no attempt to categorize these disabling injuries, it is certain that a very significant percentage involved the skeleton, muscles, or both.

When the stress or impact upon the body has been of sufficient magnitude, and these stresses include torque (twisting) compression, flexion, extension, and shear, it is reasonable to expect that injuries such as fracture, stretching or tearing of the muscle, tendon, or ligament, as well as nerve and blood vessel damage may have occurred. This would be particularly true if the victim indicates that there is pain in the area, if the part shows false motion, and if the victim suspects that a bone is broken. If there is a deformity, it is likely that the bone is broken or that the joint is dislocated. Also, if there are much pain and discoloration in the joint, consideration must be given to the possibility of a sprain, dislocation, or a fracture.

It should be kept in mind that fractures and other types of muscle-skeletal injury are not always easily detected even by competent medical personnel. Pain is a good indicator of fracture. However, the emotional stress of a fall or crash can and often does result in a situation where the victim feels little initial pain, and swelling may not be immediately evident. Multiple injuries may be present and the first-aider must be careful to perform a thorough examination to prevent seizing upon the most obvious injury and causing additional trauma to the victim by overlooking less obvious but potentially more serious injuries.

BROKEN BONES OR FRACTURES

Fractures are breaks in a bone. There are two kinds, the open and the closed fracture. The closed fracture does not involve a rupture of the skin, and frequently is referred to as a simple fracture. The open fracture implies that the skin is broken, and it is sometimes called a compound fracture. Both types of fractures are serious, but the open or compound is especially dangerous because it involves the bone, skin, nerves, blood vessels, and other tissues of the body. Because the skin has been broken, and in all likelihood the bone has penetrated or protruded to the outside, the danger of infection is great. Also, shock will be more intense, and in general the situation can be more difficult than in the case of closed fracture. A great danger with both types of fractures is the additional internal damage done to nerves and blood vessels through rough or improper handling of the victim. Arteries, the main nerves, and blood vessels are located in close proximity to the long bones of the arms and legs. Broken bone ends tend to be quite sharp and are often jagged and can cut delicate surrounding tissues.

Closed Fractures

Fractures are known as closed as long as the skin has not been broken. Such fractures are common in the arm, leg, hand, foot, collarbone, and pelvis. Some of the names given to closed fractures are greenstick, impacted, comminuted, fissure, oblique, and transverse.

Greenstick Fracture The greenstick fracture is most common in young people. It is so called because the bone bends and breaks only on one side. This type of fracture is sometimes referred to as an incomplete fracture.

[170] Bone, Joint, and Muscle Injuries

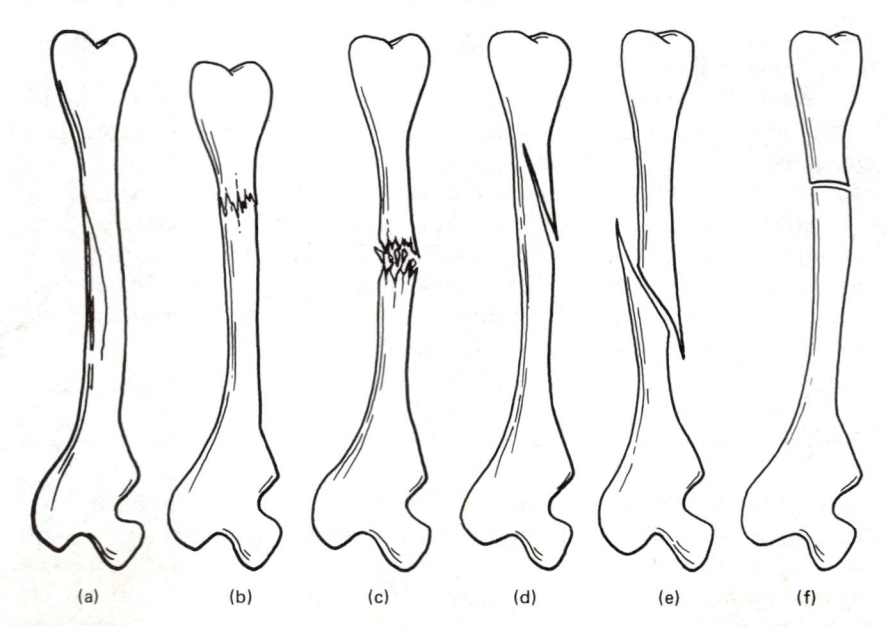

FIGURE 11.1 Types of fractures: (a) greenstick, (b) impacted, (c) comminuted, (d) fissure, (e) oblique or spiral, and (f) transverse.

Impacted Fracture The impacted fracture is one in which the bones are jammed and bone parts are forced together. Falling from a height and using the hands and arms to lessen impact are a common way to get such a fracture.

Comminuted Fracture Comminuted fractures are characterized by a splintering of the bone, as in crushing-type injuries, which break bones and in which the bone is broken into more than two pieces. This type of accident results from great force, and the motor-vehicle crash is a common cause.

Fissure Fracture The fissure fracture has only a small separation between the two broken ends of the involved bone; consequently, it is fixed in place easily and mends nicely.

Oblique Fractures or Spiral Fracture In oblique fractures the bone separation extends diagonally across the bone. The broken bone is sharp-pointed and more easily penetrates other tissues. A spiral fracture is caused by torsion when the fracture site twists.

Transverse Fractures Transverse fractures are so called because the break crosses the bone at right angles.

Broken Bones or Fractures [171]

Signs and Symptoms of Closed Fractures

The tissue overlying the break usually is tender. Other evidence of the fracture includes swelling, deformity, and pain on moving. Although the victim usually protects the fracture area from motion, often he will cautiously move parts beyond the fracture, such as wrists, fingers, or toes. Frequently a fracture is not suspected, so care for possible breaks as if they were definite.[1]

Symptoms of closed fractures include the victim's ability to

1. Hear and feel the bone snap upon breaking.
2. Feel the sensitivity to touch in the immediate area; the pain from the broken bone is more localized than in a sprain.
3. Identify the false position and false motion when attempting to move the injured part.
4. Feel the broken ends (crepitus).
5. Realize the loss of use or function of the body part.
6. Notice the difference in the corresponding part, such as the shoulder, arm, or leg. The injured part will usually appear to be shorter.

Protection of Closed Fractures

If a fracture is indicated, the victim should be protected from shock. It should be remembered that shock can be immediate or delayed; it can be slight or intense. Certainly the victim should be placed in a lying or sitting position, preferably lying, and the injured part should be immobilized and protected by splints, supports, or arm slings. A rule that should be observed and followed is, "If in doubt, splint them before you move them." Because tendons extend beyond the joints, splints should always extend above and below the adjacent joints to keep the area of the fracture immobile for maximum protection.

Inflatable splints and commercial splints of other types are preferable to makeshift devices; however, for proper use of the inflatable and commercial splints the first-aider should be completely familiar with their instructions.

Splints can best be made by padding boards of the right width and length with gauze or cloth. The splint should extend beyond the two broken ends of the bone. Splints can be quickly improvised from newspapers, magazines, umbrellas, or any other reasonably firm material.

The following are examples of simple fracture cases:

1. *Forearm and wrist.* These should be splinted with boards, magazines, or newspapers. After splinting, the arm should be placed in a sling and secured to the body.

[1] Carl J. Potthoff, "First Aid." *Today's Health,* October, 1966, p. 78.

[172] Bone, Joint, and Muscle Injuries

2. *The clavicle or collarbone.* This is painful and the victim will not want to raise his arm upward to a horizontal position. There will be a tendency to drop the injured shoulder. The best protection is to place the arm on the injured side in a sling and bind the arm to the body. The victim should be transported to medical help in a sitting position and protected against falling or fainting.

3. *Hand and foot.* These fractures do not need to be splinted.

4. *Elbow.* This is an important joint and great care should be exercised in providing protection for a suspected fracture in this area. It is suggested that the fractured elbow not be moved, that it be protected by splinting in the position in which it is found. If the arm is straight, the elbow should be left straight; if bent, it should be left in that position.

5. *Fractures of the ribs.* These can make breathing painful, more difficult and labored. Rib fractures can be protected best by binding them with several triangular bandages folded as cravats or one large cravat and by using wide strips of adhesive tape. Sharp blows to the chest from hit baseballs, kicks, or other forcible impact can cause this type of injury.

6. *Upper arm (humerus), upper leg (femur).* These are very dangerous fractures because they involve bones that are extremely important. There is a single bone in the upper part of the arm and the leg. The muscular structure in these areas is very heavy. Because there is a tendency for muscles in the area of a fracture to contract, especially where the muscles are heavy, a major danger arises when the muscles force the bones to override. This can cause the simple fracture to become compound. Such fractures can be protected by wooden splints placed carefully on either side of the fracture and bound preferably by the use of traction splinting, using the Thomas splint or improvising with wooden traction splints.

7. *The kneecap (patella).* This is commonly fractured in front-seat passengers in automobile collisions. It is a painful fracture with much swelling. This injury can be protected best by splinting with a board on the underside of the leg, from buttocks to foot, by securing with a triangular or elastic bandage. Persons with such injuries should be transported in a lying position.

8. *Neck and back.* Such fractures are very severe and most dangerous to protect. If there is a doubt, the victim should be protected as if there was a fracture. Fractures to the neck and back are frequently associated with automobile and airplane crashes, football, tumbling, wrestling, swimming, and diving activities. Severe blows and falls from heights also cause this type of injury. The possibility of neck fracture is far greater when the victim has impacted his head on the top portion when the body is rotating forward. Dislocation or fracture dislocation involving severance of the spinal cord is common in this situation. Spinal cord involvement is sometimes evident when the victim complains of a burning sensation at the base of the skull. Great care must be exercised in such cases, and medical attention should be summoned immediately. The first-aider should pay

Broken Bones or Fractures [173]

particular attention to the respiration of such persons and be prepared to provide pulmonary resuscitation if breathing stops. The victim should be placed on a rigid platform such as a door or special litter. There should be sufficient help to lift the victim and keep his head, neck, and back in good alignment. There should be no bending, twisting, shaking, or jarring. If the neck is the suspected area, it should be secured by a pillow, blankets, or padding and secured by tying. Manual traction on the head or a cervical collar should be used before attempting any repositioning of the victim. The victim should be placed on his back (supine). If the back is the suspected area, it is desirable to pad beneath the small of the back and place the victim in a supine position and literally tie the victim to the litter, with head, neck, arms, torso, legs, and ankles secured. Contrary to the foregoing suggestions, Henderson [2] says that people with back injuries should be placed in a face-down position at all times. If a blanket litter is used, the victim should always be in a face-down position. The objective is to protect by immobilizing the entire body. The result of too little protection or carelessness in this type of injury can be permanent paralysis.

9 *The hip or pelvis*. This is the location of another serious fracture which for the most part involves older persons and is associated with falling, impact or crushing blows. The fractured pelvis is a common type of automobile injury because of the great force or impact the person sustains in the front seat during collisions. These injuries are severe and tend to cause intense shock. There is the likelihood of accompanying internal injuries to the bladder, ureter, rectum, and reproductive organs because splintered bones may damage these organs along with other tissues. The urine should be checked for internal bleeding after such accidents.

If there is the slightest indication of pelvic injury, the person should be kept down, and under no circumstances other than fire or explosion should he be moved until splinting has been accomplished with the legs, hips, and torso immobilized. Suitable transportation must be secured and the victim delivered to the hospital for care.

10 *Skull and face*. These fractures commonly occur as a result of automobile accidents, football and boxing activities, and other forcible blows to the face and head. The victim may be conscious or unconscious. The person should be kept down and quiet and protected from his own secretions and from shock. Stimulants should not be given. Medical aid and hospital care are mandatory. Satisfactory transportation should be summoned immediately.

---

[2] John Henderson, *Emergency Medical Guide*, 3rd ed. New York: McGraw-Hill, 1973, p. 205.

[174] Bone, Joint, and Muscle Injuries

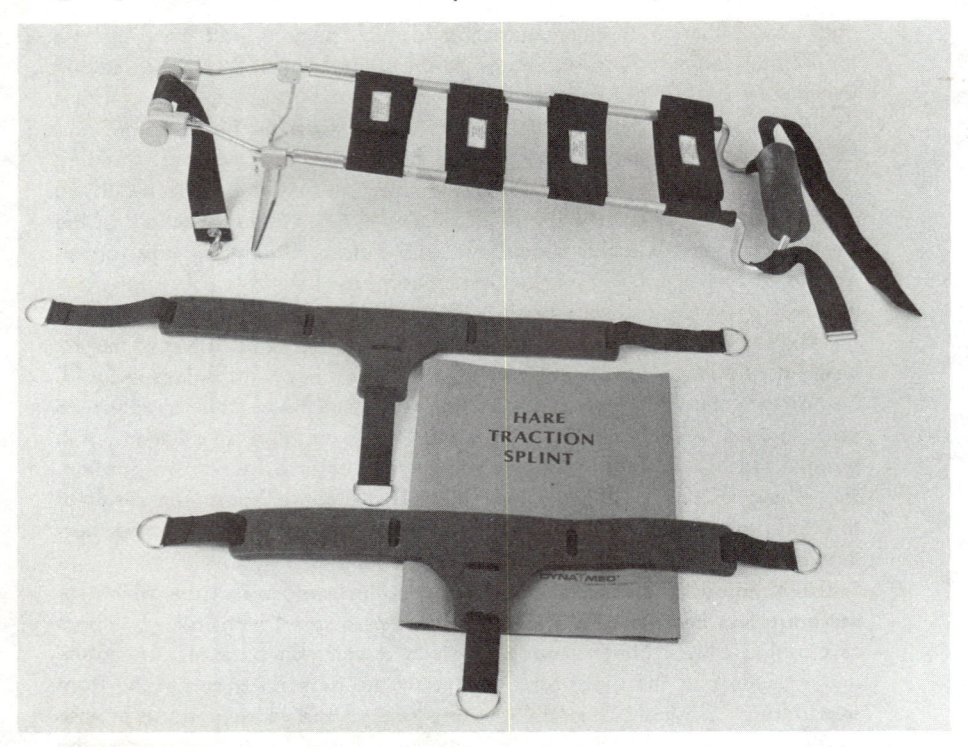

FIGURE 11.2 Hare traction splint used to transport an accident victim. (Dyna-Med., Inc., Carlsbad, California)

Open Fractures

These are fractures that were in the past called "compound." The broken bone has punctured the skin and has protruded to the outside. By the time it is examined the broken end may be withdrawn. If there is such evidence of a compound or open fracture, the part should be protected as though it were a compound fracture.

Signs and Symptoms of Open Fractures Cole and Puestow describe the open fracture:

> In general there are two types of open fractures. The first one is due to direct violence and is sometimes spoken of as having been compounded from without, i.e., by the force of the object producing the injury. In this instance the external force is so great that not only is there a fracture of the bone, but clothing, dirt, foreign bodies (such as the inflicting agents themselves—bullets, shell fragments, bomb fragments) are carried directly into contact with the fractured bone ends. The infecting organisms are carried in with the foreign material.

Broken Bones or Fractures [175]

The second type of open fracture is that caused by indirect violence, for example, the knee may be severely injured by twisting, but the twisting force is directed up the shaft of the femur (the large thigh bone) and a spiral fracture of the femur may occur. With the twisting force, one end of the spiral fracture may be pushed out through the muscles and the skin until the tip of the bone is outside the skin, several inches away from the site of the fracture itself. Such an open fracture is sometimes spoken of as having been compounded from within, one can readily appreciate that in a case of this kind there would be relatively less chance of contamination, unless the projected bone was buried in the dirt, etc. in which case the possibility and probability of infection would again be rather high. If, however, the projecting bone end were adequately protected and cleansed before drawing it back in place, the danger of infection would be lessened.[3]

Specifically, the signs of an open fracture are as follows:

1. The protruding bone comes through the skin and then becomes invisible.
2. The skin is open in the injury area, and other visible evidences of a fracture are false position, false motion, shock, and intense pain.
3. A massive injury to the arm or leg with accompanying false position.
4. The protruding bone is visible to the first-aider.

Protection of Open Fractures

This is an open wound, so there is the possibility of contamination. It is possible that much foreign matter has been forced into the wound or that the bone has penetrated the skin to the extent that it should be considered contaminated. Every precaution should be taken to lessen the chance of infection.

These victims will be suffering from intense shock. They should be kept down and warm. The use of comforting words may be helpful. The open wound should be protected with the most sterile dressing at hand. The victim should not see his wound and fracture because this could increase the shock condition, thereby making the total problem greater.

If the victim is within a few minutes of the hospital and doctor, and if his fracture involves an arm or leg, it is possible for the first-aider to maintain traction on the part by maintaining a constant and steady pull. Otherwise the part should be splinted, preferably with a traction splint.

If the victim is at a great distance and time from medical help, it is suggested that he be protected from contamination, bleeding, and shock. The fracture should be splinted, transportation should be obtained, and the injured delivered to the hospital.

It is possible for injuries of this type to occur miles from help. In this

---

[3] Warren H. Cole and Charles B. Puestow, *First Aid: Diagnosis and Management.* New York: Appleton-Century-Crofts, 1965, pp. 227–228.

[176] Bone, Joint, and Muscle Injuries

instance, a rescue squad of several persons (four to six), with the necessary first-aid supplies and splints, plus a good litter, are needed for carrying the victim the great distance to transportation. The best rescue device in remote areas is the helicopter. State police and municipalities are fast moving toward the use of them for rescue and quick delivery to hospital and medical centers.

SPRAINS

Sprains are injuries to the joints. The joints commonly receiving sprains are the ankle, wrist, finger, knee, shoulder, and elbow. Sprains result from the injury of the soft tissues about the joint, especially the

Summary of Fracture Protection

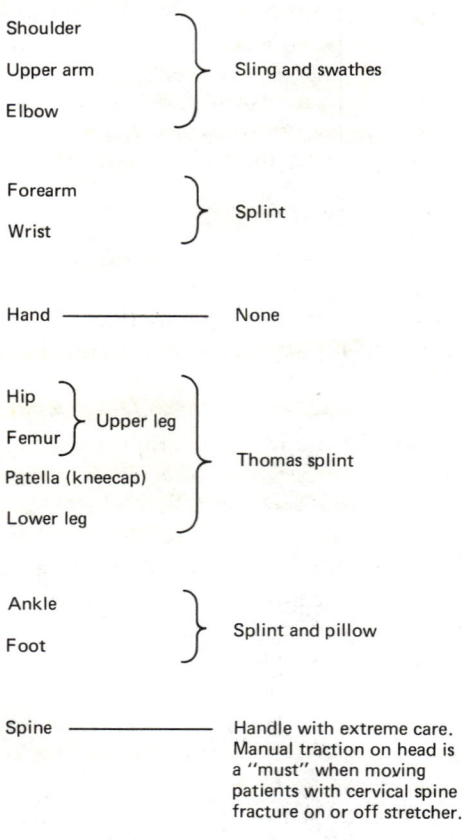

Body Part	Treatment
Shoulder, Upper arm, Elbow	Sling and swathes
Forearm, Wrist	Splint
Hand	None
Hip, Femur (Upper leg), Patella (kneecap), Lower leg	Thomas splint
Ankle, Foot	Splint and pillow
Spine	Handle with extreme care. Manual traction on head is a "must" when moving patients with cervical spine fracture on or off stretcher.

FIGURE 11.3 Fracture treatment chart. (From *Emergency Care of the Sick and Injured*, R. H. Kennedy, ed. Philadelphia: W. B. Saunders Co., 1966. Courtesy of W. B. Saunders Co. and C. Pool.)

Sprains [177]

ligaments, blood vessels, and tendons. Sometimes they include slight fractures. These injuries can be severe and result in immediate swelling and pain, or they can be of a minor nature. The ligaments are bands of connective tissue and are slightly elastic. They bind the ends of the bones to help form the joints. It is when too much pressure or force is applied, or a sudden twist or jerk occurs, that the ligament is torn or pulled loose from its attachment. When this happens, blood vessels and tendons may also be injured. This is a sprain.

Sprains are common injuries, especially to the ankle joint and the wrist. Such injuries tend to become progressively aggravating. If the ankle is sprained once, it seems to be more easily sprained a second time. Each successive sprain may be worse. It is advisable to permit the sprain to become fully recovered or mended.

Signs and Symptoms of Sprains

There are several rapidly appearing symptoms that result from sprains. It is difficult for the first-aider or even the physician to make a positive determination because the injury could be a sprain, dislocation, or fracture. Only an x-ray can help the doctor make a more positive diagnosis. It is advisable that all severe joint injuries be x-rayed and that the x-ray be read by a radiologist.

In the event that a joint is injured and does not respond within a reasonable time, then again the x-ray should be the determinant.

> Sprain must be studied carefully. If the tear is extensive, surgical repair is indicated. It is for this reason that the authors object to treatment of sprains with novocaine injections. Motion prevents healing, and the possibility of an unstable joint is enhanced.[4]

The following should be helpful to the first-aider and the athletic coach in the identification of sprains:

1 Swelling in the area of the joint. This may indeed be rapid.
2 Tenderness to the touch. The tenderness may be general and over a larger area than for a fracture.
3 Discoloration in the area. This will be caused by the leakage of blood and other body exudates. Discoloration may be intense (black and blue) or slight.
4 Pain upon attempted motion or movement of the part, disabling the joint or part.
5 Pain upon weight-bearing. The victim will protect this part and will not want to use the ankle or wrist. He will need to be assisted or he will hobble on one foot usually.

[4] Ibid., p. 225.

[178]   Bone, Joint, and Muscle Injuries

Protection of Sprains

The kind of protection that the first-aider gives to the sprain victim depends upon where the injury takes place and what supplies are available.

If the injury takes place on the school ground, gymnasium floor, practice field, or even in the home, it will be somewhat easier to protect the victim. If the injury involves the farmer in the field, the hunter some distance from help, or the mountain climber or skier, the circumstances will be quite different, and the problem will be greater.

Protection at School and at Home Many sprains happen at school in connection with play, physical education, and athletics. Schools especially need to have plans for taking care of sprains. In the event that there is a sprain observe the following guidelines:

1. The victim should put the part at rest by immediately relieving the weight. He should be carried if it is an ankle or knee injury.
2. The injured part should be elevated. This will help to reduce bleeding and pain. Pillows or folded blankets can best provide elevation.
3. Cold applications—ice bag, cold towel, or bucket of cold water—should be continued until bleeding has stopped. This should be kept up for a period up to 24 hours, depending upon the severity of the sprain.
4. The injured part should be bandaged to further reduce bleeding. The elastic bandage, because of its elastic nature, is preferred to the ankle wrap or cotton webbing. The bandage should not be applied too tightly. A bandage that is too tight will cut off circulation, and there will be severe pain.
5. Either cold applications of ice water or the practice of ice massage at intervals of approximately four hours combined with movement of the affected part to the point just short of pain will stimulate recovery by increasing circulation in the injured area.
6. The victim should stay down, keep the part elevated and at rest, and provide sufficient time for recovery. The physician can best tell the victim when he should again use the part.
7. A crutch or cane should be used for support when beginning to use the part. The part should be wrapped with an elastic bandage, which will be a good reminder that healing requires time.

A person should remember that these are the only joints he will ever have. If abused by repeated injuries and poor care, a person may become a partial cripple. Loose joint capsules, bone spurs, and arthritis are all possible consequences of repeated or poorly cared for joint injuries. The one basketball game missed will be forgotten. However, a person cannot forget the knee or ankle that will hinder him throughout life—so take care!

Protection in the Field, Some Distance from Help Accidents resulting in sprains away from help and with limited supplies present a grave problem. Farmers, hunters, and others can help to protect themselves by

1. Lying down and elevating the part immediately.
2. Remaining in a resting position for a reasonable time to permit bleeding to stop.
3. Improvising a wrap by using a piece of clothing and bandaging the injured part if it is essential that he walk to help.
4. Waiting for help or signaling for help if he has a sounding device such as a gun.
5. Hunting or fishing with a companion. He should use the "buddy system" and be prepared with reasonable supplies.
6. Advising others as to where he will be working, hiking, hunting, or camping.

STRAINS

Strains are muscle injuries and are caused by stretching the muscles beyond a reasonable limit. Individual muscle fibers or entire muscles may be torn from their attachments, and the tendon and fascia that fasten or attach the muscle to the bone may be ruptured or even pulled loose.

> Strains are caused by a violent, unexpected movement such as may occur when one is attempting to lift a heavy weight and slips. The result is a wrench, which is violent enough to produce some degree of tearing in the muscle groups upon which the brunt of the force is thrown. This kind of accident may occur also as the result of attempting to lift a heavy weight improperly, so that the force being exerted by the muscles themselves is great enough to produce a tear in the muscle or in its tendon.[5]

Lifting too much weight and not knowing how to lift are common causes of strains. The lower back muscles are frequently strained. It is important that the one who is lifting squarely places his feet, and that the lifting for the most part be done with the great muscles of the thigh. The lifter's back should be straight, with knees bent. The lift should be gradual and not jerky or forced. One should not make a repeated effort to lift. One or two efforts are sufficient. If the weight is too great to lift, then it is obvious that the person needs to get additional help or give up the idea of moving the object.

Muscle strains can result also from overexertion such as in running. The trackman who does not sufficiently warm his muscles before an event or the runner who everextends himself may strain muscles of the legs. Strains are painful and necessitate emergency care and protection.

[5] Henderson, op. cit., p. 210.

[180] Bone, Joint, and Muscle Injuries

Signs and Symptoms of Strains

There are several helpful signs or indications for the first-aider to follow in making this determination:

1. A sharp pain (a catch or stitch) at the time of or shortly following the muscle exertion.
2. A tendency for the injured part (back or leg) to become sore and stiff and for this soreness to become progressive.
3. A feeling of intense pain in the injured part when attempts are made to use the area.
4. A spasm in the muscle of the injured area and the inability to use the part without being assisted.

Protection of Muscle Strains

The following are several steps to follow in giving first-aid protection to the victim of the strain (muscle) injury:

1. If the strain involves the muscles of the lower back, the victim should be placed in a lying position on his back, preferably on a hard surface, such as a very hard mattress or the floor.
2. The victim should be made comfortable, allowed to rest. Cold wet applications should be applied to the area of the injury to help relax the muscle spasm.
3. If the victim is uncomfortable on his back, he might be propped up with his knees elevated, if this would be restful.
4. The injured area could be massaged with ice to help relax the muscles and ease pain.
5. The victim should be permitted to assume a standing position when the muscles ease their continuous contractions or spasm.

DISLOCATIONS

The movement of a bone end or of two bones from their joint is a dislocation. Dislocations and fractures have similar indications. However, a dislocation always has marked evidence of deformity, with a noticeable enlargement in the injured area. The fingers and the thumb are dislocated frequently, although it is not uncommon for a person to dislocate the shoulder, jaw, toes, elbow, or knee joint. When there is a dislocation, the muscles, blood vessels, and nerves are injured in addition to the joint and the two ends of the involved bones. If the injury involves one of the ball-and-socket joints, such as the shoulder, the ball will have been forced from its socket. Falls and blows are the most common causes of this type of injury.

Dislocations [181]

It is the responsibility of the first-aider to protect, so when a dislocation occurs it should be immobilized as quickly as possible and the victim taken to medical help. It appears to be customary for coaches and industrial nurses to apply a steady pull to dislocated fingers to cause them to be repositioned. This should be avoided if possible. Dislocations should be restored to their normal position without undue delay because the swelling and contraction of the associated muscles will continue and can make the task more difficult.

Signs and Symptoms of Dislocations

There are several helpful indications for making this determination:

1. Intense pain in the joint.
2. Sudden swelling and discoloration.
3. A noticeable deformity in the joint.
4. The presence of shock, which may come suddenly or be somewhat delayed.
5. Rigidity and loss of use in the injured joint.
6. The injured part is longer or shorter than the corresponding part. It is usually shorter.

Protection of Dislocations

As previously mentioned, it is important that the rescuer take immediate action to protect the injured part and the victim and get medical help. Specifically the following steps are suggested:

1. The joint should be immobilized and the victim placed in the most comfortable position. This can be done with splints or, in the case of the shoulder, an arm sling.
2. Cold applications, especially ice bags or packs, should be used to help reduce the swelling and pain.
3. The victim should be protected against shock. He should be kept warm if need be with blankets or covering.
4. Medical help should be sought as soon as possible.
5. An attempt should be made to realign the part, if medical help cannot be obtained.

Protection of Specific Dislocations Dislocations can occur at any movable joint; however, there are several joints where this type of injury is most likely, such as the shoulder, hip, jaw, elbow, finger, thumb, and knee. The first-aider can provide protection as indicated:

1. *The lower jaw.* It is not too difficult to dislocate this joint. Until medical help is obtained, the dislocated jaw can be protected by using a four-tailed bandage or the triangular bandage folded as a cravat to support. A bow knot should be used so the bandage can be removed rapidly in the case of

Bone, Joint, and Muscle Injuries

vomiting. If there is intense pain in the jaw at the joint and if the teeth do not meet properly (occlusion), it is reasonable to conclude that the jaw is dislocated. The first-aider should not attempt to realign this joint.

2. *The shoulder.* These injuries are painful. The doctor, preferably an orthopedic surgeon, should do the setting. Protection can be given by placing the arm in a sling and binding the arm securely to the body. The victim will be more comfortable in a sitting position.

3. *The finger.* This is probably the most common site for dislocations. The first-aider should not attempt to reposition this injury if medical help is at all available. He will probably save himself from possible liability. This injury is not as simple as it first appears and is often accompanied by fractures and bone chips.

4. *The elbow.* The elbow should be protected by splinting as if it were broken or fractured. No attempts should be made to straighten the elbow. There will be intense pain, so the first-aider should protect for shock.

5. *The thumb.* This will be very noticeable because the thumb joint may appear to be near the palm. Because of the structure and complexity of this joint, the first-aider should not attempt to realign it. He can only protect and take the victim to medical help.

6. *The knee.* This is a very serious dislocation. However, the first-aider can protect the injury by padding and bandaging and by using a splint down the back or dorsal side of the leg for support. Only a medically trained person should attempt to reposition the knee.

7. *The patella or kneecap.* The kneecap can be dislocated laterally. The leg should be immobilized and medical attention sought. The first-aider should splint from the side and should not attempt to straighten the leg by force.

ACTIVITIES

1. Prepare a variety of splints, padded plywood or some other reasonably firm material, and demonstrate fixation splinting for the lower arm, wrist, upper arm, and lower leg.

2. Prepare wooden splints of the correct size and width and show by improvising how to place the leg or arm in traction to prevent the simple fracture from becoming a compound fracture.

3. Build a wooden litter for protecting and transporting neck and back injury victims. Demonstrate to the class how to splint and transport the victim of a neck or back injury.

4. Secure a set of plastic splints from the local rescue squad or undertaker and demonstrate their use and effectiveness.

5. Prepare to explain and demonstrate the protection of a dislocation and a severely strained back muscle.

QUESTIONS TO ANSWER

1. Fractures are described in several ways. What do the terms *open, closed, simple,* and *compound* mean?
2. What is the difference between a greenstick and a fissure-type fracture? Why is the greenstick called an incomplete fracture?
3. What are the usual signs or indications of a simple fracture? A compound fracture?
4. How can the first-aider distinguish between a severe sprain and a fracture?
5. What first-aid protection should a first-aider give for a badly sprained ankle?
6. How should a rescuer splint a fractured kneecap or patella to give the best immediate protection?
7. What checks should a first-aider make to determine the location and extent of injury or damage in neck and back injuries. What checks should he make if the victim is unconscious?
8. What indications or signs should one look for in suspected pelvic injuries? Why do pelvic fractures require a high degree of protection?
9. In what position should a first-aider transport a person with a broken neck? A broken back? Explain why these positions are necessary for the protection of the accident victim.
10. What equipment, splinting material, and assistance would one need to traction-splint a broken leg (femur)? The upper arm (humerus)?

SELECTED REFERENCES

AMERICAN NATIONAL RED CROSS, *Standard First Aid and Personal Safety.* New York: Doubleday, 1973.

COLE, WARREN H., and PUESTOW, CHARLES B., *First Aid: Diagnosis and Management,* 6th ed. New York: Appleton-Century-Crofts, 1965.

CUTTER, W., and ELSTEIN, L. H., *Accident Prevention and First Aid.* New York: Cornerstone Library, 1965.

HAFEN, BRENT Q., and PETERSON, BRENDA, *First Aid For Health Emergencies.* St. Paul, Minn.: West Publishing Co., 1977.

HAFEN, BRENT Q., and KARREN, KEITH J., *First Aid and Emergency Care Workbook.* Denver, Colo.: Morton Publishing Co., 1977.

HENDERSON, JOHN, *Emergency Medical Guide,* 4th ed. New York: McGraw-Hill, 1978.

KENNEDY, ROBERT H., *Emergency Care,* Committee on Trauma, American College of Surgeons. Philadelphia: Saunders, 1966.

POTTHOFF, CARL J., "First Aid." *Today's Health,* October, 1966, p. 78.

PART III
SPECIFIC EMERGENCY CARE PROBLEMS

This section of the book is concerned with a number of specific emergency care problems. Knowledge of the protection to be rendered for each problem is important to the first-aid person.

Included in Part III are the following chapters:

12   Psychological First Aid
13   Poisonous Bites and Stings
14   Poisonous Plants
15   Special Problems
16   Disaster Preparedness

12. PSYCHOLOGICAL FIRST AID

Psychological first aid is based on the principle of establishing and maintaining effective rapport with accident or disaster victims. The first-aider should provide understanding, reassurance, encouragement, assistance, and direction in order to help the victims function. Normally, psychological first aid is discussed with reference to natural or man-made trauma situations, but psychological first aid also applies to recreational, automobile, school, home, and work accidents. Establishing an effective relationship with those persons who have experienced an emergency or trauma is important. It will aid in more rapid recovery and emotional stability, whereas ignorance of first-aid measures or assistance may lead to an increase of severity of the problem and less chance of future recovery.

PRINCIPLES

In providing psychological first aid, there are four fundamental principles for dealing with the psychologically disorganized person.[1] It is important for the first-aider to understand and apply these principles.

Accept a Stressed Person's Limitations as Real

In time of a disaster or personal emergency, emotional stress may be extreme. Some persons will condition and organize themselves to the

[1] American Psychiatric Association, *First Aid for Psychological Reactions in Disasters*. Washington, D.C.: American Psychiatric Association, 1964, pp. 16–22.

[187]

situation. However, there are those persons who will more deeply experience emotional trauma. The same experience can have tremendously different meanings and implications for different individuals. Those who can quickly find composure should be understanding and helpful to those who are less emotionally composed. The first-aider should not show frustration or resentment when the victim cannot be as readily competent as others.

The inability to function normally is very real to the person. He does not want to react this way, but he has no control over his reaction to the incident. It is the job of the first-aider to help the person gain confidence and effectiveness. The first-aider should assist the person to discover some tasks he can do which will increase his trust in others and himself.

Acceptance of One's Own Limitations

The person who attempts to be of assistance and aid those who are emotionally distressed must realize that he is as susceptible to personal anxieties as anyone else. Natural concerns in cases of disaster are family and friends. The person in an assistance role must be prepared to handle his own emotional problems immediately. His own weaknesses should be recognized and dealt with. Giving psychological first aid can be a trying and an exhausting job. It is important not to overextend one's own limits because one may develop an emotional disorder as a result of stress from exhaustion. The first and most important job in giving psychological first aid is to endure and control one's own feelings, and then one can successfully give reassurance and assistance to others.

Evaluate the Disturbed Person's Abilities Quickly and Accurately

For an individual to be of assistance and aid to a disturbed person, it is necessary to immediately and accurately evaluate his behavior and select the best approach to the problem. In speaking with him it is important to observe any abilities, interests, or skills that may be utilized in helping him reorganize his emotions. Asking him what happened and giving him a chance to reply in his own way can be beneficial. Just talking about the experience can greatly relieve feelings of despair and hopelessness and will develop a rapport between the victim and the first-aider. It is important to seek information about his identity, family and friends, and how those who are close to him can be contacted. Also, inquiring about his occupation and interests will give a hint as to some type of therapeutic work that he can do. Displaying interest and kindness and helping the victim find a way to use his skills to help overcome the emotional trauma are objectives of giving psychological first aid.

Accept Every Person's Right to His Own Feelings

It is important never to tell a person who is emotionally disrupted how he should feel. It is the duty of the individual who wishes to be of assistance to help the person accept and deal with his feelings. He does not want to react severely, but he cannot help himself; he responds on the basis of past experience and his own personality make-up. One must help him understand his feelings and give guidance in coping with the problem. To give psychological first aid the first-aider must let the victim know his feelings are understood and he is not blamed for them. This should be the first step toward helping him. Once he trusts the first-aider he will respond more freely to discretion and assistance.

REACTIONS TO EMERGENCIES

In the event of an emergency or a disaster, individuals will have varied responses psychologically. The psychological reaction of an individual to an emergency will depend on the individual's own personal psychological resources, the nature and severity of the emergency or disaster, and the extent to which he and his loved ones may be involved. An awareness of the types of reactions that can be expected and some suggestions for assistance will be of great value to anyone who may experience any emergency. The American Psychiatric Association has identified five different reactions to disaster, ranging from normal to severe emotional and bodily responses. The five reactions are (1) normal, (2) individual panic, (3) depressed, (4) overactive, and (5) physical (conversion).[2] These five areas will be discussed in addition to what the first-aider should or should not do in regard to each reaction. It must be stressed that even though the five areas are categorized, the victim may show responses in several areas at one time or he may jump from one reaction to another. For example, an individual may show signs of individual panic in addition to overactive responses. A second person may reveal depressed reactions and suddenly demonstrate the opposite, overactive responses.

Normal Reactions

Whenever anyone experiences a personal emergency, some reactions are considered normal. It is important to understand and expect some obvious signs of disturbance. There will be an increase in heartbeat, more rapid breathing, and increased anxiety. The person may feel his heart pounding. There may be perspiration, nausea and even vomiting, mild diarrhea, and frequent urination. Muscular tension increases which readies

[2] Ibid., pp. 12–15.

[190]   Psychological First Aid

the body for quick action, but this is followed by a feeling of trembling and weakness. Sometimes the person may remain confused for a time, but soon recovers and is able to take some action. These are natural and usually temporary psychological reactions to stress.

Protection Giving reassurance and talking to the victim are the best psychological first aid that can be given those in stress situations. Helping them in conversation will assist them to regain composure. A few words of sympathy and encouragement may help them regain control of their emotions. Usually, no special assistance is necessary. However, the help of a physician may be required if the symptoms persist or increase in severity.

Individual Panic

Individual panic is sometimes referred to as blind flight or hysterics. This response is not too common but the danger lies in the fact that it is so contagious. A few persons can initiate panic in a crowd. Such situations may occur when a fire breaks out in a building where there are many people. The whole crowd may blindly rush to one exit. Some may be crushed to death or smothered in the panic.

The single most important element of panic is its blindness to reality. Individual panic may be manifested by the unreasoning attempt to flee and a lack of judgment. It may also result in uncontrolled weeping or wild running about. Moving away from a source of danger in a rapid and orderly fashion is the typical reaction. In panic the person exhibits uncontrolled, purposeless motor behavior that may lead to additional danger and destruction.

Protection The person experiencing individual panic is difficult to assist because of his explosive physical activity. It is important that the first-aider not use brutal restraint, strike the person, or douse him with water. In individual panic, controlling the victim and isolating him from others will help curb contagion of this reaction to stress. The first-aider should try kind firmness at first, encourage the person to talk; it may help to give him something warm to eat or drink. Sedatives should not be given unless by physician's orders. If the person is unmanageable, he should be restrained firmly but patiently. It may require two or three persons to do this. However, it may be necessary to prevent general panic, if isolation is not possible.

Depressed Reactions

Depressed reactions are slowed down, numbed, dazed, unresponsive reactions to a stress situation. The individual draws back into himself as a protection against more stress. The person may stand or sit without

Reactions to Emergencies

moving or talking. He may have a vacant expression and seem puzzled or preoccupied with the disaster situation. The victim will lack any emotional display and is unable to help anyone. He cannot take on responsibility and cannot react constructively unless guidance is given. An example of a depressed reaction is when someone's home burns and he just sits in a dazed condition and watches it, unable to function. On receiving news of the death of a loved one, a person experiencing depressed reactions will just sit numbed and unable to respond.

Protection Usually, the person will respond as he gains confidence and trust in the first-aider. The first-aider should try to gain contact gently and attempt to develop a rapport. It is best not to tell the person to "snap out of it." But the first-aider should handle the victim with patience, understanding, and kindness. He should try to get the victim to tell what happened. His own and the victim's feelings of resentment should be recognized. After rapport has been established the first-aider should assign the victim a simple routine job and give him warm food and drink.

Overactive Responses

The overactive response is the opposite of the depressed reaction. This person explodes into a flurry of activity which is meaningless and serves no realistic purpose. He may be very argumentative, talk rapidly, try to take over the situation, and refuse assistance from others. Also, he may joke inappropriately, make endless suggestions, and criticize other persons. He may have an unreal confidence in his abilities which causes him to be intolerant of others and interfere with organized leadership. He may jump from one activity to the other without any real purpose. The problem in this response is that, like panic, it may spread throughout a group.

Protection To help this type of person regain composure, the first-aider should encourage the person to talk about what happened. His need for keeping busy with physical activity should be a guide to helping find him jobs that are purposeful and require physical effort. Supervision is necessary to control these responses. The first-aider should not suggest that this person is acting abnormally or argue with him. Sedatives should never be given without a physician's order, but warm food or drink may be given to help the overactive person gain composure once again.

Bodily Reactions

It is normal for an individual to experience some physical reactions, but these should subside fairly soon. It is when the physical reactions persist and increase in severity that a more serious concern must be shown. Severe nausea and vomiting are common reactions and can be very painful and disabling. Many times the bodily reactions take the form of conversion hysteria where the victim will experience blindness, deafness, or paralysis. He unconsciously converts his fear into the belief that some part of his body has ceased to function. He is not faking and is completely unaware that there is no physical basis for his handicap. He is as disabled as if it were a physical injury.

Protection The victim should never be told that there is nothing wrong with him, because he realizes there is. The first-aider should not blame or ridicule the person but show kindness, assurance, and interest in him. Also, the first-aider should make the victim comfortable, find something for him to do that will take his mind off his disability, and get help. He will need assistance, whether it be psychiatric or medical.

GENERAL GUIDELINES FOR PSYCHOLOGICAL TRAUMA

There are several basic guidelines of psychological first aid that should be followed in case of a situation where assistance is required. The first-aider should

1. Be able to recognize emotional injury in the victim as quickly as possible.
2. Be understanding, kind, patient, and try to establish rapport to show that he wants to help the victim.
3. Establish as much contact with the victim as possible, calmly and sympathetically.
4. Encourage the person to talk out his feelings and fears.
5. Encourage an exhausted person to rest and sleep. Sleep is an excellent measure to help bring strength and self-control.
6. Not give sedatives. A physician should administer them.
7. Encourage several hours of physical activity if the person is too emotionally excited to sleep. This will give him an outlet and calm the person so that sleep will come naturally.
8. Do not get emotionally involved with the victim in relation to his problem.
9. Be honest.

SUICIDAL TENDENCIES

One very real problem today is attempted and successful suicides. Read and Greene[3] state that about 20,000 suicides are reported every year, but that this figure is much less than the actual total, which could be an estimated 100,000. One could say that once every minute (or even

[3] Donald A. Read and Walter H. Greene, *Health and Modern Man.* New York: Macmillan, 1973, p. 405.

more often) someone in the United States either kills himself or tries to kill himself with conscious intent.

Situations that can lead to suicidal attempts include withdrawal, bereavement, depression, alcoholism, feelings of failure, and economic or employment problems. Any person who feels unworthy is usually depressed. He feels guilty about something and believes that he should be punished; he may think that success is impossible; he may think the future is hopeless and the best solution is death. Anyone who exhibits open signs of severe depression, threatens suicide, and speaks about how he cannot go on, should be taken seriously. Many potential suicide persons wish to be saved; hence a threat of suicide or an attempt at suicide should be considered as a cry for help. A potential suicide should not be left alone, neglected or ignored. He needs help as soon as possible. Someone who is close to him, family or friends, should talk to him and get professional help or counseling for him. There is little psychological first aid that the layman can give except to encourage him and get him to talk about his feelings. Professional help in the form of the family physician, psychiatrist, psychologist, or other qualified person should be obtained. To provide potential suicide victims with proper aid, "crisis centers" have been established in many cities. The experience of these centers suggests that suicide is more preventable than many other causes of death and that most persons can be shown better ways than suicide to resolve their problems, crises, and conflicts.

The following six items may provide guidelines for the first-aider in determining the potentially suicidal state of an individual:

1 Feelings of loss, aggression, and depression are an important precondition of a suicide. Depression is probably the only one of the three items aforementioned which can be recognized by a first-aider.
2 Many suicides have an antecedent history of emotional and physical illness.
3 There is an overwhelming pattern of preoccupation with death and the desire to die, frequent and recurrent communications of suicidal ideas and fantasies, specific statements of intent and repeated attempts.
4 The incidence of suicide increases precipitously with increasing age.
5 Susceptibility to suicide is lowest among those who have strong family ties, church, work, and community relationships. The unmarried (single, widowed, and divorced) generally have higher suicide rates than married people.
6 Time, season, and weather conditions appear to influence suicide rates. For people in depression, the early morning hours may be critical from a suicidal point of view. A drop in barometric pressures and other weather conditions are often associated with an increased incidence of suicide.[4]

[4] Joseph Hirsh, "Suicide, Part 4: Predictability and Prevention," *Mental Hygiene*, July, 1960.

ACTIVITIES

1. Write a paper on the similarities and differences of symptoms and emergency care for the five reactions to a trauma.
2. Contact the American Psychiatric Association and request their material on psychological first aid. Read, study, and report to the class or group on their materials.
3. Visit a local trauma center and report on the provisions included for psychological first aid.
4. Develop a series of posters depicting the five different reactions to a disaster.
5. Contact the local general hospital and discuss with the resident psychiatrist the cases of suicide attempts during the past year. Report to the class as to the types of people, occupations, etc., that were most prevalent.

QUESTIONS TO ANSWER

1. Define psychological first aid as it applies to a trauma or emergency.
2. Discuss the normal reactions to a disaster. What are the symptoms and necessary first-aid measures?
3. What are the symptoms and first-aid protection for individual panic reaction?
4. Discuss the depressed reaction to a disaster.
5. What is the difference between the depressed reaction and overactive reaction?
6. How does a person with a physical reaction differ from those reactions in questions 2 through 5?
7. Identify the basic guidelines of psychological first aid.
8. Discuss "Accepting a Stressed Person's Limitations as Real."
9. Discuss "Accepting Every Person's Right to His Own Feelings."
10. What situations can lead a person to commit suicide? Why?

SELECTED REFERENCES

AMERICAN INSTITUTE FOR RESEARCH, *Psychological and Social Adjustment in a Simulated Shelter*, A Research Report. Reprinted by the Office of Civil and Defense Mobilization, November, 1960.

AMERICAN PSYCHIATRIC ASSOCIATION, *First Aid for Psychological Reactions in Disasters*. Washington, D.C.: American Psychiatric Association, 1964.

GILLESPIE, DARWIN K., "Psychological First Aid." *Journal of School Health*, Vol. 33, No. 11 (November, 1963).

GRANT, HARVEY, and MURRAY, ROBERT, *Emergency Care*. Bowie, Md.: Robert J. Brady, 1971, p. 11.

KATZ, BARNEY, *Understanding People in Distress*. New York: Ronald Press, 1955, pp. 56–59, 212–214.

MCGONAGLES, L. C., "Psychological Aspects of Disaster." *American Journal of Public Health*, April, 1964.

MAHONEY, ROBERT F., *Emergency and Disaster Nursing*, 2nd ed. New York: Macmillan, 1969, pp. 198–209.

MATTHEWS, ROBERT A., and ROWLAND, LLOYD W., *How to Recognize and Handle Abnormal People*. New York: The National Association for Mental Health, Inc., 1965.

READ, DONALD A., and GREENE, WALTER H., *Health and Modern Man*. New York: Macmillan, 1969, pp. 422–429.

ROGERS, JACK M., "Transportation of the Emotionally Disturbed Patient," *Emergency Care*. Robert H. Kennedy (ed.). Philadelphia: Saunders, 1966, pp. 78–81.

13. POISONOUS BITES AND STINGS

There is usually much interest among first-aid class members when dealing with the bites of animals and the stings of insects. It is true that a small percentage of persons experience a venomous snake bite or have a severe allergic reaction from the venom of a stinging insect; however, it is a certainty that when one does have such an experience it is a severe traumatic problem. It is important to be able to recognize the problem and to know what to do to protect the victim.

Associated with animal bites is the problem of rabies. Although the incidence of rabies infection has lessened greatly in recent years, the disease is still dreaded and remains incurable. However, the treatment after exposure has greatly improved. It continues to be important that animals be immunized against rabies and that medical help be sought in the event of exposure to rabies. Dogs and cats continue to increase in number, and in many areas of our country wild animals are plentiful; they will always be a problem from the standpoint of rabies.

The number of estimated snake bites and resultant deaths varies among authorities.

> Dr. Parrish estimated that between 6,500 and 7,000 persons in the United States were bitten each year.[1] A more recent estimate (1975) by Amerex Laboratories in San Antonio, Texas, put the number at 8,000 and the same source stated that "during the past five years, the number of deaths from snake-venom poisoning in this country has not exceeded 12 each year." Dr. Watt's estimate is eight to 18 deaths a year.[2]

[1] Henry M. Parrish, *Medical Tribune*, March, 1963.
[2] Charles Elliott, "Snakebite! What to Know—What to Do." *Outdoor Life*, September, 1977, p. 85.

Poisonous Bites and Stings [197]

Snakes and lizards usually are considered to be the most dangerous of the venomous animals. They are widespread throughout the United States, especially the snakes. The one dangerous member of the lizard family, the venomous Gila monster, is found only in the Southwest.

The bites and stings of venomous animals were responsible for at least 460 fatalities for the period 1950 through 1959 in the United States, according to Dr. Henry M. Parrish, of the University of Missouri School of Medicine. An analysis of the original death certificates of the 460 venom victims by Dr. Parrish, who is an Associate Professor of Community Health and Medical Practice showed that bees killed more persons in the United States during the decade than did rattlesnakes. Deaths from bee stings totaled 124, those from rattlesnake bites totaled 94.[3]

Parrish also describes the speed at which the different venoms act and the relative danger of some of the particular venoms. This is discussed later in this chapter.

Several of the major animal groups have poisonous species from the standpoint of being toxic to other animals and man. Although there is no poisonous mammal, all mammals are capable of transmitting the virus of rabies (hydrophobia), one of the world's oldest and most feared diseases. It is the bite of the infected animal that, in most cases, transmits the infection to the victim.

Reptiles, including snakes and lizards, in the eyes of most people, present the greatest problem from the standpoint of venomous animals. There are many species and they are spread throughout the world, except in the colder regions. The amphibians are not considered a problem group, although there are some species, such as the very warty toads and the salamanders, that are poisonous to touch.

The arachnids include several poisonous and troublesome animals—scorpions, spiders, ticks, mites, and chiggers. These animals bite, sting, and suck, with the human being the most likely victim.

There are several species of ticks in the United States and two or three of them attack man. For example, Rocky Mountain fever is spread by one such tick.

The insects, especially the Hymenoptera (bees, wasps, bumblebees, yellow jackets, and hornets), present a problem with their stings and venoms to those individuals especially who are sensitive or allergic to the venoms. It is the great rapidity at which these venoms act when injected that makes them so lethal. This is why it is said, "The sting of the honeybee can be more dangerous than the bite of the rattlesnake." Indeed it is if a person is hypersensitive to the bee venom.

[3] Parrish, op. cit., *Medical Tribune*, March, 1963.

[198]   Poisonous Bites and Stings

MAMMALS

The problem to be considered is the animal bite and the danger of rabies or hydrophobia. The term *mad-dog* is commonly used because the animal may become vicious and readily attack other animals including man. Other infected animals may seem to be quite docile and friendly and may not want to fight. This form of rabies is described as "dumb."

The infection of rabies is associated with the bites and licks of mammals. These include primarily the dog, cat, fox, skunk, raccoon, possum, and bat; however, it could be caused by the bite or lick of any mammal infected with the disease at a given time. Rabies is caused by a virus present in the saliva of the infected mammal, so the lick into or upon a body opening, such as a break in the skin, could be the means by which the virus enters the body.

Rabies in humans has decreased from an average of 22 per year in 1946–1950 to 1–3 cases per year since 1960. The number of cases of rabies in domestic animals has decreased similarly. In 1946, for example, there were more than 8,000 cases of rabies in dogs, compared with 129 in 1975. Thus, the likelihood of humans being exposed to rabies by domestic animals has decreased greatly, although bites by dogs and cats continue to be the reason for giving the majority of antirabies treatments.

The disease in wildlife—especially skunks, foxes, raccoons, and bats—has become increasingly prominent in recent years, accounting for more than 70 percent of all reported cases of animal rabies every year since 1968. Wild animals constitute the most important source of infection for humans and domestic animals in the United States today. In 1975 only Idaho, Vermont, Hawaii, and the District of Columbia reported no wildlife rabies.[4]

Rabies, if untreated, continues to takes the lives of 100 percent of its victims. If an animal or man develops the symptoms or if the disease has its onset, it is always fatal. The disease can reach epidemic proportions and does among the Eskimos, wildlife, and dogs of the Far North.[5]

There is a very effective and widely used vaccination for dogs and cats which is good for up to three years. In some states the vaccination is required; however, this is a difficult law to enforce.

There are also effective vaccinations for man in the event of exposure, and these are described in *Rabies Prophylaxis* by the U.S. Public Health

---

[4] *Rabies Prophylaxis*. U.S. Department of HEW, Public Health Service, Center of Disease Control, Atlanta, Ga., December, 1976. (Distributed by Illinois Department of Public Health.)

[5] Christian McCain, "One Man's Battle Against Rabies." *Today's Health*, December, 1964.

Mammals [199]

Service as (1) the Duck Embryo Vaccine (DEV) which is a killed vaccine prepared from embryonated duck eggs infected with a fixed virus and inactivated with beta-propiolactone, and (2) the Rabies Immune Globulin (RIG) which is antirabies gamma globulin concentrated by cold ethanol fractionation from plasma of hyperimmunized human donors. RIG, the passive antibody, is administered only once at the beginning of the therapy. DEV should be given in 23 doses beginning the day RIG is administered. Twenty-one of the DEV doses may be given in 21 daily doses, 14 doses may be given in the first seven days (two injections a day) followed by seven daily doses. The remaining two doses should be administered as boosters. The first booster will be given ten days after the twenty-first dose and the second booster ten days later.

Only the physician can determine the need for vaccination. If the animal is wild it will be considered as being rabid, and the RIG-DEV treatment probably will be given. If the dog or cat is healthy it is unlikely that the treatment will be administered; however, if it is rabid or if rabies is suspected, the RIG-DEV treatment most likely will be administered.

The Rabid Animal—Signs to Watch For

There are indications to look for and to understand in the animal suspected of having rabies. Persons who have dogs, cats, or domestic animals should be familiar with these signs or symptoms:

1   The animal may appear to be docile during the early stages or the animal may be very nervous, even aggressive and then become docile.
2   The animal may develop a cough and act as if it had a bone fast in its throat. This is an indication that the animal's throat is becoming paralyzed.
3   The animal may be very nervous and tear and destroy its bedding, chew on wood or other items.
4   The animal may be or become vicious and attempt to fight any and all.
5   The animal may show evidence of paralysis, especially in the hind legs.
6   If the animal escapes, it may travel for 10 to 15 miles or until it dies. During this travel it may attack other animals while in flight such as horses, cows, hogs, as well as dogs and cats or wildlife. This is a common means of spreading the disease and, of course, the manner in which the wild animal in particular spreads it.
7   Carnivorous animals (especially skunks, foxes, coyotes, raccoons, dogs, and cats) and bats are more likely than other animals to be infected with rabies.[6]
8   An UNPROVOKED attack is more likely to mean that the animal is rabid.[7]

---

[6] *Rabies Prophylaxis*, op. cit., p. 2.
[7] Ibid.

Poisonous Bites and Stings

Protection for Rabies Bites or Infection

It is important that animal bites receive emergency care, that the bite be reported, and that a physician be consulted. Steps to remember are as follows:

1. The wound should be cleansed carefully with soap and water and flooded to help wash away the virus. It should be remembered that the virus is in the animal's saliva.
2. A physician should be consulted. He will want to see and treat the wound, advise the victim concerning further treatment, and help decide the course of action to follow.
3. The animal, if secured, should be watched carefully for at least ten days. The veterinarian should have the dog or cat confined in an escape-free place.
4. The physician will without doubt indicate the need for beginning the immunization if the animal cannot be found and there is evidence of rabies in the area.
5. If the bite or bites are about the face or neck and there is strong evidence of rabies in the animal that inflicted the bites, the physician will usually indicate the need for the immunization to begin at once. He may even suggest two injections daily for a week.
6. The local health authorities should be notified. If such is not available, law enforcement officials should be informed. It is important that the animal be taken alive and secured.
7. If the animal must be killed during capture, then care must be taken not to damage the head and brain. The brain is used for making the laboratory examination. If the head has to be transported and a time element is involved, the head should be packed in ice to preserve it. The brain should be delivered at the earliest moment to the health laboratory for examination.
8. Sick animals and strange animals, especially wild animals, that appear to be too friendly should not be handled. They should be avoided and/or destroyed.
9. All dogs and cats should be vaccinated to protect them from rabies. If an animal is exposed to the disease, it should either be destroyed or be confined for a period of up to six months.

Animal bites about the face and neck are extremely dangerous. The closer the bite is to the brain or spinal cord, the shorter the incubation period. The incubation period is the time between the bite and the onset of the disease. It is said that the infective virus travels by way of nerves rather than the bloodstream; if so, this may be the explanation for the great variation in the incubation period.

Reptiles [201]

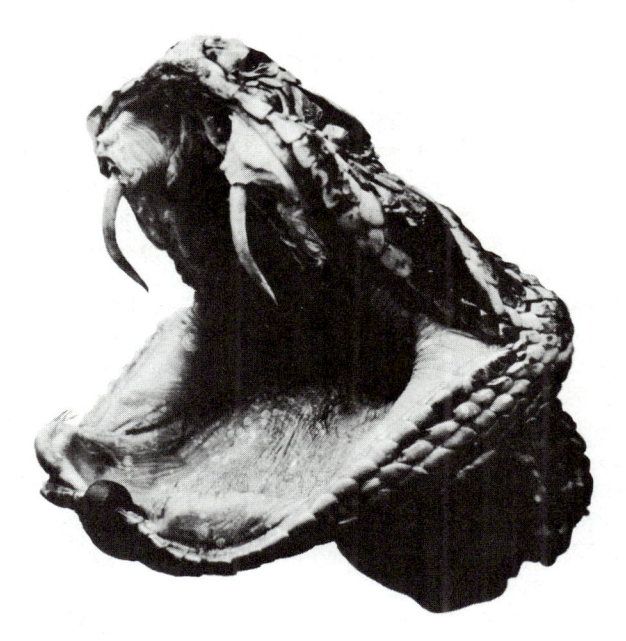

FIGURE 13.1 Head of a pit viper. (Wyeth Laboratories)

REPTILES

The highest snakebite frequency a year from all species of poisonous snakes was reported from North Carolina, Arkansas, Texas, Georgia, West Virginia, Alabama, and Louisiana. In recent years each of these states had ten or more persons bitten for every 100,000 population, with North Carolina having the highest rate of 18.79 bites per 100,000 population. The

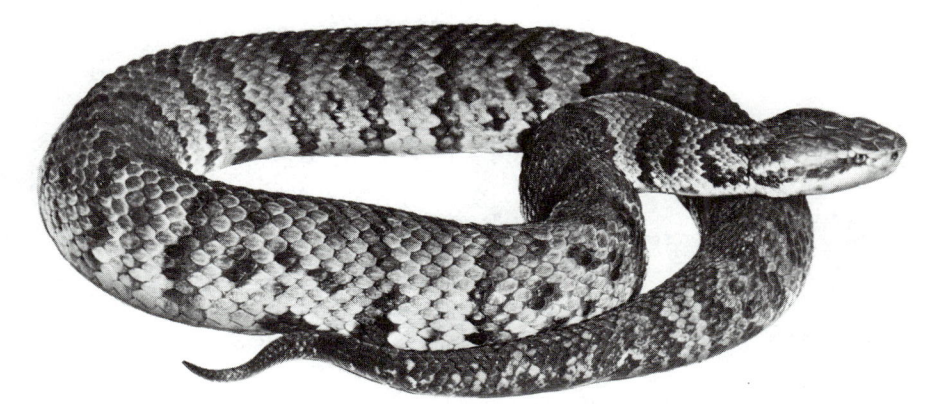

FIGURE 13.2 Cottonmouth moccasin (*Agkistrodon piscivorus*). (Wyeth Laboratories)

three states with the most snakebite deaths were Georgia, Florida, and Arizona, and these latter two states had only a death rate of 0.6 per 100,000. This does not mean that the poisonous snake is not a serious threat to our safety in the out of doors.[8]

Rattlesnakes account for 75 to 85 percent of all human deaths from snakebite. Forty-nine percent of the snakebites occur in persons under 20 years, and 48 percent were in children of school age or younger. Of these, 37 percent were bitten in close proximity to their homes.[9]

It should be understood that poisonous snakes are widely distributed over the United States. The cottonmouth moccasion (*Agkistrodon piscivorus*) is distributed over the Southwest, the Gulf States area, and the Mississippi Valley as far north as southern Illinois. Of all poisonous snakes, the copperhead (*Agkistrodon contortrix*) probably is more commonly found throughout the United States. The copperhead is one species with several subspecies. The states of North and South Carolina, West Virginia, Pennsylvania, Missouri, Oklahoma, Arkansas, Illinois, and others have a substantial population of this reptile. Missouri claims to have the "Copperhead Capital," located in a small village in the Ozarks, close to the Arkansas border.

Rattlesnakes (*Crotalus*) are said to be found throughout the continental United States with the exception of Maine, and they have probably crossed this state line too. In several areas of the United States, rattlesnakes abound in great numbers and they seem to maintain their population, even though there have been concerted efforts to eliminate them. Some 15 or more species of rattlesnakes are found within the U.S. borders. All of these species are dangerous because they possess fang and poison gland and have troublesome dispositions. No other species of snake has rattles. The rattlesnake's rule of behavior seems to be, "Let me alone and I won't bother you. Violate that rule, and watch out."

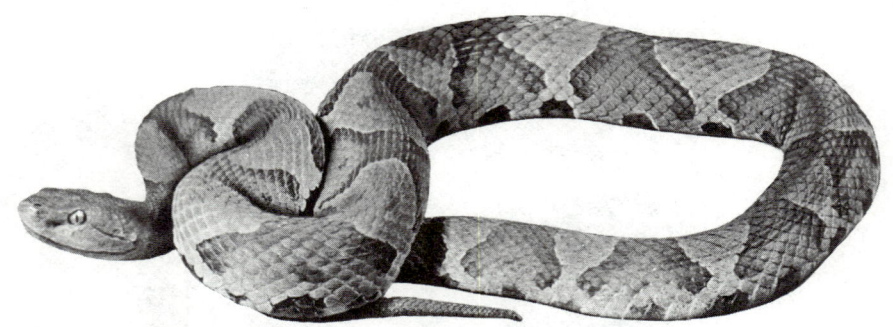

FIGURE 13.3 Copperhead (*Agkistrodon contortrix*). (Wyeth Laboratories)

[8] Elliot, op. cit., p. 85.
[9] Wyeth Laboratories, *Antivenin*. Philadelphia: Wyeth Laboratories, 1965, p. 19.

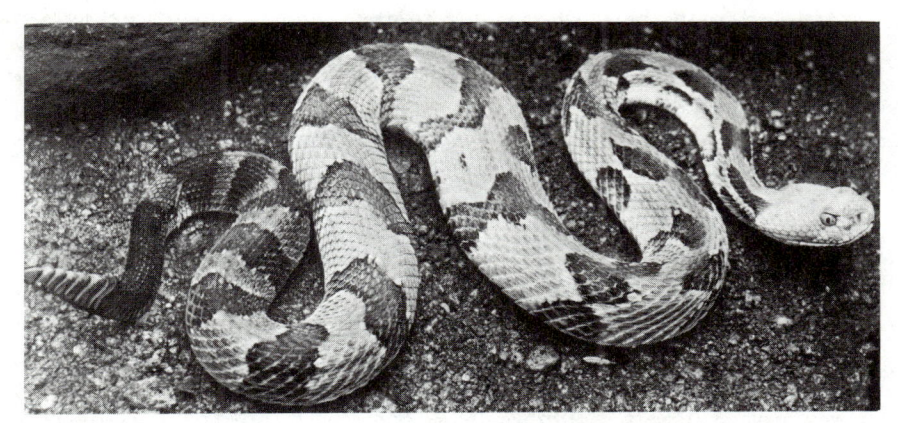

FIGURE 13.4 Timber rattlesnake (*Crotalus horridus*). (Wyeth Laboratories)

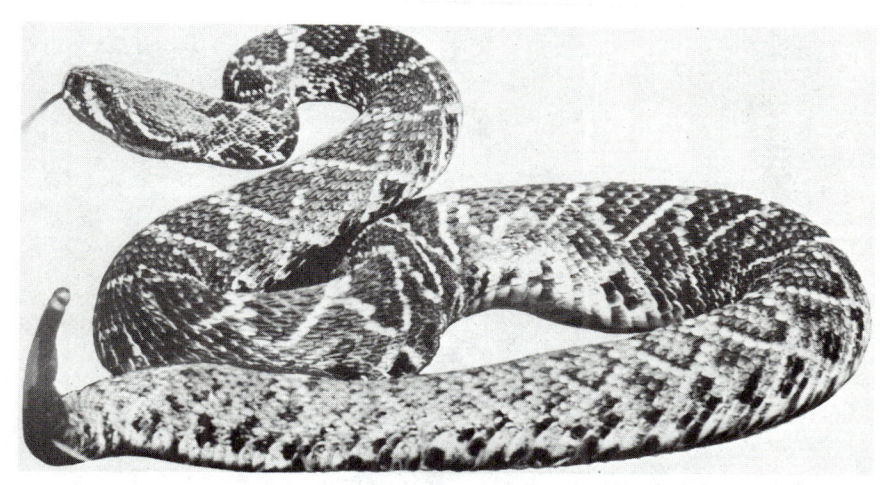

FIGURE 13.5 Florida rattlesnake (*Crotalus adamanteus*). (Wyeth Laboratories)

The eastern (Florida) and western (Texas) diamondback rattlesnakes are the largest and most dangerous venomous snakes in the United States. This is because of their large size, the length of their fangs, the quantity of venom, and the nature of the venom. The Texas diamondback is found from Arkansas through Oklahoma and Texas to southern California. It is responsible for more serious and fatal bites than any of our other snakes. This is a bold snake, commonly found in the open country and very often around or near farm and ranch homes. The Florida or eastern diamondback is the larger of the two and is found in the eastern United States and Gulf States.

The coral snake is usually associated with the southern United States.

[204] Poisonous Bites and Stings

It has a striking color pattern, due to the banded "red on yellow on white." The red bands are wider and they are bordered by narrower bands of either yellow or white. This is a small snake, but its bite is very dangerous. The venom of the coral snake is neurotoxic rather than hemotoxic as in the case of the pit vipers.

Prevention of Snakebite

The best way to be protected against snakebite is to be able to identify venomous snakes on sight. It is important to know of their habits and the habitat that is most suitable for them. The pit vipers—rattlesnake, cottonmouth water moccasin, and copperhead—for the most part are nocturnal, that is, they are more likely to travel and feed at night. They seem to be more sensitive after the sun goes down. It has been the experience of most persons that the rattler is much more prone to use his rattles in the dark.

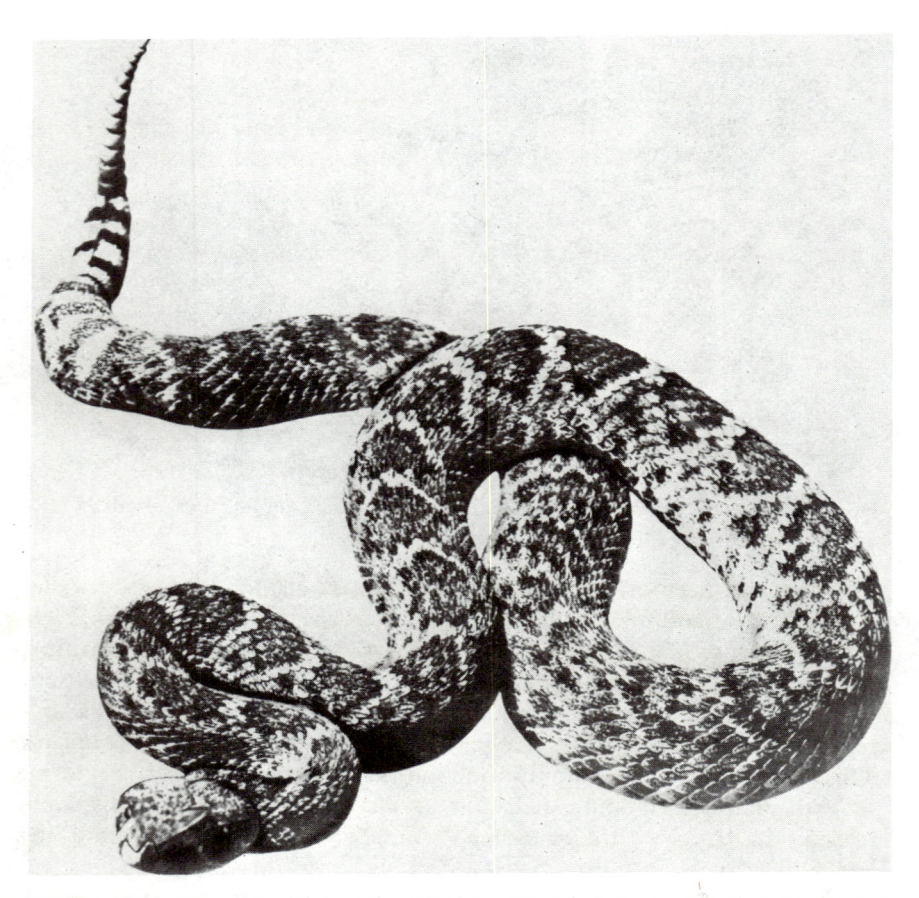

FIGURE 13.6 Texas diamond-back rattlesnake (*Crotalus atrox*). (Wyeth Laboratories)

Reptiles [205]

He can see but a person cannot see him, so the advantage is with the reptile.

Persons who enjoy collecting snakes and handling them should use suitable equipment and should exercise great care in holding the snake. The snake should be held correctly behind the head so that it cannot move the head to the side, open its mouth, and bite. The other hand should grasp the snake's body, midway or below, so the snake cannot coil about the arm. Heavy cloth bags are good for transporting snakes. Snake cages should be secure and kept locked. When in snake country, whether a person is collecting snakes or hunting, he should concentrate on his task and avoid trouble.

Persons hunting, hiking, camping, or working in snake-infested areas should wear protective clothing—boots, heavy pants, or leggings with the pants being worn on the outside of the boots. Since about half of all snake strikes are below the knee, this is an important area to protect.

Special Precautions If persons who work, live, or play in areas where the poisonous reptile lives are to protect themselves, they must understand the snake and the protection problem. Helpful precautions follow.

1. *Season.* Snakes are more dangerous during the early spring. They have been storing venom, getting ready for the first big feed. The poison glands are loaded. This may be different in the West and South.
2. *Time of day.* The pit viper is nocturnal, so the twilight and dark hours are the most dangerous. The chance of encountering the snake is best at night.
3. *Hiding place.* Snakes have dens and also like rocks, ledges, wood piles, heavy covers, caves, and old buildings.
4. *Person's action.* A person should be careful where he sits, climbs, places his hands, walks, and sleeps. Sleeping on the ground in snake country can be very dangerous.
5. *Clothing.* A person should wear protective clothing about the lower legs.
6. *Buddy system.* A person should use the buddy system when hunting, fishing, camping, hiking, or collecting snakes. If there is an accident, help will be needed.
7. *Snake.* If possible, the snake should be killed. It is important to know and be sure the snake was venomous. The dead snake should be taken for identification.
8. *Obstacles.* A person should step over logs, branches, and other objects with care, as these are good hiding places for snakes.
9. *Area around water.* A person should watch carefully about stumps, logs, and low branches near water. He should check a boat before entering it and be careful where he ties the boat.
10. *Car.* A car should be parked in a cleared open area. The doors should be closed and the windows rolled up most of the way. A person should sleep in a car rather than on the ground.
11. *Handling snakes.* A person should avoid any unnecessary handling of

[206] Poisonous Bites and Stings

snakes and should not frighten others with snakes. He should beware of the freshly killed snake; it may strike and the separated head can bite.

12 Preparation. A snake kit, preferably a first-aid kit, should be carried. A person should know the recommended procedure for snakebite and how to use the kit.

Symptoms of Snakebite

The following are the signs or symptoms of the venomous snakebite:

1. Fang marks are present; teeth marks will probably be noticeable.
2. An immediate burning pain which spreads rapidly, especially from the pit viper's bite.
3. Sudden swelling beginning soon after the bite in the bite area and then spreading toward the body. This is especially true for bites on the arm or leg.
4. Shock, nausea, weakness, and numbness. The muscles may twitch and the skin may tingle.

Protection for Snakebite

In no area of emergency care is there as much confusion and disagreement as this. Much of the conflict is about the matter of protection or treatment. The medical person is trained to treat, whereas the first-aider is limited to protective measures. Dr. Herbert L. Stahnke, Director of the Poisonous Animal Research Laboratory, Arizona State University, has said, "The treatment of venomous bites or stings cannot wait while the therapist studies his lesson, whether he be a layman or physician." Certainly this is a major part of the problem. The physician in his routine practice will not encounter many such victims. It is more likely to be the hunter, outdoorsman, rancher, forester, or farmer who comes face to face with this emergency. There are several methods suggested for the protection and treatment of the snakebite victim. Each of these is based upon considerable research.

The greatest conflict in the protection of a snakebite has to do with the cold or cooling treatment. This difference of opinion in the protection methods should be noted as they are presented in this chapter.

Ligature-Cold Technique This method was developed by Dr. Stahnke. In his book, *The Treatment of Venomous Bites and Stings*, this method is discussed in great detail. The following are the steps recommended for the snakebite victim. A person giving aid should

1. Stop all muscular activity.
2. Place a ligature (constricting band) between the bite and the heart.
3. Place the bitten area and the area well around the bite in ice water.
4. Remove the constricting band after about seven minutes in the ice water.

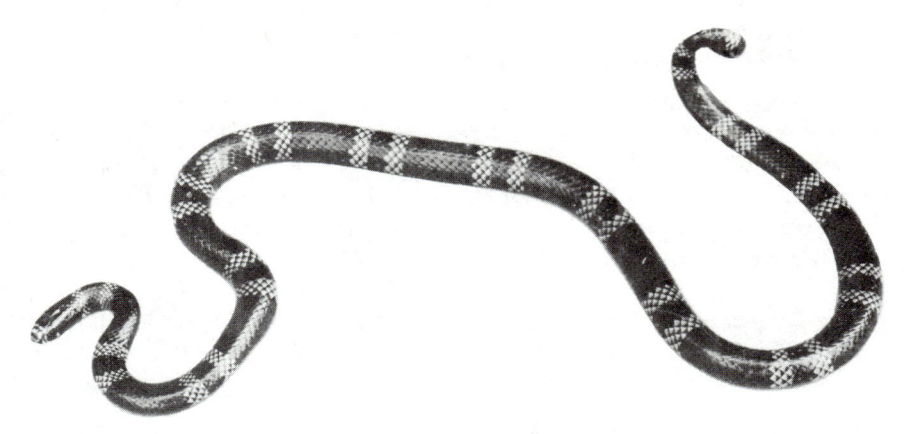

FIGURE 13.7 The poisonous coral snake (*Micrurus lemniscatus*).

5 Keep the victim warm.
6 Get the victim to medical help.

Dr. Charles Watt-Dr. Bruce Means Method The following procedures for the emergency treatment of snakebite are based upon research and experience of Dr. Charles Watt of Thomasville, Georgia and Dr. Bruce Means of the Tall Timber Research Station in Florida. Their work contradicts some of the earlier findings. According to their method, in the event of a snakebite a person should

1 Get to a doctor as soon as possible, no matter what else he is forced to do.
2 Get away from the snake. If possible have someone else kill the snake so that it can be taken for identification.
3 Put a light tourniquet (constricting band) above the bite. It should be so loose that a finger can easily be inserted beneath it.
4 If possible without wasting time, immobilize the bitten limb with a splint and make sure the bindings are loose. Have others move him immediately.[10]

If time away from medical help is longer, a more complex procedure should be followed. A person should

1 Wash the wound with water, soap, or alcohol.
2 Mark a short, straight incision between and slightly beyond the fang marks but no deeper than the fatty tissue under the skin (usually about one eight of an inch).
3 Suck the wound with his mouth if he has no cuts in the mouth. If available, a suction cup can be used, especially if the wound is in an area he cannot reach with the mouth and he is alone.

[10] Elliot, op. cit., p. 86.

[208] Poisonous Bites and Stings

4   Apply a tourniquet and a splint as directed previously.
5   Get to the doctor at the earliest moment.

Dr. Watt is opposed to the use of cold on the snakebite. He has found in reviewing many cases that no deformity or loss of limb resulted except in the cases when some cooling had been used. He is as much against using one ice cube as a ton of ice. Dr. Watt and Dr. Means have found that many persons who underwent the cooling process and lived, either lost limbs or were deformed.

Dr. Thomas Glass Procedure   Dr. Thomas G. Glass says, "Crippling from pit viper envenomation is caused by too little *treatment*, too much *first aid*, or both." Dr. Glass recommends the following first aid for all snakebites:

1   Apply a constricting band above and below the bite site. Do not obstruct the blood supply.
2   Apply crushed ice in plastic bags to the bite site or apply some other cooling agent such as chemical cold packs.
3   Obtain the snake and bring it to the hospital (preferably dead).
4   Transport the victim to a medical facility as soon as possible in a safe manner and do no harm.
5   Do not skin test for antivenin and do not make any cuts.[11]

These three methods of protecting snakebite are presented for your consideration. There are other methods including that of the American National Red Cross.

The doctor's first task is to identify, if possible, the kind of snake that inflicted the bite. More than one person has been given both first-aid and medical treatment for a bite that was harmless. If the snake itself is not available for identification, the fact that it was venomous (there are only four poisonous species in the United States) can usually be determined by the fang marks, pain, swelling, discoloration, and shock.

Antivenin is the only effective medical treatment, though the possibility of allergy to horse-blood serum always must be reckoned with.

ARACHNIDS

Arachnids are insectlike animals with two body regions and four pairs of legs. They do not have wings. Scorpions, ticks, spiders, and chiggers are arachnids.

---

[11] Thomas G. Glass, "Early Debridement in Pit Viper Bites." *JAMA*, Vol. 235, No. 23 (June 1976), p. 2513.

Scorpions

These animals inject venom into their victims by means of a stinger located at the base of the tail. There is a poison gland with a duct that leads to the stingers. The sting is painful, and there are swelling, discoloration, and usually a burning sensation. There are many species of scorpions, two very dangerous species in the Southwest.

The stricken person may become restless, nauseous, and have abdominal cramps. The first-aid protection consists of the following, as described by Dalrymple. Dalrymple describes the L-C technique as developed by Stahnke.[12]

1. A tight tourniquet is placed between the sting bite and the body, as close to the puncture as possible. Ice is then placed directly on the sting. A bath of crushed ice and water is prepared quickly and the entire member is immersed well past the tourniquet. Immersion continues steadily for five minutes before the tourniquet is removed, then is resumed for at least two hours. No incisions, on-off refrigeration, hot packs, morphine, or alcohol should be allowed.
2. The idea is to slow down venom absorption as drastically as possible. Stings of common scorpions should respond readily to this treatment. But a doctor should be summoned immediately if one of the deadly species is identified, or symptoms indicate it was the culprit, or if a person has been stung several times in widely separated sites, is very young, or has been stung around the head, back of neck, backbone, or genitals.

Scorpion antivenin is available free to any licensed physician from the Poisonous Animals Research Laboratory, Arizona State University, Tempe, Arizona 85281.

Spiders

The black widow, the brown recluse, and the tarantula are three problem spiders. All spiders possess some poison, but the amount is usually quite small. The bite does present an emergency situation.

The black widow, about a half-inch long, can be identified by its shiny black body with the red hourglass on the underside of the abdomen. Only the female is dangerous.

The brown recluse is medium brown in color, about an inch long, has a mark on its back that resembles a fiddle. Both the male and female brown recluse are dangerous. The black widow is widely dispersed, and the brown recluse seems to be spreading rapidly. The first aid for spider bites is to

[12] Bryon W. Dalrymple, "The Zodiacs Noxious No. 8." *Field and Stream*, May, 1962, p. 100.

[210] Poisonous Bites and Stings

1. Place a constricting band above the bite immediately and leave it in place for five to ten minutes.
2. Pack the area with ice. The extremity affected should be kept low.
3. Keep the victim comfortable.
4. Obtain medical help as soon as possible.

Ticks

These insectlike arachnids are flat, hard, and brown with four pairs of legs and no wings; their habitat is the woods and fields. They live as blood-sucking parasites on warm-blooded animals. Rabbits, squirrels, dogs, cats, human beings, and other mammals make suitable hosts. They are especially troublesome in the spring and early summer.

Tularemia, Rocky Mountain spotted fever, Q fever, and Colorado tick fever are all spread by ticks. It is possible for the tick bite to cause an infection of the skin as well as one of the diseases mentioned. Persons can help keep ticks off the body through the use of several commercial products that are available, and by wearing tight clothing around their wrists and ankles. It is very important to know what to do to protect against ticks. The following procedure is helpful.

1. Search the body including the scalp as soon as possible after the possible exposure. The longer ticks are attached, the more likely they are to transmit disease if infected.
2. Remove the tick by covering its body with an oily substance or exerting a steady pull with tweezers and perhaps first sliding a knife partway under its body from the rear or bringing a heated object close to the animal, if this can be done safely. Do not squash it.
3. Wash the bite wound gently with soap and water, and apply an antiseptic after the tick has been removed. Afterward, the hands are to be washed thoroughly.
4. Consult a physician regarding the advisability of vaccination against spotted fever if exposed often to ticks. If allergic to eggs, the victim should be advised that the vaccine is prepared from egg culture.

Chiggers

Chiggers are mites. They are common in the South and Midwest. The early summer is the usual time to have a chigger problem. If the chigger enters a hair follicle and injects his fluid, an irritation will persist for several days.

The best solution is to prevent the chigger's invasion by clothing, repellents, bathing promptly, and changing one's clothing completely.

A repellent that works very well for many is powdered sulfur, thoroughly dusted over the body. One should consult his physician or pharmacist for additional recommendations.

Once the chiggers have made their attack, some comfort can be had from the application of calamine, alcohol, ammonia water, or baking soda solutions. The irritation usually persists for several days and there is much discomfort.

INSECTS

Every summer, especially during the month of August, a large number of people are endangered by the teeming world of insects. A generalized systematic reaction to a single insect sting can present a medical emergency that can result in death within 10 to 15 minutes. Since eight of every thousand persons are allergic to insects and that four of these eight are extremely sensitive, the potential for trouble is great.[13] Unless the hypersensitive person is prepared for the emergency, he may not be alive when he reaches medical help.

Dr. Claude A. Frazier says that the insect sting kit is an insurance measure for the vulnerable patient. But it should be more than that since it can provide vital time to get the patient in shock to medical assistance. It should be a standard item in first-aid supplies wherever the public might encounter the Hymenoptera. Dr. Frazier gives the following instructions to avoid stings. A person should

1. Have Hymenoptera nests periodically destroyed while still manageable around the home and yard.
2. Do not go barefoot or wear sandals outdoors from April to October.
3. Do not wear bright, flowery clothing. Bright colors attract bees especially.
4. Do not wear floppy clothing to entangle and madden Hymenoptera.
5. Wear long pants, long-sleeved shirts, and gloves if working among flowers or fruits. Cover up.
6. Avoid wearing anything bright such as jewelry or buckles.
7. Do not use scented lotions, soaps, shampoos, or perfumes.
8. Wear light colors such as white, light green, tan, or khaki.
9. If Hymenoptera are encountered, do not swat. Retreat slowly. If retreat is is impossible, life face down and cover the head with the arms.[14]

ACTIVITIES

1. Visit a local hospital or physician and discuss the treatment of snakebite and other venomous bites in your area and report to the class.
2. Prepare a paper on ticks of the United States and the problems they present.

[13] Claude A. Frazier, "Insect Stings—A Medical Emergency." *JAMA*, Vol. 235, No. 22 (May 1976), p. 2410.
[14] Ibid.

3 Prepare a first-aid kit for camping, hunting, and other outdoor activities and give special emphasis to the protection of venomous bites and stings.
4 Research the new developments in the treatment of rabies for both man and animal.
5 Prepare a paper on the two dangerous spiders, the brown recluse and the black widow.

QUESTIONS TO ANSWER

1 What precautions should a person take to protect himself against snakebite?
2 Describe the Ligature-Cold technique for the protection of snakebite.
3 How do the insects and the arachnids differ? Which presents the greatest problem from the standpoint of emergency care?
4 Defend the statement, "The sting of the honeybee is more dangerous than the bite of the rattlesnake."
5 What are the signs or symptoms that indicate that an animal may be rabid?
6 Which animal bites are the most dangerous and why? What is significant about the virus of rabies being present in the saliva of the infected animal?
7 Discuss the general distribution of venomous snakes in the United States. When are snakes the most dangerous? Why?
8 What emergency protection can the first-aider give the victim of a black widow or brown recluse spider bite?
9 What emergency protection can the first-aider give the victim of a scorpion sting?
10 How can the person who is hypersensitive to the sting of the Hymenoptera protect himself? What precautions should he take?

SELECTED REFERENCES

BAHMANYAR, MAHNWULD, et. al., "Successful Protection of Humans Exposed to Rabies Infection." *JAMA*, December 13, 1976.
COREY, LAWRENCE, and HATTWICK, MICHAEL A. W., "Treatment of Persons Exposed to Rabies." *JAMA*, April 21, 1975.
EAST, BEN, "Warning: Death May Not Rattle." *Outdoor Life*, November, 1975.
ELLENBOGEN, CHARLES, "Postexposure Antirabies Therapy." *AFP*, Vol. 15, No. 3 (March, 1977).
ELLIOTT, CHARLES, "Snakebite! What to Know—What to Do." *Outdoor Life*, September, 1977.

FRAZIER, CLAUDE A., "Insect Stings—A Medical Emergency." *JAMA*, May 31, 1976.

GARNER, WALTON R., and JONES, DAVID O., "Problems Associated with Rabies Preexposure Prophylaxis." *JAMA*, March 15, 1976.

GLASS, THOMAS G., "Early Debridement of Pit Viper Bites." *JAMA*, June 7, 1976.

PARRISH, HENRY M., "460 Die of Snake-Bite in 10 Years." *Medical Tribune*, March 13, 1965.

PUBLIC HEALTH SERVICE, *Rabies Prophylaxis*. Atlanta, Georgia: U.S. Department of HEW, Public Health Service, Center for Disease Control, 1976. (Distributed by Illinois Department of Public Health.)

PUBLIC HEALTH SERVICE, "Rabies Risk, Management, Prophylaxis and Immunization." *Annals of Internal Medicine*, April, 1977.

14. POISONOUS PLANTS

Each year thousands of Americans in one way or another are poisoned by common hazardous plants. In practically every section of the United States, one or more of the many species of poisonous plants can be found. Many of these poisonous plants are being brought into the yards, gardens, and homes and are raised without knowledge of their potential danger. A great number of them are moderately poisonous, possibly producing mild illness or irritation, whereas others will result in serious consequences. Some plants cause dermatitis (inflammation of the skin), hay fever, or other allergic reactions owing to the sensitivity of the person. Other plants are very decorative flowers or shrubs praised for their beauty, but these too are very poisonous when touched or ingested.

SKIN IRRITATION PLANTS

In the United States there are over 60 kinds of plants that may cause skin irritation. Most persons are immune to a vast number of these plants. However, some plants such as poison ivy, poison oak, and poison sumac affect almost every person who comes in contact with them. Immunity in one situation does not necessarily indicate that a particular person will be immune at a later time. Some individuals are more prone to the plant irritation after having once suffered from it.

Poison Ivy, Oak, and Sumac

Poison ivy and poison oak plants grow in abundance in almost every part of the United States. Each year these attractive looking vines and shrubs (including poison sumac) cause nearly 2 million cases of skin

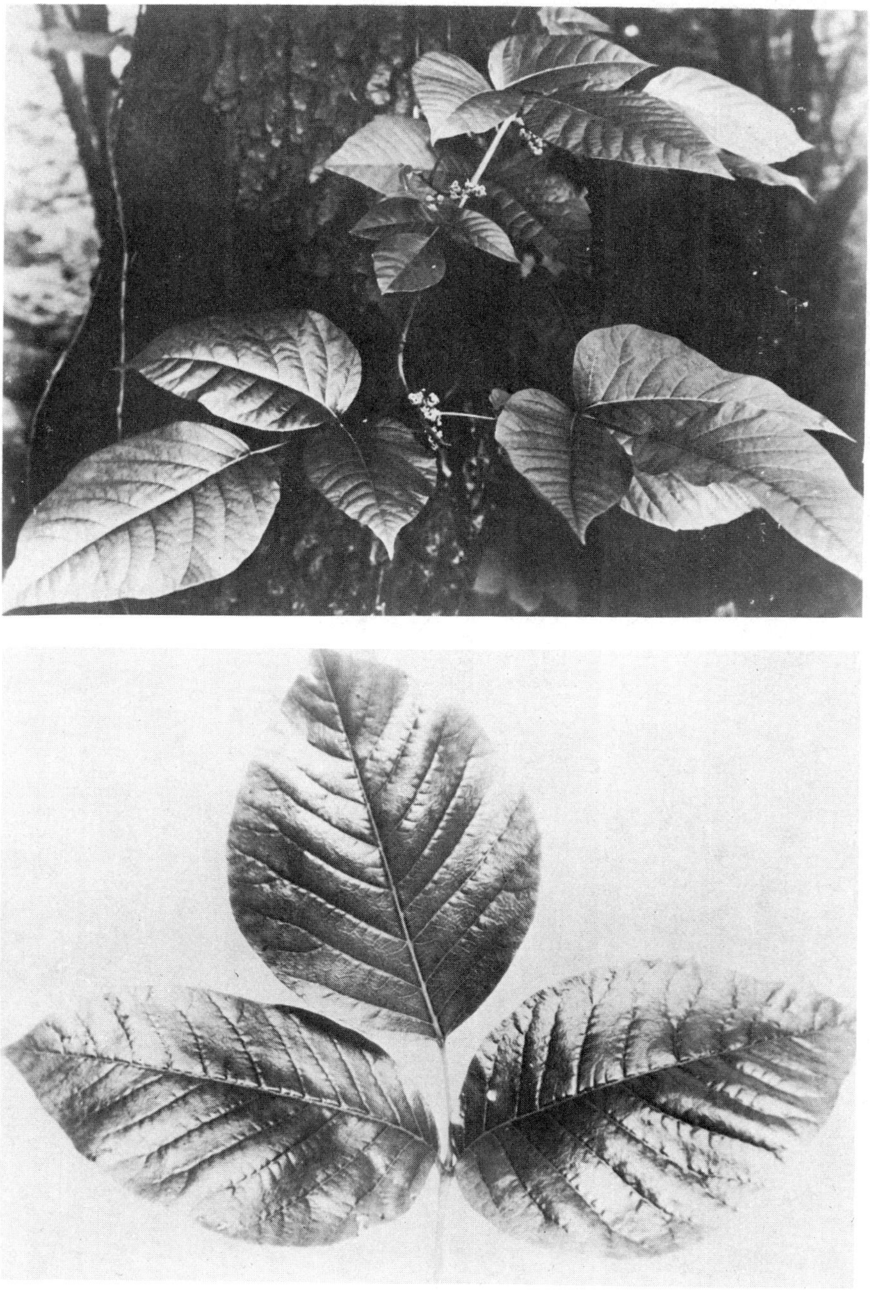

Skin Irritation Plants [215]

FIGURE 14.1 Top: common poison ivy vine with cluster of flowers at the axis of each leaf. Bottom, and next page: less common leaf forms that may occur on the same plant or on different plants of common poison ivy. (U.S. Department of Agriculture)

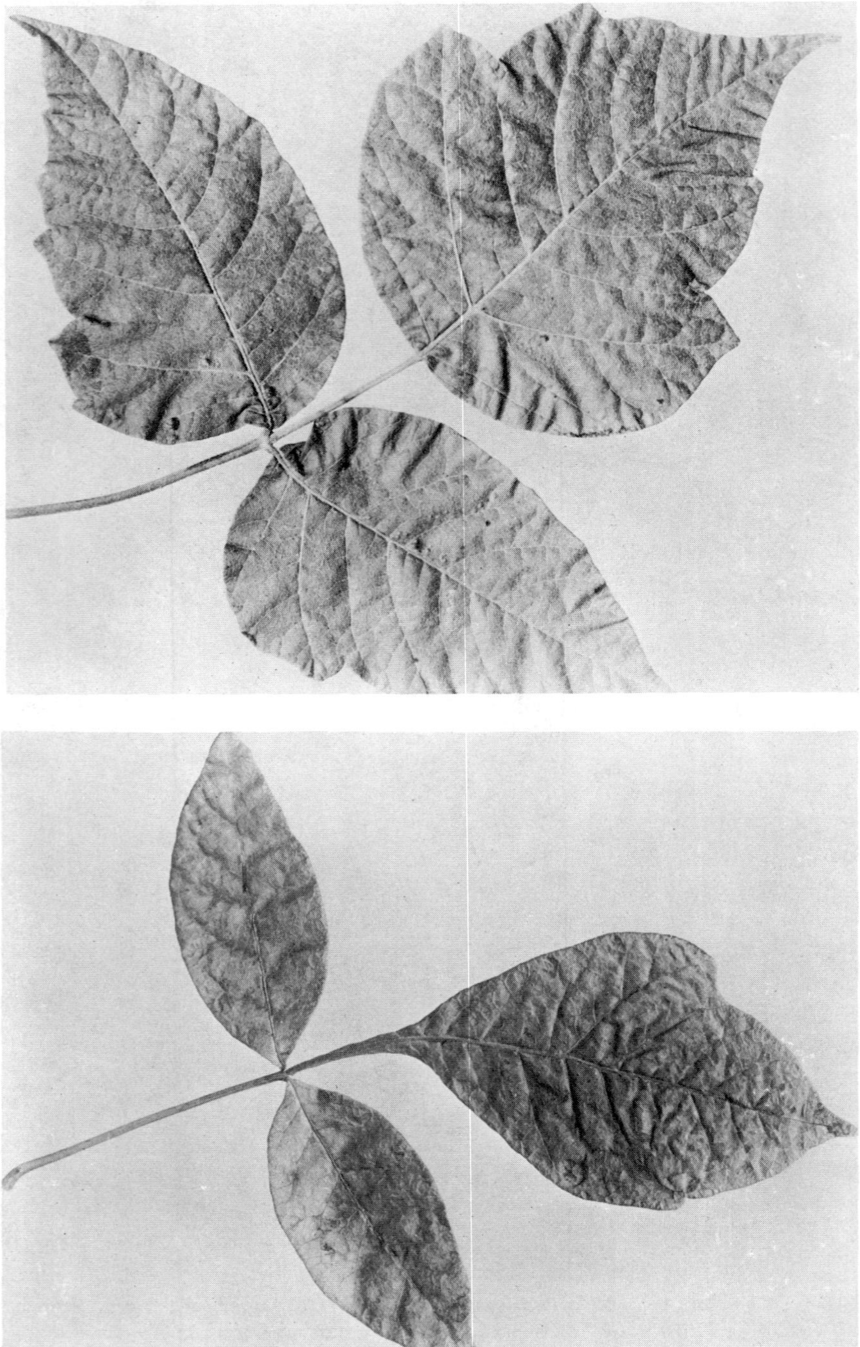

[216] Poisonous Plants

FIGURE 14.1 (continued) Less common leaf forms of poison ivy. (U.S. Department of Agriculture)

Skin Irritation Plants [217]

poisoning serious enough to require either medical attention or at least one day of restricted activity, or both. Although active, roaming youngsters are the most frequent victims, no age group and few individuals are immune.

The skin irritant of poison ivy, poison oak, and poison sumac is a toxic agent which can be found in all parts of the plant—not just the leaves, but in the fruit, stem, and roots as well. This toxic agent is called urushiol. Urushiol is ample in the sap of the plant, so that the greatest danger from this type of plant poisoning occurs in the spring and summer.

According to the National Institute of Allergy and Infectious Diseases,[1] reactions to poison ivy, oak, or sumac do not occur if an individual simply gets near the plants. The skin must make contact with the urushiol from the plant. Smoke that contains droplets of urushiol may cause skin, nose, throat, and lung irritation. Occasionally, a person may contact poison ivy, oak, or sumac through some intermediate object—a tool, clothing, or a pet—that has been contaminated by the toxic agent urushiol. Cases have been reported of persons being poisoned from the changing of tires on an automobile that had been driven through poison ivy many months

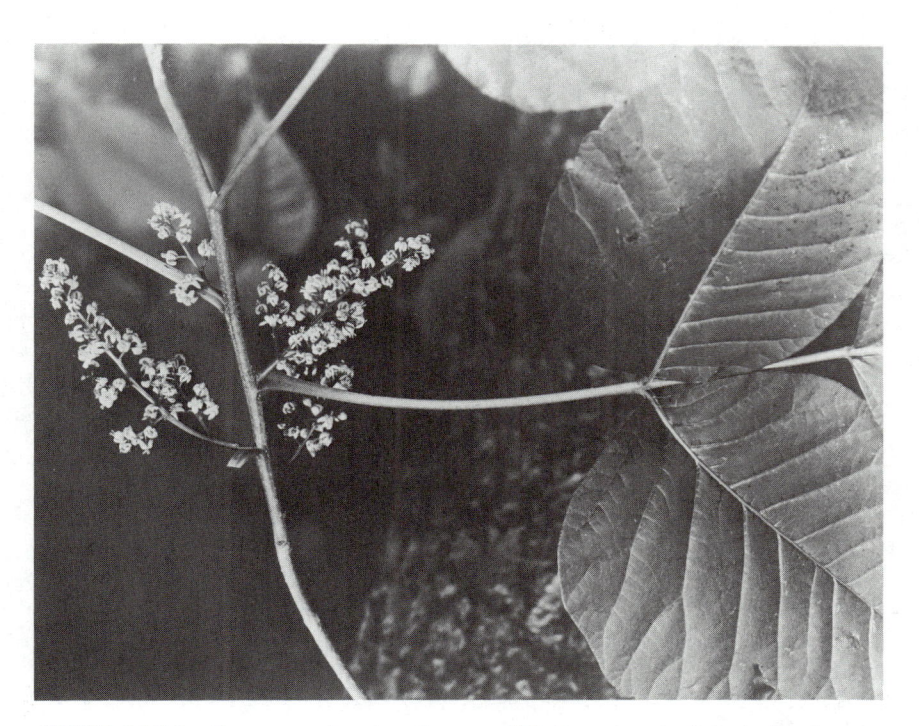

FIGURE 14.2A Common poison ivy: flowers. (U.S. Department of Agriculture)

[1] National Institute of Allergy and Infectious Diseases, *Poison Ivy, Oak and Sumac*. Washington, D.C.: U.S. Government Printing Office, 1967.

[218] Poisonous Plants

before. Other cases have been cited where individuals who had not left the house contacted poison ivy because of a household pet that was permitted to venture outdoors.

Poison Ivy   In all probability, poison ivy has caused more suffering and unpleasant experiences than any other plant. Poison ivy is best characterized by its cluster of three green leaflets, with each leaflet being usually oval with pointed tips (see Figure 14.1). The green color of the leaflets is present in the spring and summer months; during the fall they change to colorful scarlet orange and russet shades. The leaf forms among poison ivy plants are as variable as their growing habit. The flowers and fruit of this plant are always in clusters which originate in the axis of the leaves, usually on the smaller branches. The flowers are yellowish green to white

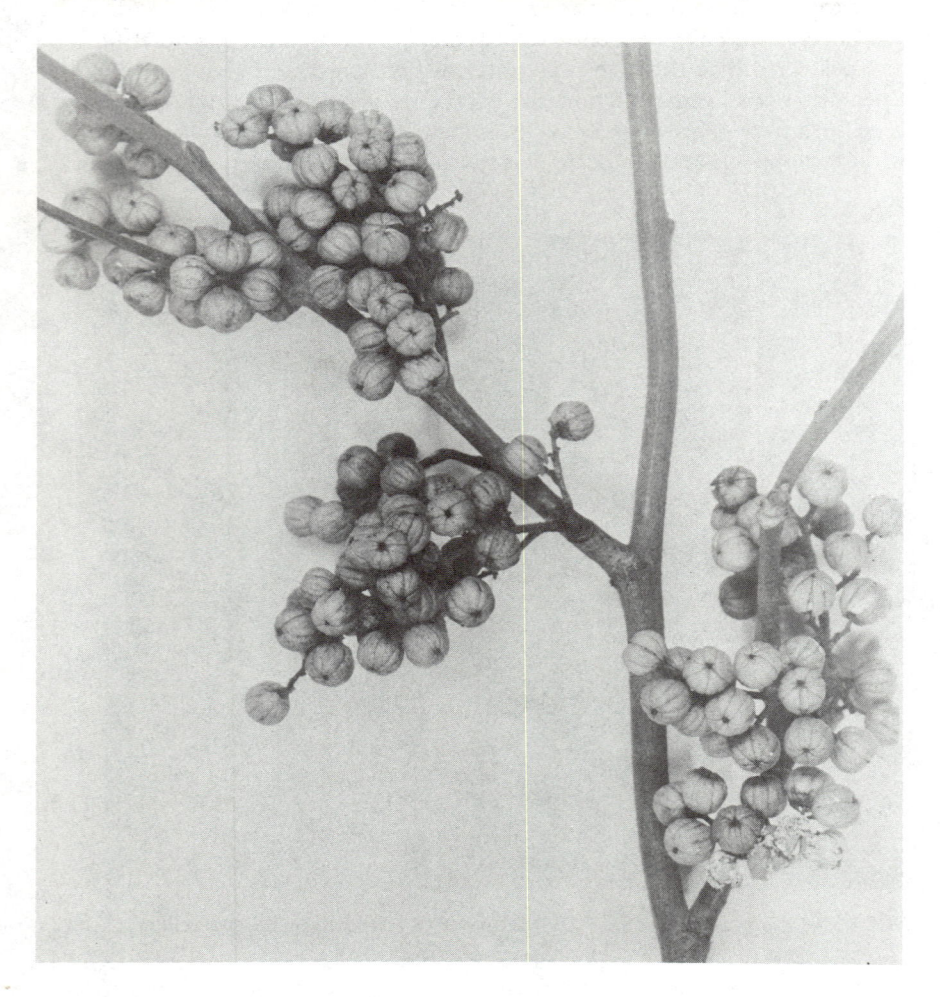

FIGURE 14.2B   Common poison ivy: fruit. (U.S. Department of Agriculture)

Skin Irritation Plants [219]

in color. The fruits have a white, waxy appearance in the shape of a berry. Poison ivy can be found growing in one of three ways: (1) woody vines attached to objects for support, (2) trailing shrubs on the ground, or (3) taking a shrub or treelike appearance.

Poison Oak There are two types of poison oak plants found in the United States: oakleaf poison ivy and western poison oak. The oakleaf poison ivy is commonly found in the Southeast and the eastern part of the country. Oakleaf poison ivy grows as a low shrub. Leaflets of this plant occur in multiples of three, as does poison ivy, but are lobed like the leaves on some varieties of oak trees (Figure 14.4). The center leaflet usually has the oakleaf look, and the side leaves may have uneven edges. The flowers and fruit (sometimes velvety) look and grow like those on the common poison ivy plant.

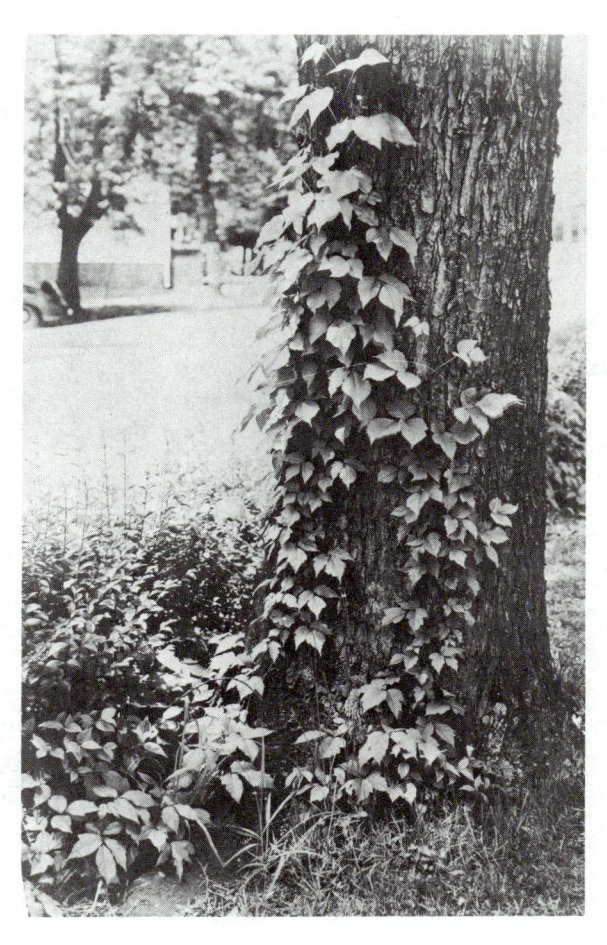

FIGURE 14.3A Common poison ivy growing in a hedge and on a shade tree. (U.S. Department of Agriculture)

[220]   Poisonous Plants

The western poison oak grows all along the Pacific Coast, from southern California to Washington. This plant's leaves are also identified by three leaflets (Figure 14.5). Each leaf is shiny green when mature and

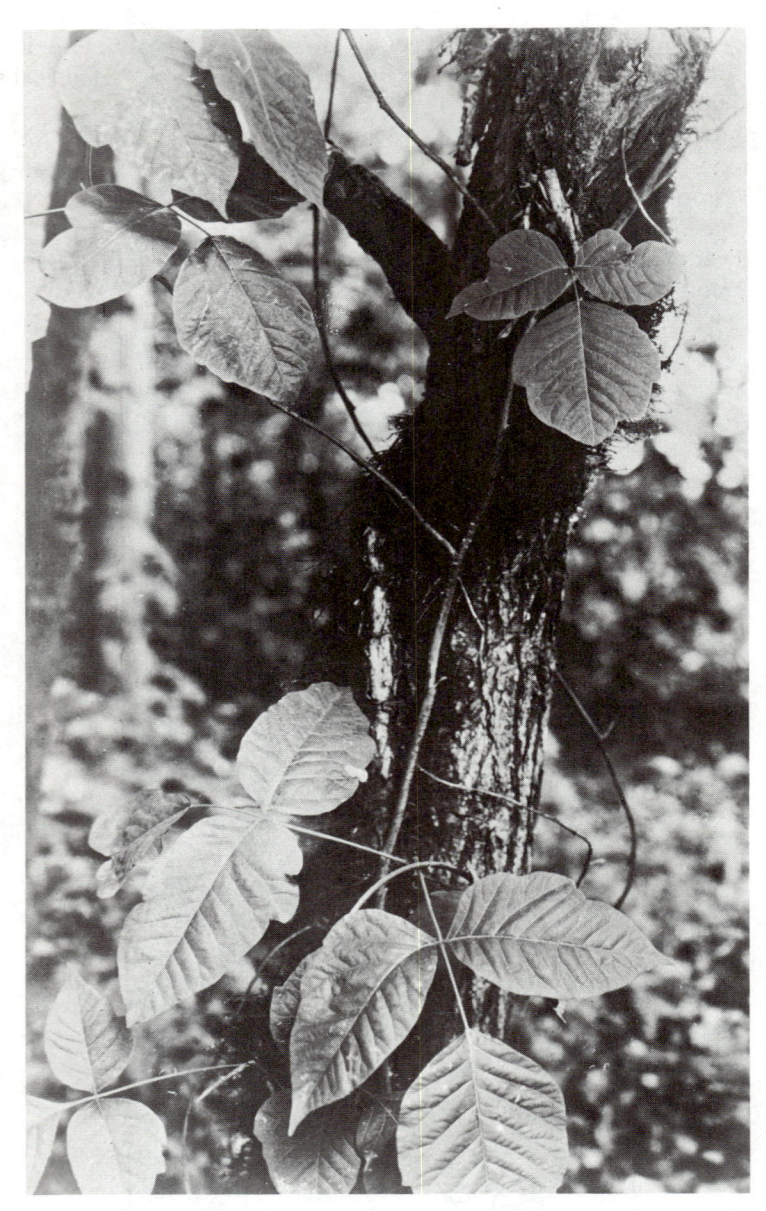

FIGURE 14.3B   Common poison ivy vine, showing leaves and roots that attach to a tree. (U.S. Department of Agriculture)

Skin Irritation Plants [221]

turns yellow or red when the soil begins to dry out in late spring or early summer. Usually, western poison oak grows as an upright shrub with many stems in the ground. It may also grow as a climbing vine reaching heights of up to 30 feet. A person can locate this poisonous plant growing up to 6 feet in a spreading cluster in open fields. Its flowers are shaped like the poison ivy flowers and are usually greenish white and about one-quarter inch in diameter. The fruit is normally greenish white and approximately the size of a raisin.

Poison Sumac Poison sumac grows in swampy areas as a coarse woody shrub or a small tree ranging in height from 5 to 25 feet. This poisonous plant is basically found east of the Mississippi River. The leaves of poison sumac may have from 7 to 13 leaflets ranging from 3 to 4 inches long and 1 to 2 inches wide. The edges of the leaflets are smooth. The leaves of poison sumac are bright orange during the early spring. Later the color of the leaves changes to a dark green on the upper surface and a light green on the lower surface. In the fall, the leaves turn to a brilliant red-orange or russet color. The flowers are yellowish green and they hang in long clusters from the axis of the leaves. The fruit grows in the same manner and is ivory white or green-colored.

Symptoms As discussed earlier in this chapter, reaction to poison ivy, oak, and sumac is caused by the irritating substance urushiol. The first symptoms of poisoning are itching and a burning sensation, which commonly occur within 24 hours but may develop in a few hours or be delayed for several days. These first symptoms will be followed by inflammation and swelling and then the appearance of blisters. In situations where the irritation is on the face near the eyes, the eyelids may be red and swollen. In extreme cases, fever, swollen lymph nodes, nausea, and other symptoms may occur. The reaction of the individual, the season of the year, the stage of development of the plant, and the amount of urushiol contacted affect the severity of the aforementioned symptoms. Presence of the poisoning over a long period of time is probably due to continued contact with the poisonous plant.

Protection Where possible, the skin should be washed with soap and water. Washing is effective for this type of plant poisoning. However, those persons who are highly sensitive to urushiol are not protected by soap and water from severe reactions. The cases of poisoning that do develop will usually clear up by themselves within two or three weeks. Calamine lotion helps dry the skin and also helps relieve the itching sensation. Most ointments, creams, and other lotions being advertised as keeping urushiol from the skin have been judged of little value. Baths in warm (body temperature) water may help relieve itching. For severe cases it is recommended that the person contact a physician, who in turn

[222] Poisonous Plants

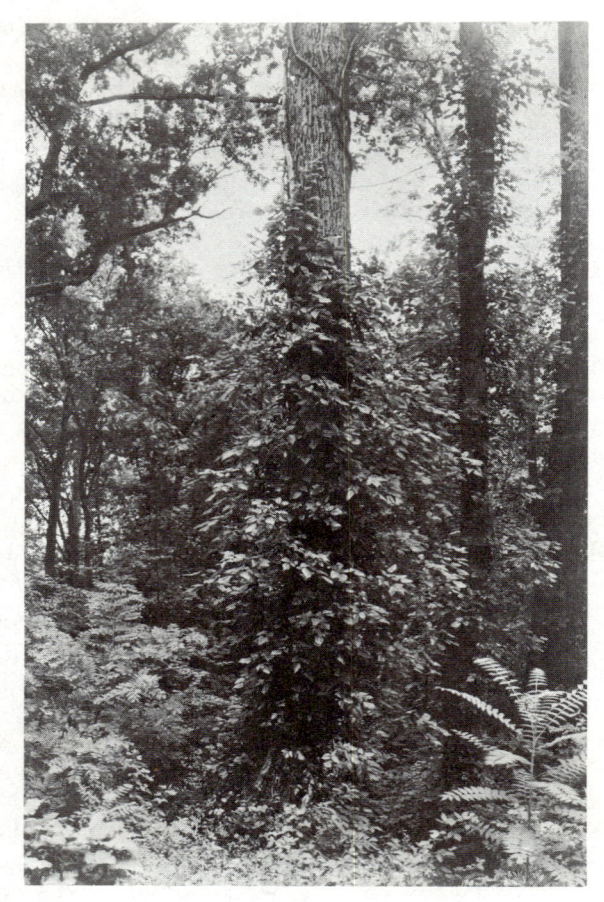

FIGURE 14.3C Common poison ivy growing up the trunk of a tree. (U.S. Department of Agriculture)

will normally prescribe drugs for reducing the itching and swelling and helping to prevent infection.

Preventive Measures

The best way of preventing skin irritation from poisonous plants is to stay away from the plants. But poison ivy and poison oak will grow almost anywhere—from the woods and glades to the backyards. The following are suggested as ways of preventing plant poisoning:

1   Be able to identify the various types of poisonous plants. The numerous varieties will be discussed in a later section of this chapter. A person can avoid these plants if he knows how to identify them.

Skin Irritation Plants [223]

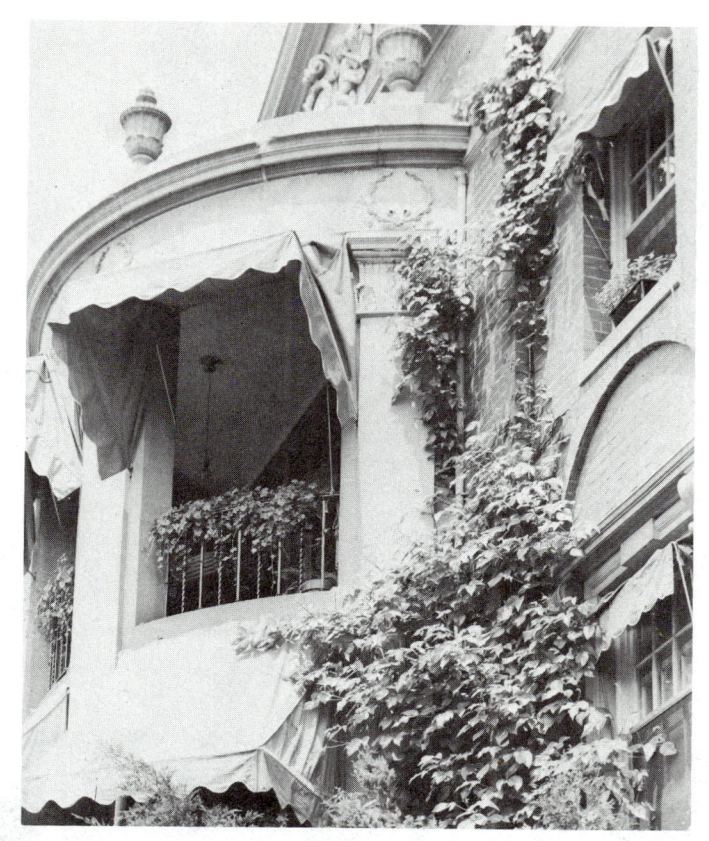

FIGURE 14.3D Common poison ivy growing up the side of a house with ornamental shrubs. (U.S. Department of Agriculture)

2. Know how to protect yourself when in an area where the poisonous plants are growing. Long shirtsleeves, long trouser legs, and gloves will help guard against possible irritation. Directions should be given so that clothing will not be touched after use. Urushiol has been known to remain on clothing for as long as a year. Clothing should not be washed in soap and water, but should be dry-cleaned. The person doing the dry-cleaning should be aware of the poisonous plant exposure.
3. Never burn poisonous plants, particularly poison ivy, oak, and sumac, even though the plants are dead and dry. Smoke from the burning plants may contain droplets of urushiol and cause severe poisoning to the skin.
4. Never handle family pets that have been running out of doors, particularly in wooded or weed areas. If the pet is suspected of having had contact with poison ivy, oak, or sumac, it is suggested that a bath be given. The pet itself is in no danger of the urushiol poisoning.

[224] Poisonous Plants

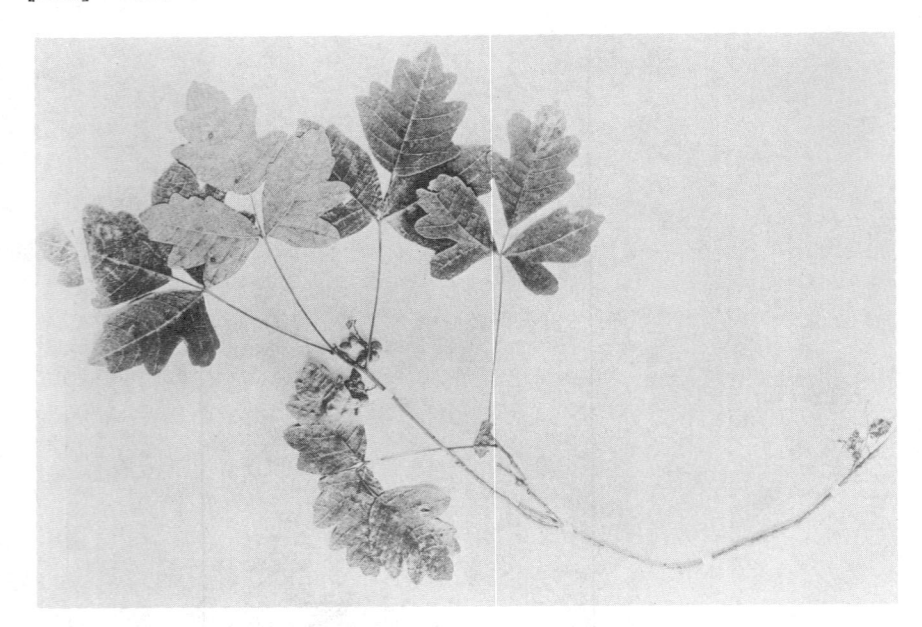

FIGURE 14.4 Eastern oakleaf poison ivy. (U.S. Department of Agriculture)

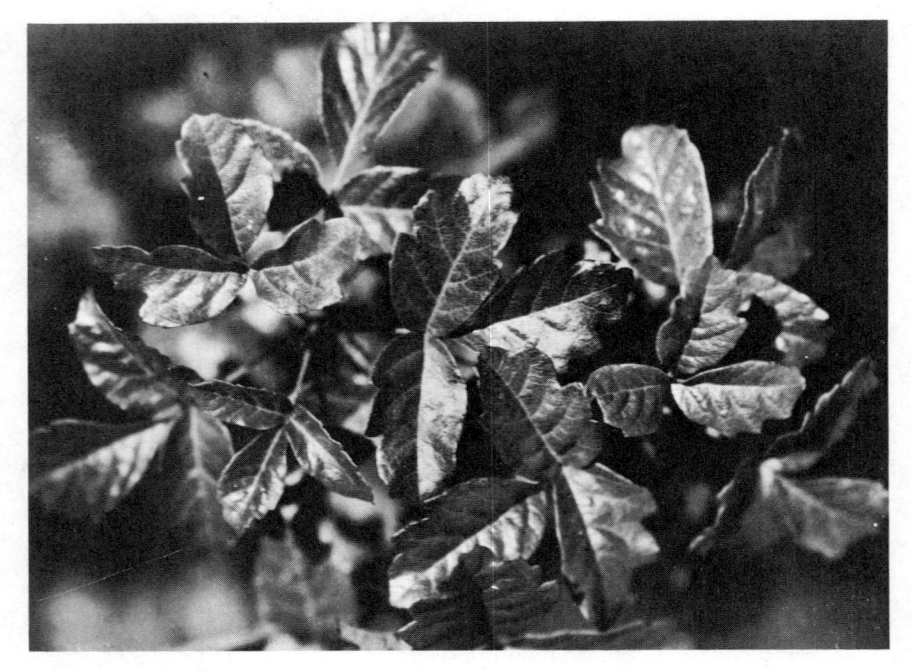

FIGURE 14.5 Western poison oak. (U.S. Department of Agriculture)

ORAL POISONING PLANTS

Some of the plants that decorate our homes and communities each year are potentially dangerous because of poisonous substances. The present popularity of plants also has resulted in an increase in occurrence of plant poisoning. During a recent year, cases reported to the National Clearinghouse for Poison Control Centers indicated that plants were the leading category of substances most frequently ingested by children under five years. The tendency of young children to put things into their mouths is a real problem for parents. It should be the responsibility of parents and other persons to know those plants that poison. In addition they should have the knowledge to decide what protective measures should be taken, and should teach their children how to identify poisonous plants. Some of the more common types of plants that result in oral poisoning are identified and discussed in the following sections.

Castor Bean

The oil of the castor bean plant has many commercial uses and can be used in small amounts for medicinal purposes. The seeds of the castor bean plant and, to a certain extent, the foliage are poisonous (Figure 14.8). The castor bean plant is found in the warm regions of the United States, but can be found as a home plant in all parts of the nation.

Symptoms Oral ingestion of one chewed castor bean seed has been known to be fatal. Normally if the seeds are swallowed whole, poisoning will not occur. When chewed, the seeds produce a burning sensation in the mouth. Depending on the amount of beans chewed, the symptoms of nausea, vomiting, diarrhea, and circulatory collapse will appear immediately, within a few hours, or several days later.

Protection As stated in the previous paragraph, if the seed was swallowed whole, there is little danger of poisoning. As there is no known antidote available for castor bean poisoning, one should immediately induce vomiting. If respiratory failure does occur, apply mouth-to-mouth artificial respiration. Medical attention is necessary in this type of plant poisoning.

Mushrooms

Mushroom hunting is definitely not a hobby for an amateur. There are many different types of mushrooms, some of which are deliciously edible and others of which are deadly poisonous. There is no single rule, characteristic, or procedure to simplify the task of identifying poisonous or

[226] Poisonous Plants

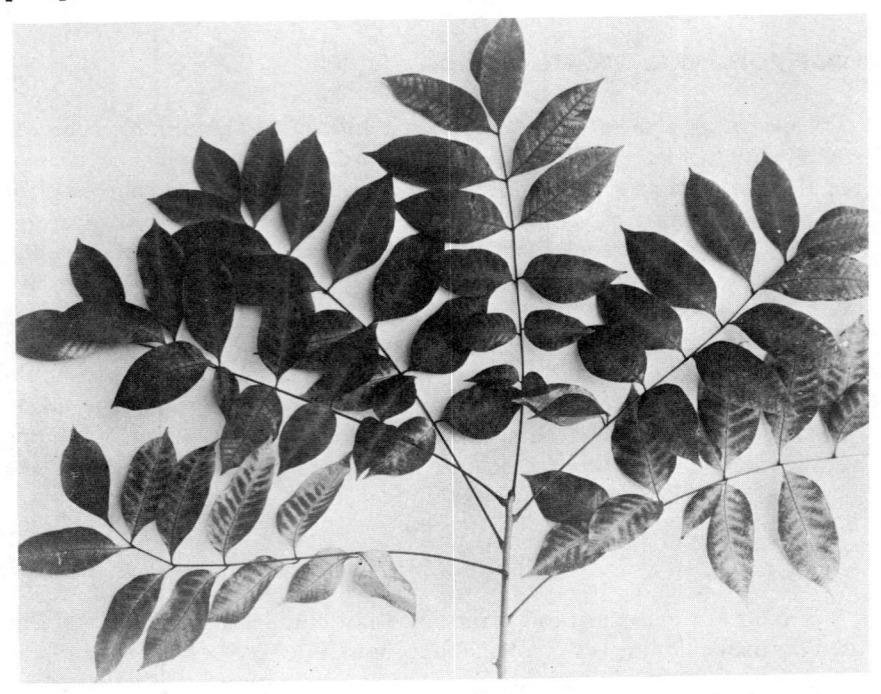

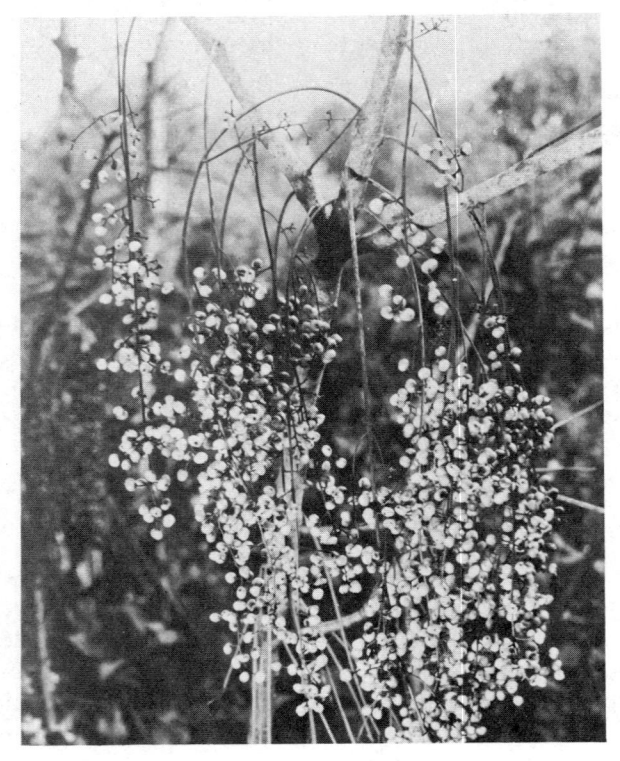

FIGURE 14.6 Poison sumac with compound leaves (top), and plant with poison fruit (bottom). (U.S. Department of Agriculture)

Oral Poisoning Plants [227]

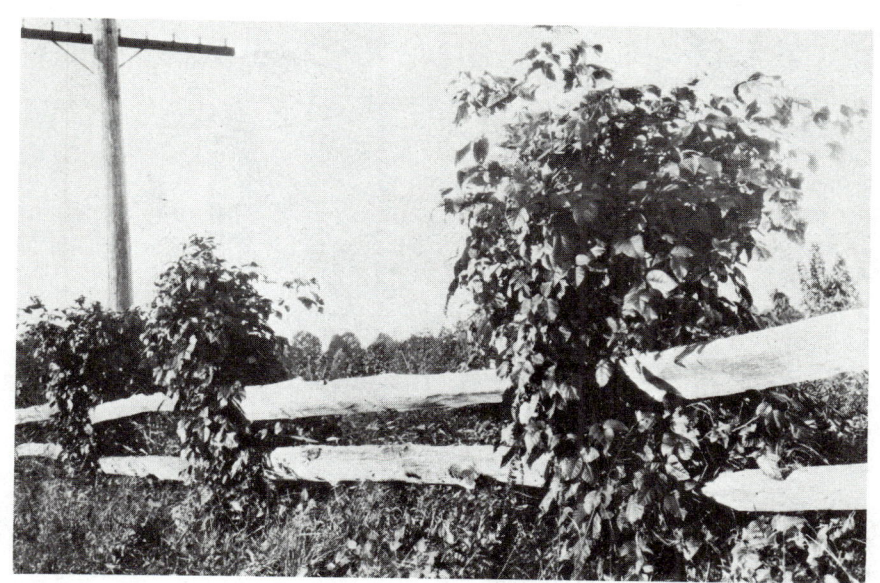

FIGURE 14.7 Common poison ivy growing along a fence row. (U.S. Department of Agriculture)

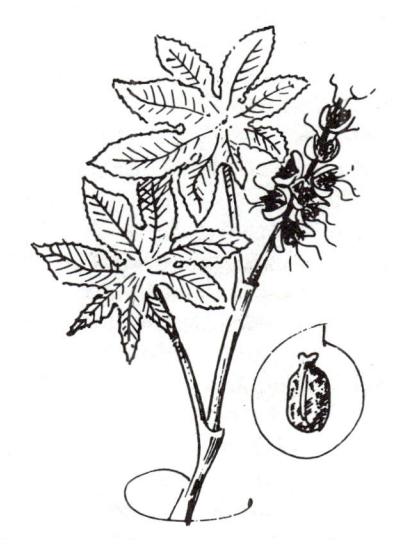

FIGURE 14.8 Castor bean plant (*Ricinus communis*). (Wyeth Laboratories)

nonpoisonous mushrooms. Only a person experienced and learned in positive identification of mushroom varieties can judge mushrooms. Commercially grown mushrooms are certain to be safe because there are strict

[228] Poisonous Plants

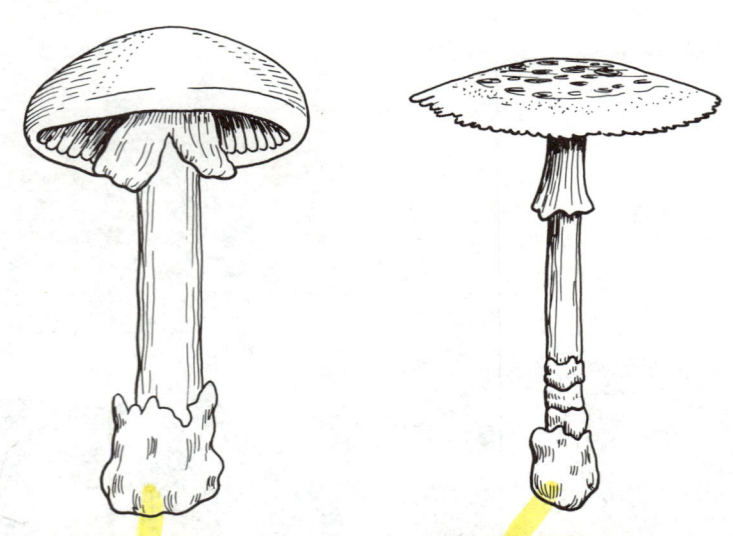

FIGURE 14.9 Fly agaric (*Amanita muscaria*) and destroying angel (*Amanita phalloides*) mushrooms.

regulations governing their production and sale. It is wise to use the commercial brands if one is not an expert in mushroom identification.

There are two dangerous mushrooms that will be briefly discussed. These are the fly agaric (*Amanita muscaria*) and the destroying angel (*Amanita phalloides*) (Figure 14.9). Ingestion of just a small part of one of these mushrooms is sufficient to cause death.

The *Amanita muscaria* is characterized by its large three- to eight-inch-broad orange red to bright yellow cap which is usually rough with white or buff wartlike scales. This mushroom is found throughout the United States in open woods from July to October.

Symptoms of *Amanita muscaria* poisoning will normally occur rapidly, usually within one to two hours. Increased secretions of the salivary glands and profuse perspiration take place first, followed by vomiting, diarrhea, labored breathing, slow pulse, and a confused state of mind. Death is rare, but may result from respiratory failure.

Removal of the ingested *Amanita muscaria* mushroom is a necessity. Shock protection may be needed if shock symptoms are present. The victim should receive medical attention.

Amanita phalloides is the deadliest of all the mushrooms. This plant stands about six inches high with a shiny, white cap which has a diameter varying from two to five inches. The most recognizable feature of this mushroom is the stem. Directly beneath the cap is a membrane encircling the stem, which is connected to a cup-shaped membrane. These two membranes separated as the plant developed. Therefore, an inverted cup-shaped membrane is located on the upper part of the stem, and an upward cup-shaped membrane at the lower stem. From this came the name "death's cup." When gathering mushrooms make sure that care is taken to remove the surrounding soil to determine if there is an upward cup. The *Amanita phalloides* is commonly found in wooded areas from June to September.

Physical symptoms of *Amanita phalloides* poisoning will not be present for ten hours. Symptoms are sudden and are characterized by abdominal pain, vomiting, and diarrhea. Death may occur within two days. Medical help is needed immediately. Giving an emetic to cause vomiting and protecting against shock are the only emergency first-aid procedures that should be utilized until medical help is available.

Mistletoe

Mistletoe is a woody parasite (primarily on oak trees) which is used in an ornamental way in many homes in the United States. This plant infests many trees in the southeastern states. What most people do not realize is that the small, white berry growing on the plant is very toxic (Figure 14.10). Mistletoe is easily recognizable to most people because of its popularity and commercial value in relation to Christmas.

It is extremely important to keep the berries, and the plant as well, out of the reach of small children. The berries may be attractive and inviting to them and they may be tempted to taste the berries.

Symptoms Common characteristics of mistletoe plant poisoning are vomiting, diarrhea, slow or irregular pulse, cardiac irregularities, and possibly symptoms of acute gastroenteritis. Death has resulted from ingestion of the mistletoe berry.

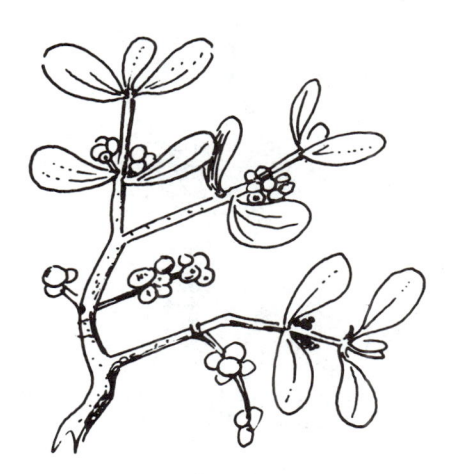

FIGURE 14.10 Mistletoe (*Phoradendron*). (Wyeth Laboratories)

[230] Poisonous Plants

Protection Water or milk should be given to dilute and help delay absorption of the poisonous substance. Syrup of ipecac or other emetic should follow to remove the poison from the stomach.

Oleander

The oleander is an evergreen shrub that primarily is ornamental in use. This plant may reach a height of 20 feet and is commonly found in the southern United States. Oleander may also be found as a potted plant in the northern states. Large white, pink, or red flowers are produced by the oleander in the summer. All parts of the plant are extremely toxic, be they dried or green. The leaves are leathery in appearance and 4 to 12 inches in length.

Symptoms The symptoms that appear from ingestion of oleander are similar to the symptoms of digitalis poisoning. That is, cardiac arrest may result. Other effects include drowsiness and dizziness, nausea, vomiting, and bloody diarrhea.

Protection The first aid necessary in this situation is primarily the same as that for mistletoe: an emetic should be given to remove the poisonous material and medical attention is needed.

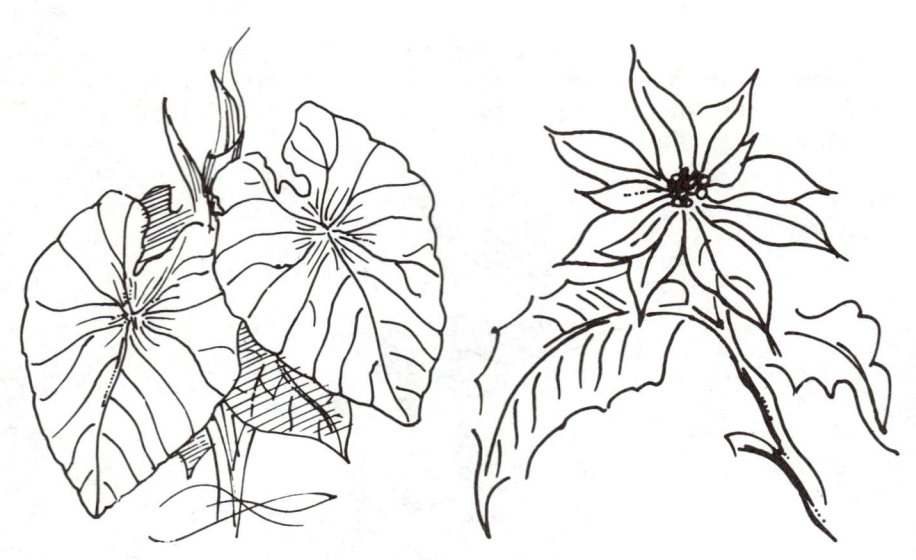

FIGURE 14.11 Common house plants that are toxic. Left: elephant's ear; right: poinsettia. (Wyeth Laboratories, Philadelphia, Pa.)

Oral Poisoning Plants [231]

Other Toxic Plants

In addition to the preceding there are other toxic plants considered dangerous which are found about the home, in wooded areas, and in the community. It would be impossible to list every plant that has the potential to cause oral poisoning. A good principle to follow is to never put any plant into the mouth.

Wyeth Laboratories has categorized common poisonous plants into the following eight groups: (1) House plants, (2) plants in the flower garden, (3) vegetable garden plants, (4) ornamental plants, (5) trees and shrubs, (6) forest plants, (7) plants of the marshes, and (8) field plants. Figure 14.14 summarizes the eight groups by plant name, toxic part, and poisonous symptoms.

Protection   In general when a person ingests a toxic part of a plant, the first-aider should immediately contact the poison control center if possible. Syrup of ipecac should be given along with water for removing the poison from the stomach and diluting the substance in the stomach, respectively.

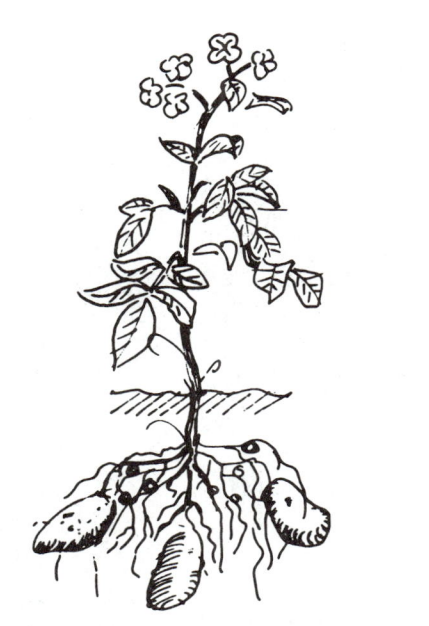

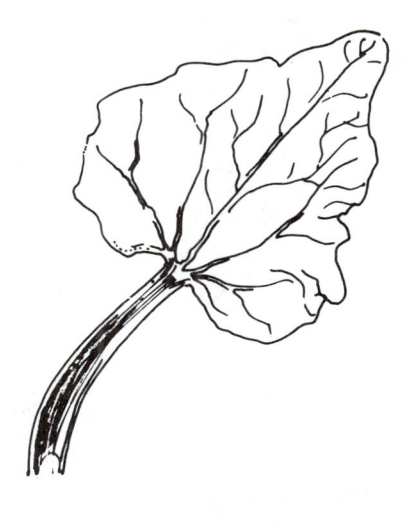

FIGURE 14.12 Common vegetable garden plants that are toxic. Left: potato; right: rhubarb. (Wyeth Laboratories, Philadelphia, Pa.)

[232]   Poisonous Plants

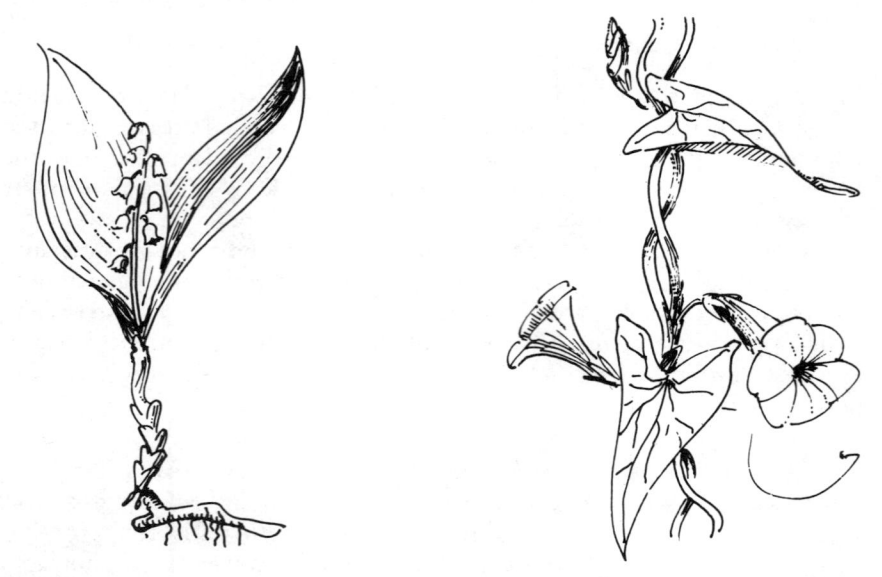

FIGURE 14.13   Common flower garden plants that are toxic. Left: lily-of-the-valley; right: morning glory. (Wyeth Laboratories, Philadelphia, Pa.)

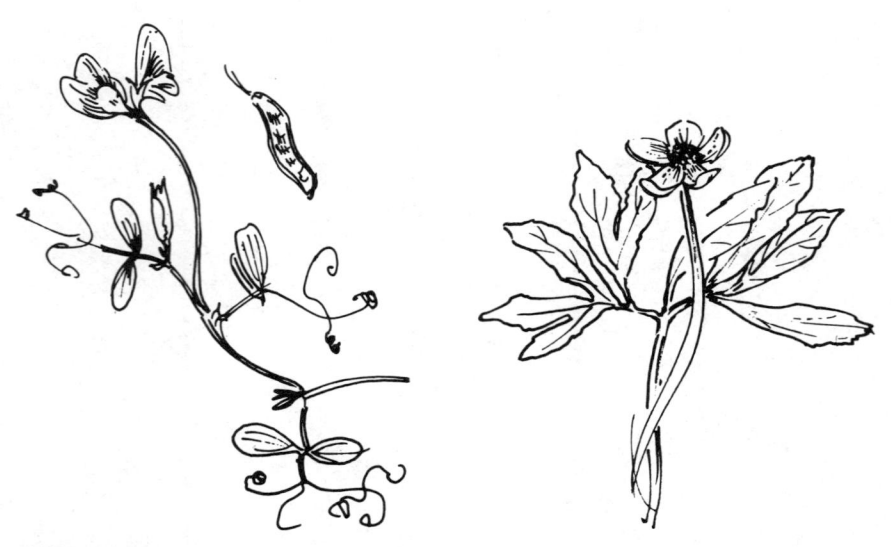

FIGURE 14.13 (continued)   Common flower garden plants that are toxic. Left: sweet pea; right: Christmas rose. (Wyeth Laboratories, Philadelphia, Pa.)

Activities [233]

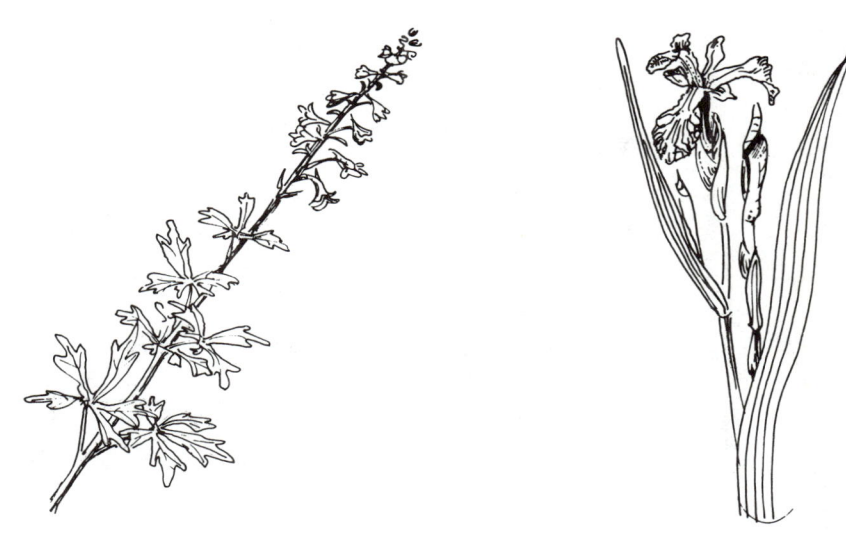

FIGURE 14.13 (continued) Common flower garden plants that are toxic. Left: larkspur; right: iris or blue flag. (Wyeth Laboratories, Philadelphia, Pa.)

Prevention There are many ways to avoid plant poisoning problems. A person should

1. Know plants. One should learn their scientific names and find out from the florist or librarian if they are poisonous.
2. Keep poisonous plants out of the reach of children.
3. Educate children at an early age of the danger of putting any plant or part of any plant into their mouths.
4. Not bite or chew an unknown plant.
5. Avoid chewing on jewelry made of seeds or beans. Care must be taken when buying jewelry that contains the jequirity bean. For the best preventive care, jewelry containing poisonous substances should never be brought into the home and definitely not bought at all.

ACTIVITIES

1. Determine what poisonous plants are located about your home, place of work, or favorite recreational area.
2. From activity number one, ascertain the proper steps in emergency care for each of the poisonous plants found.
3. Talk to a botanist (plant specialist) about the differences between edible and poisonous mushrooms.
4. Organize a plant identification program so that you and your friends will become more aware of the hazardous common plants.
5. Write a paper on the benefits of preventive care when working around poison ivy, poison oak, or poison sumac.

FIGURE 14.14 SUMMARY—PLANTS THAT POISON

Plant	Toxic Part	Symptoms
HOUSE PLANTS		
Hyacinth, Narcissus, Daffodil	Bulbs	Nausea, vomiting, diarrhea. May be fatal.
Oleander	Leaves, Branches	Extremely poisonous. Affects the heart, produces severe digestive upset and has caused death.
Dieffenbachia (Dumb cane) Elephant ear	All parts	Intense burning and irritation of the mouth and tongue. Death can occur if base of the tongue swells enough to block the air passage of the throat.
Rosary pea, Castor bean	Seeds	Fatal. A single rosary pea seed has caused death. One or two castor bean seeds are near the lethal dose for adults.
Poinsettia	Leaves	Vomiting, diarrhea, abdominal cramps.
Mistletoe	Berries	Fatal. Both children and adults have died from eating the berries.
PLANTS IN THE FLOWER GARDEN		
Larkspur	Young plant, Seeds	Digestive upset, nervous excitement, depression. May be fatal.
Monkshood	Fleshy roots	Digestive upset and nervous excitement.
Autumn crocus, Star-of-Bethlehem	Bulbs	Vomiting and nervous excitement.
Lily-of-the-valley	Leaves, Flowers	Irregular heart beat and pulse, usually accompanied by digestive upset and mental confusion.
Iris	Underground stems	Severe, but not usually serious, digestive upset.
Foxglove	Leaves	One of the sources of the drug digitalis, used to stimulate the heart. In large amounts, the active principles cause dangerously irregular heartbeat and pulse, usually digestive upset and mental confusion. May be fatal.
Bleeding heart (Dutchman's breeches)	Foliage, Roots	May be poisonous in large amounts. Has proved fatal to cattle.
VEGETABLE GARDEN PLANTS		
Rhubarb	Leaf blade	Fatal. Large amounts of raw or cooked leaves can cause convulsions, coma, followed rapidly by death.
ORNAMENTAL PLANTS		
Daphne	Berries	Fatal. A few berries can kill a child.
Wisteria	Seeds, Pods	Mild to severe digestive upset. Many children are poisoned by this plant.
Golden chain	Bean-like capsules in which the seeds are suspended	Severe poisoning. Excitement, staggering, convulsions and coma. May be fatal.

Plant	Parts	Symptoms
Laurels, Rhododendron, Azaleas	All parts	Fatal. Produces nausea and vomiting, depression, difficult breathing, prostration and coma.
Jessamine	Berries	Fatal. Digestive disturbance and nervous symptoms.
Lantana camara (red sage)	Green berries	Fatal. Affects lungs, kidneys, heart and nervous system. Grows in the southern U.S. and in moderate climates.
Yew	Berries, Foliage	Fatal. Foliage more toxic than berries. Death is usually sudden without warning symptoms.

TREES AND SHRUBS

Plant	Parts	Symptoms
Wild and cultivated cherries	Twigs, Foliage	Fatal. Contains a compound that releases cyanide when eaten. Gasping, excitement, and prostration are common symptoms that often appear within minutes.
Oaks	Foliage, Acorns	Affects kidneys gradually. Symptoms appear only after several days or weeks. Takes a large amount for poisoning. Children should not be allowed to chew on acorns.
Elderberry	Shoots, Leaves, Bark	Children have been poisoned by using pieces of the pithy stems for blowguns. Nausea and digestive upset.
Black locust	Bark, Sprouts, Foliage	Children have suffered nausea, weakness and depression after chewing the bark and seeds.

FOREST PLANTS

Plant	Parts	Symptoms
Jack-in-the-pulpit	All parts, especially roots	Like dumb cane, contains small needle-like crystals of calcium oxalate that cause intense irritation and burning of the mouth and tongue.
Moonseed	Berries	Blue, purple color, resembling wild grapes. Contains a single seed. (True wild grapes contain several small seeds.) May be fatal.
Mayapple	Apple, Foliage, Roots	Contains at least 16 active toxic principles, primarily in the roots. Children often eat the apple with no ill effects, but several apples may cause diarrhea.

PLANTS OF THE MARSHES

Plant	Parts	Symptoms
Water hemlock	All parts	Fatal. Violent and painful convulsions. A number of people have died from hemlock.

FIELD PLANTS

Plant	Parts	Symptoms
Buttercups	All parts	Irritant juices may severely injure the digestive system.
Nightshade	All parts, especially the unripe berry	Fatal. Intense digestive disturbances and nervous symptoms.
Poison hemlock	All parts	Fatal. Resembles a large wild carrot. Used in ancient Greece to kill condemned prisoners.
Jimson weed (thorn apple)	All parts	Abnormal thirst, distorted sight, delirium, incoherence and coma. Common cause of poisoning. Has proved fatal.

[235]

[236] Poisonous Plants

QUESTIONS TO ANSWER

1 Compare and contrast poison ivy and poison oak.
2 What is the poisonous toxic substance found in poison ivy, oak, and sumac?
3 Does a person have to come into direct contact with the plant in order to get poison ivy? Why?
4 List four measures for preventing skin irritation caused by plants.
5 Discuss the three ways that poison ivy can be found growing.
6 Name the two types of poison oak plants found in the United States.
7 What parts of the castor bean plant are poisonous?
8 Differentiate between the two poisonous mushroom plants discussed in this chapter.
9 Which of the two poisonous mushroom plants is the more deadly?
10 What part of the mistletoe plant is particularly dangerous when ingested.

SELECTED REFERENCES

HAFEN, BRENT Q., and PETERSON, BRENDA, *First Aid and Health Emergencies*. St. Paul, Minn.: West Publishing Co., 1977.

KINGSBURY, JOHN M., *Poisonous Plants of the United States and Canada*. Englewood Cliffs, N.J.: Prentice-Hall, 1964.

MUENSCHER, W. C., *Poisonous Plants of the United States*. New York: Macmillan, 1951.

NATIONAL INSTITUTE OF ALLERGY AND INFECTIOUS DISEASES, *Poison Ivy, Oak, and Sumac*. Washington, D.C.: U.S. Government Printing Office, 1967.

NATIONAL SAFETY COUNCIL, *Poisonous Plants*. Safety Education Data Sheet No. 8. Chicago: The Council, 1970.

U.S. DEPARTMENT OF AGRICULTURE, *Poison Ivy, Poison Oak and Poison Sumac*. Farmers' Bulletin No. 1972. Washington, D.C.: U.S. Government Printing Office, 1967.

WYETH LABORATORIES, *The Sinister Garden*. Philadelphia: Wyeth Laboratories, 1966, pp. 5–42.

YOUNGKEN, HEBER W., JR., *Common Poisonous Plants of New England*. Washington, D.C.: U.S. Government Printing Office, 1964.

15. SPECIAL PROBLEMS

Many problem conditions can occur suddenly. It is important that emergency care, rescue, and first-aid persons have training concerning these emergencies so they can better protect the victims. Particularly, teachers, coaches, rescue squads, civil defense volunteers, firemen, and policemen need to be familiar with the special problems in first aid. Because of the lack of medical service in the small community and on the farm and ranch, persons in these areas especially can profit from emergency care or first-aid training.

UNCONSCIOUSNESS

There are many causes of unconsciousness, such as asphyxia, shock, heatstroke, heat exhaustion, heart attack, convulsions, epilepsy, fainting, intoxication, diabetic coma and insulin shock, hemorrhage, electric shock, and overdoses of drugs and barbiturates.

The causative factor may be an injury, illness, or an act of nature. If possible, the first-aider should determine the cause in order to give appropriate protection to the victim.

It is helpful if the person who is to give the protection was present at the time the victim became unconscious. If he were not, it would be helpful if he could talk to someone who was. It is very important to know the condition that could have caused the particular unconsciousness; without this information the problem is more complex. In special problem situations such as asphyxia, heatstroke, heart attack, diabetic coma, and insulin shock, it is most important that the rescuer understand the problem.

[237]

[238]   Special Problems

Unconsciousness has been classified by some as red, white, and blue. This is due to the fact that under certain conditions the skin will change its color. The skin always becomes blue in asphyxia; red in sunstroke, apoplexy, drunkenness, skull fracture, concussion, and epilepsy; and pale or white in severe hemorrhage, shock, heat exhaustion, fainting, freezing, convulsions, and poisoning. This index without doubt has some shortcomings; on the other hand, it can be helpful to the first-aider.

If the victim is hanging by the neck or is in water in contact with electricity, and the skin is blue, his problem is asphyxiation. If the victim falls in the street, slumps and collapses elsewhere and is unconscious, it could be lack of blood in the brain or fainting. Fainting can be easily determined if the person is kept down, with head lowered or feet elevated. In this position, if the problem is fainting, consciousness will return in a few minutes.

The heart attack victim will usually indicate specific symptoms, as will the person suffering from apoplexy. The heatstroke victim will have a high temperature with a red, hot, and dry skin. The intoxicated may have his bottle; if not, certainly the odor of alcohol will suggest the nature of his condition. However, it is very important to remember that it takes a large quantity of alcohol to produce unconsciousness. The victim may have had a few drinks and then an accident. His problem could be much more serious than alcoholic intoxication. Confusing intoxication with severe injury or illness is a common mistake made in first-aid care.

It is important that the victim of unconsciousness be kept quiet and reasonably warm. In most cases, it is unwise to attempt to arouse the victim with smelling salts, water, or physical manipulation.

It is suggested that the following procedure be followed for the unconscious:

1. Quickly control the hemorrhage if any. Give artificial respiration if breathing slows. This occurs in only a small share of unconsciousness cases.
2. Lay the victim flat if the face is pale; if it is flushed, raise the head and shoulders on pillows.
3. If diabetes or anaphylactic shock is a possibility, the victim may carry a direction card. If found, follow the stated advice.
4. It is usually best to summon medical help, or at least to secure medical advice by telephone before attempting other measures. If the cause was an accident and transportation is necessary, always check first for all injuries and give proper first aid. Gentle, not hasty, transportation is indicated. Even though recovery soon occurs spontaneously, secure follow-up study unless the case is clearly one of simply fainting.[1]

---

[1] Carl J. Potthoff, "First Aid—Unconsciousness." *Today's Health*, November, 1962, p. 76.

APOPLEXY

Apoplexy is more commonly referred to as a stroke, although the death certificate will probably indicate cause of death as cerebral vascular lesion. The usual cause is a ruptured blood vessel in the brain and the bleeding or hemorrhage that follows. High blood pressure (hypertension), arteriosclerosis (hardening of the arteries), and emboli (blood clots) are referred to as the three stroke villains.[2]

Stroke, or apoplexy, most frequently occurs in older people. Strokes can occur in middle life and, upon occasion, earlier. Strokes occur in some persons in their thirties and forties striking suddenly at night or passing almost unnoticed as a sudden dizzy spell or a momentary blackout.[3]

It is important to understand the causes of stroke and to be aware of its telltale indications.

The little strokes are of special significance; frequently, the minor strokes are advance warnings to which persons must be alert, especially among the older members of our families, acquaintances, and friends. These minor strokes may occur in a series over a relatively short period of time.

> The medical profession is indebted to Dr. Walter Alvarez for emphasizing the frequency with which "little strokes" occur. The knowledgeable patient or his family may be able to identify "little strokes" by changes in the patient's behavior, including degeneration of table manners and the appearance of poor social and business judgment. Dizzy spells and attacks of forgetfulness are common. These and a host of other physical and personal aberrations often can represent repeated episodes of "little strokes" and herald a more ominous occurrence.[4]

If the aforementioned signs, such as memory failure, blackout, and change of personality appear, it is of extreme importance that such information be made available to the physician at once. It may be possible to postpone for an indefinite period the more massive and possibly the fatal stroke which can follow.

Apparently, it is possible for the victim to have a massive or severe stroke without earlier indications; however, the belief is that the victim usually has the "little stroke" or some previous evidence that a severe stroke problem is impending. If the stroke is massive with considerable brain damage or bleeding, there will be definite indications.

---

[2] Alfred Soffer, M.C., "What You Should Know About Strokes." *Today's Health,* August, 1968.

[3] American Medical Association, *Today's Health Guide.* Chicago: AMA, 1965.

[4] Soffer, op. cit.

[240] Special Problems

Symptoms

There are signs of apoplexy which are important to the first-aider:

1. The victim may be unconscious or semiconscious. His speech may be unintelligible. Also, it is difficult to know if the victim understands the speech of another person.
2. The victim's breathing may be heavy or labored.
3. The victim's extremities may be paralyzed, usually on one side.
4. The victim's pupils may be dilated unevenly, one large and one small.
5. The victim's face may be distorted; usually the mouth will appear to be drawn to one side.
6. The victim's face may be flushed (red in color) and congested. The veins of the neck appear prominently.
7. The victim's condition will appear suddenly with little or no warning.
8. The victim may experience a severe headache and possibly a dizzy spell.
9. The victim's mouth may be drooling. He may be nauseous and may vomit.
10. The victim may experience convulsions.

Protection

It is hoped that this severe problem will occur in the home where provisions for care will at least be minimal. Even better, if the forewarning was recognized and action taken, the victim could be resting in bed. The stroke may occur when the victim is resting in bed normally, or it might occur during sleep.

The first-aider or a member of the family can provide the following protection before the physician arrives:

1. Immediately summon medical help.
2. Keep the victim down and flat. It may be helpful to raise the head and shoulders, also to remove or loosen the clothing.
3. Turn the victim to one side so that the secretions and/or vomitus will not make breathing difficult or block the breathing passages.
4. Provide reasonable and moderate covering to protect against shock but don't overheat.
5. Give no liquids, medication or food by mouth because the victim is unconscious.
6. Apply cold applications about the head, face, and neck. This could help reduce bleeding.
7. Make no effort to transport the victim to the hospital until an ambulance is available.

A person with a family history of strokes or hypertension should take protective action before danger strikes. He should have an annual health examination, watch his diet, and control body weight, get plenty of physical exercise regularly, and live moderately. The use of tobacco and alcohol should be considered carefully, and the physician's advice concerning their use should be followed.

> Those who suffer from migraine headaches may experience sensations resembling those which occur in a stroke: a numbness and weakness in one side of the body, trouble with shock and vision. However, these sensations disappear in a few minutes and are followed by the sick headaches.[5]

Certainly a pounding headache and the rising or elevated blood pressure are frightening signs and possible indications of a stroke, but a person should not get so concerned that he becomes a victim of hypochondria.

CONCUSSION

Concussion is an injury to the brain, usually caused by a blow to the head. Knowledge of the circumstances surrounding an injury can be very helpful to a rescuer in making a judgment of concussion. The victim may be dazed, semiconscious, or unconscious. He may speak, but his speech may be profane and the rationality of the spoken words may be questionable.

The brain is surrounded by a protective fluid (cerebrospinal fluid) and membranes (meninges); and it is completely encased by bone. A sharp blow, however, can still jar or shock the brain and cause injury (i.e., concussion). When the brain is so injured, it tends to swell. Because the space within the skull is limited, the danger of impaired circulation arises, accompanied by the possibility of resultant brain damage. If there is damage to the brain and bleeding, the injury could prove fatal.

Some individuals, such as boxers and football players, experience repeated concussions. This is dangerous and the customary recommendation is to give up the sport if the individual wants to live and enjoy life. Certainly it is most essential that persons engaged in contact sports, motorcycle riding, race car driving, outer space activities, and others protect their head to the maximum with the best protective head gear available.

Symptoms

It is important that the first-aider be familiar with the symptoms or signs of concussion, such as the following:

1. Bump on the head and other indications of a blow to the head.
2. Headache—mild to severe.

[5] Soffer, op. cit.

[242]   Special Problems

3. Inability to sense the activity, time, place, day, and to answer simple questions.
4. Pupils of the eye dilated unequally.
5. Semiconscious to unconscious.
6. Possible paralysis of legs or arms.
7. Pulse varying from being full to slow, with heartbeat from weak to rapid.
8. Eyes varying from unequal pupils to widely dilated to small in extreme cases.

Protection

There are several guidelines to follow:

1. The victim should be kept in a lying position.
2. The victim should be kept quiet until a doctor sees him.
3. If the victim's face is red, his head and shoulders should be elevated with a folded blanket or pillows. If the victim's face is white or ashen in color, the head should not be elevated.
4. If it is necessary to move the victim, he should be moved or carried in a flat position. Preferably, the ambulance should be brought to the victim.
5. The victim should not be given stimulants as they can increase the circulation of the blood. If a cerebral lesion is possible, such stimulation could make bleeding more severe, consequently enhancing the danger.
6. The victim of a suspected concussion should be examined by competent medical personnel as soon as possible.

CONVULSIONS

Convulsions are sudden attacks, usually in children, with unconsciousness, muscular twitching and other convulsive acts.

The convulsion is not as common as it was a decade or two ago. Because there is better understanding of foods and nutrition, many convulsions have been prevented through proper nutritional habits. It is felt that most of the convulsions today are caused by fever and infection. The convulsion usually follows an illness in which fever is or was a problem, and this contributes to the cause of the seizure. Other possible causes are low blood calcium, rickets, poisoning, congenital defects, concussion, and lack of oxygen. When the convulsion occurs a physician should always be called, especially for the first seizure; they should never be ignored. Certainly, the first convulsion will cause a greater impact on the parent. If the attacks continue to come, it is extremely important to seek the most complete medical help and assistance available. There is no doubt that continued and repeated convulsive seizures can cause a child to become retarded and possibly have other problems. Children's research hospitals offer help for such troubled children and their parents.

Symptoms

Several indications that can prove helpful to the parent or first-aider should be understood and learned. Some symptoms of convulsions are

1. Twitching, jerking, and violent and sudden disturbance of muscular energy.
2. Foaming of the mouth if the facial muscles are involved, and bleeding or foamy blood if the victim bites himself.
3. Unconsciousness.
4. Breathing that is loud and heavy.
5. Holding of the breath until the skin turns blue.
6. Neck muscles may bulge and cause an interference in the venous circulation and thus cause the skin to become blue.
7. Complete exhaustion and stuporous state.

Protection

It has been suggested that medical help be called in every such situation. While waiting for medical help a first-aider or parent should

1. Never panic. Once the convulsion has started, little can be done to stop it. An attack will usually end in a few minutes. The first-aider should not restrain the victim's movements, give him liquids, or slap and try to wake him. If possible, the victim should be lowered gently to the floor or a bed so he doesn't fall. Any furniture that he might strike during the convulsion should be moved.
2. Give artificial respiration if the victim becomes blue from breathing stoppage. This is rarely necessary, though breathing often stops for some seconds.
3. Provide bed rest and quiet and call the doctor when the convulsion is over.
4. Discuss the problem with the physician if it is thought that the convulsion was mimicked. Meanwhile, although children need affection, the first-aider should be casual about the "convulsion." [6]

It is also suggested that the child be put to bed and kept as quiet as possible. The victim should be covered to conserve body heat, but he should not be overheated. If it is felt that the child is putting on a show, this should be discussed with the family doctor or child psychologist.

EPILEPSY

Epilepsy is a disorder of the nervous system. The word itself is derived from the Greek word for seizure, which is the chief characteristic of this disorder. Epilepsy is defined as recurrent loss or impairment of con-

---

[6] Carl J. Potthoff, "First Aid—Convulsions in Children." *Today's Health*, March, 1969, p. 80.

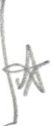

sciousness which may or may not be accompanied by muscular movements ranging from slight twitching of the eyelids to convulsive shaking of the body.[7]

Epilepsy is classified from the standpoint of origin or from the standpoint of seizure. The cause is unknown, although a disorder of brain cell metabolism is usually given as the cause. If the seizure is classified by origin, it is either idiopathic or symptomatic. If it is classified by seizure, it is grand mal, petit mal, or psychomotor.

In 1977 it was estimated that approximately 2 million of our fellow citizens were suffering from this neurological disorder. This should constitute a public health problem or concern to every American. Epilepsy occurs in every part of the United States among all age groups and races. No individual is immune.

Epilepsy is one of man's oldest afflictions. Much progress has been made in the medical treatment of epilepsy. But it remains today as one of the problems that the average person does not understand, and many misconceptions still exist among our population concerning epilepsy. Presently it is estimated that 80 percent or more of our epileptic population can live a normal life. They can and should participate in physical activities. This is good for the epileptic physically as well as mentally, for keeping the body in good physical condition tends to ward off seizures.

A review of the existing laws concerning epilepsy will convince any knowledgeable person that they are antiquated. Some states deny epileptics the right to marry, to produce children, to drive a car, or to even seek a position or employment.

From the standpoint of emergency care, it is important that epilepsy be understood. Persons must be able to recognize the seizure and know how to protect the victim. They must understand the problem from the standpoint of the victim and do their utmost not to embarrass or offend the victim of such an attack.

Symptoms

In a fair percentage of cases epileptics can recognize some type of warning of an oncoming seizure. *Aura* is the term given to a sensation that gives warning of an impending seizure. The aura differs from person to person. It may be a queer feeling in the stomach, an odd smell, a visual disturbance, or just a "feeling funny." Auras often indicate the area of the brain from which a seizure originates. Unfortunately, auras are not experienced by all epileptics or before every seizure by those who sometimes experience them. Thus, a victim should not be blamed for not

---

[7] Epilepsy Association of America, *Facts*. Washington, D.C.: The Association, 1968.

Appendicitis [245]

knowing when a seizure will occur.[8] An aura is meaningful to the victim. There are several symptoms that are important to the first-aider or rescue person:

1. The victim may sense the seizure and request help or have a prearranged plan.
2. The victim may fall and lose consciousness.
3. He may froth at the mouth.
4. There may be convulsive acts; he may defecate, urinate, or even vomit. The seizures may be quite general, involving all of the muscular systems, or quite local and involving only a part.
5. The veins in the neck may become distorted and swollen.
6. The victim's breathing may become loud and difficult.

Protection

The first-aider can help provide protection for the epileptic seizure victim by following these guides:

1. Help the victim to the floor to prevent a fall and loosen all clothing, especially collar, shirt, belt, pants, and shoes, also brassieres.
2. Use gentle restraint, not force, to keep the victim from hurting himself.
3. Place the victim on his side so that all mouth secretions can get away from the mouth.
4. Place something soft, like a folded handkerchief, in the victim's mouth only if his mouth is open. Nothing should ever be forced into the patient's mouth.
5. Keep the victim reasonably warm and provide a quiet resting place after the seizure has passed. The victim should be allowed to rest and sleep, as he will be exhausted.
6. If the seizure has been mild, permit normal activity. If the victim shows aftereffects, he may be taken home but should not be left unattended.
7. Notify the parents if the victim is a child. Teachers at school must assume the role of the parent (in loco parentis).
8. Use the seizure as a lesson for others, especially at school or at work.
9. Do not over-react and create a socially embarrassing scene for the victim.
10. Do not seek medical care for the victim unless the seizures occur in a rapid series or a seizure lasts an unusually long time.

APPENDICITIS

The appendix is sometimes referred to as the "blind gut." This projection of the gut from the large intestine (ascending colon), just below the junction of the large and small intestine (cecum), is known as the

[8] Epilepsy Foundation of America, *National News*. Washington, D.C.: The Foundation, Vol. 1, No. 2, April–May, 1968.

[246] Special Problems

appendix. There is an opening from the large intestine into the appendix, but the other end is blind or closed. When an infection occurs in the appendix there are an acute pain, nausea, and the possibility that the appendix will become inflamed, swollen, and even perforated. If the appendix is perforated, it is known as ruptured appendix and the condition is extremely serious. Appendicitis cannot be prevented; the only cure is surgery.

Appendicitis is a common but important surgical problem. Any surgery that involves going into a body cavity is serious; however, appendicitis when discovered early is rarely dangerous. If the appendix has ruptured and severe infection (peritonitis) has occurred, appendicitis is then a very dangerous problem and can be fatal.

> Acute appendicitis not treated by a doctor is as deadly as it was 50 years ago. Each year appendicitis kills 2000 Americans. Unfortunately, in an age of automation, it is a forgotten killer. Surgery for the removal of the appendix (appendectomy) follows only the removal of tonsils and adenoids among the most frequently performed nonobstetrical-gynecological operations.[9]

It has been pointed out that everyone with the exception of the lucky individuals who have had appendectomies is subject to this sudden and serious illness. There is doubt about the role of the appendix, but it is a certainty that a person can do very well without it.

> Appendicitis is difficult to diagnose because of its location. Part of the intestines, the infected appendix triggers intestinal symptoms. Because it moves around, the appendix can cause chest pains similar to those of pneumonia or ulcers. Because the appendix lies near the pelvis which is crammed with vital and sensitive organs, appendicitis can mimic diseases of these organs, while pelvic diseases can masquerade as appendicitis.[10]

Symptoms

It is important that the first-aider be familiar with the signs or indications of appendicitis:

1. A sudden and intense abdominal pain in the lower right quadrant of the abdomen. The abdominal muscles may also be rigid. The pain may be more generalized in the abdominal area or even on the left as occasionally the organs of an individual are reversed.
2. Nausea and even diarrhea.
3. Loss of appetite and possible vomiting.
4. Constipation.

---

[9] Theodore Berland, "Appendicitis, The Forgotten Killer." *Today's Health*, Chicago: AMA, May, 1964, p. 22.

[10] Ibid.

Fainting [247]

5 Fever.
6 Fatigue and tiredness.

Protection

If a person complains of pains in the abdomen, regardless of age, and especially if there is nausea and vomiting, appendicitis is a possibility. Teachers responsible for students at school should remember this. If such a problem or situation arises, the following protective procedures should be followed. The teacher or other first-aider should

1 Get the victim down and quiet.
2 Call the doctor.
3 Apply cold applications over the problem area, the abdomen.
4 Never give water or food. Anything placed in the mouth will stimulate muscular activity (peristalsis) in the gut and may cause perforation.
5 Never, under any circumstances, give a laxative or anything to stimulate a bowel movement. This can help to cause a perforation or rupture.
6 Provide suitable transportation.

FAINTING

Fainting is a form of simple unconsciousness that does not usually indicate a serious problem or disease. The cause relates to too little circulation of blood to the brain, probably a reflex between the circula-

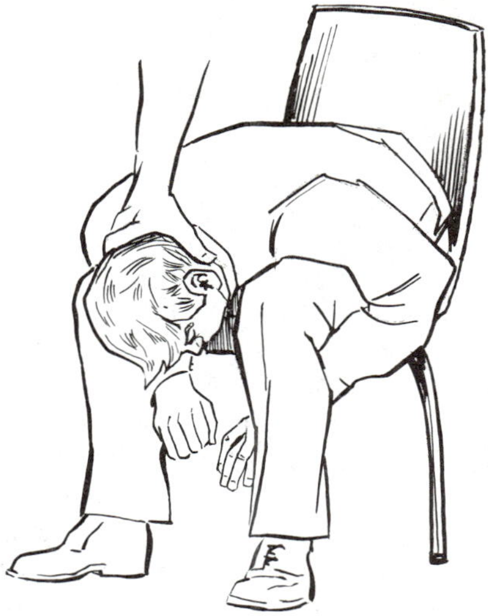

FIGURE 15.1 Position for prevention of fainting.

[248] Special Problems

tory and nervous system. However, the causes of fainting may vary considerably. Apparently a physical, emotional, or psychic factor can trigger this reaction. An unpleasant sight, bad news, standing too long, pain, the sight of blood, the taking of a blood sample, or giving blood may be the causative factor. This is actually a mild form of shock.

Fainting is not serious and the victim usually returns to consciousness in a few minutes after being placed in the reclining position. The greatest danger is the fall and the possibility of an injury resulting from the fall.

Symptoms

There are several signs or indications of fainting. It is important that the first-aider become familiar with them.

1. The person may be nauseated and even vomit.
2. There may be a feeling of lightheadedness with yawning.
3. Color may leave the individual's face and he may attempt to lie down.
4. The face becomes white and pale.
5. He may break out in profuse perspiration.
6. He becomes cold and numb.
7. The so-called blackout follows and the victim becomes unconscious.

Protection

The first-aider can provide protection from fainting by following these guides, which should be understood and learned:

1. Get the victim down, lower the head or raise the feet.
2. Cover to maintain body heat but do not overheat.
3. Use spirits of ammonia or smelling salts if available.
4. Bathe the face with cool water; however, no water throwing.
5. Keep the victim down for a reasonable period after consciousness returns.
6. Call a physician if consciousness does not return within a few minutes.

INTOXICATION

There is no doubt but that the first-aider, rescue worker, fireman, and policeman will at some time encounter the person who has been drinking and has had an accident. About one half of all motor-vehicle accidents involve drinking drivers, and one half of the pedestrians struck by motor vehicles are under the influence of alcohol.

Alcohol and its influence upon the individual is one of the most important accident-producing factors. There is the danger that rescue people and others will make the assumption that the victim was drunk. There may be broken bones, severe internal injuries, a fractured skull, or other injuries which may need protection more than the condition of too much alcohol.

Another problem that relates to alcohol is the conflict between social drinking and alcoholism. The victim has been placed in jail without being seen by a physician only to be found dead the next morning. This is a problem that needs careful consideration, and without doubt most enforcement officials need to be better prepared for it. The smaller the person, the less alcohol required to create a serious intoxication problem.

Symptoms

Intoxication is closely associated with the accident problem; consequently, it is important that the first-aider, police, rescue squad, and others understand the symptoms relating to this condition, such as:

1. *The signs of drunkenness.* These are the bottle, the odor, the unsteady gait, the lack of balance, and the thick tongue.
2. *The alcohol test.* This is a test of the breath, blood, or urine which tells how much alcohol is present in the blood. It is the only accepted proof of intoxication.

Protection

The following suggestions are for giving first aid and protection to the individual who is intoxicated:

1. The stomach should be emptied by vomiting or by artificial means.
2. If the person is unconscious, he must be kept warm.
3. If the person ceases breathing, he should be given mouth-to-mouth artificial respiration or CPR if heart beat ceases. (See Chapter 8.)
4. The victim should have medical help and receive hospital care.

HERNIA

Hernia, or rupture, relates to weak places in the abdominal wall, especially the inguinal openings or rings and about the navel. The hernia can be inherent or it can be induced.

The accidental rupture is associated with heavy work, especially with lifting and straining. It is possible for hernias to occur on many parts of the body as a result of tears to muscle facia or ligament damage.

Symptoms

There are definite signs of hernia. The first-aider should be familiar with these symptoms:

[250] Special Problems

1. A bulge in the abdominal wall in the area of the groin or navel.
2. Tenderness on digital examination.
3. Possible vomiting and nausea.
4. Possible stiffness of protrusion.
5. Pain in groin, back, or scrotum.

Protection

The following suggestions should be followed in bringing first-aid protection to the hernia victim:

1. Place the victim in a lying position.
2. Elevate the knees.
3. Use cold applications to reduce circulation and swelling.
4. Call a physician or deliver the victim to medical help.

HIVES

Hives, or urticaria, are caused in the human body by sensitizations. The causative factor usually is a food that the individual is sensitive to, especially seafoods. The problem may begin within an hour or two after the intake of the food, or the reaction may be delayed for a few days. The skin usually breaks out and itches, commonly upon the face, and the lips and eyelids tend to become swollen.

Some individuals also have allergic reactions to pollen, animal hair (dog, cat, rabbit, horse, cow), or the feathers of birds.

Symptoms

The first-aider can learn to recognize hives when they occur. The signs to look for are

1. An eruption of welts upon the skin.
2. Sensitivity and severe itching of the skin.
3. Swelling of the lips and eyelids.

Protection

The first-aider can help to provide protection and relief from hives by adhering to the following suggestions:

1. Use alcohol and calamine for reduction of itching and discomfort.
2. Use a laxative, epsom salts, or milk of magnesia.
3. Gently bathe with baking soda solution.
4. Get medical help and suggested medication.

EMERGENCY CHILDBIRTH

The birth of a child under emergency conditions is a somewhat frequent occurrence in American life. During times of stress, disaster, or a sudden traumatic experience the labor process can be stimulated and the childbirth is under way.

If a first-aider, rescue worker, policeman or others are faced with such a situation emphasis should be given to the importance of cleanliness and to assisting and comforting the mother. But most of all keep in mind that one should allow nature to take its course. When the baby is ready to come, in most cases it will.

Figure 15.2 show those stages that normally occur during childbirth. Study the stages for more complete information and what assistance that can be given. In all instances call for a physician immediately.

ACTIVITIES

1. Make a study of the football accidents in several selected high schools or colleges of the area and report on the accidents involving the head. Find out, if possible, the cause of the accident and how it could have been prevented.
2. Contact the Epilepsy Association of America and request their materials on the legal rights of epileptics. Study and report to the class or group.
3. If possible, visit the intensive care unit in the local hospital and observe the care being given to stroke, head injury, and heart attack victims. Make a report to the class.
4. Have a panel discuss epilepsy. Be sure to include the problems of an epileptic and people's attitudes toward them.

QUESTIONS TO ANSWER

1. What are the common causes of unconsciousness? Under what circumstances does the skin turn red, blue, and white?
2. What is meant by the term *little stroke?* What are the usual indications of these strokes?
3. Describe a concussion. When does it occur? How dangerous are concussions?
4. What is the difference between a concussion and a cerebral lesion?
5. What are the causes of convulsions? What can be done to protect the victim? What is the danger from frequent convulsions?
6. What is the appendix? Where is it located? What is appendicitis?

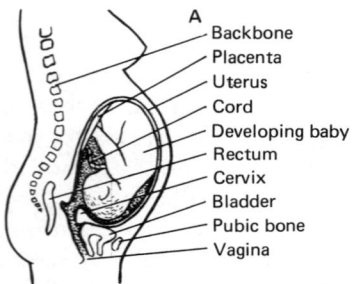

[252]   Special Problems

A

- Backbone
- Placenta
- Uterus
- Cord
- Developing baby
- Rectum
- Cervix
- Bladder
- Pubic bone
- Vagina

At full term, or after 40 weeks of pregnancy, the baby is ready to be born. The cervix, through which the baby must leave the uterus, is shown clearly here, still closed. The contractions of the muscles of the uterus will open the cervix and force the baby down through the vagina, or birth canal, to the outside.

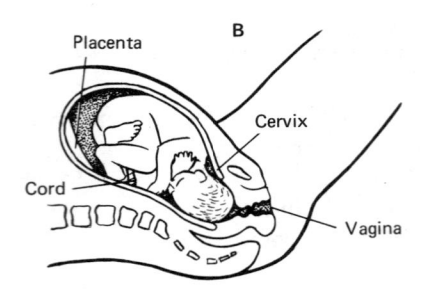

B

- Placenta
- Cervix
- Cord
- Vagina

At the end of the first stage of labor the cervix is completely open and the baby's head is beginning to come down through the vagina. Contractions begin in the lower back and later are felt in the lower abdomen. At the time shown here contractions are probably coming every 2 minutes, lasting 40–60 seconds and very strong.

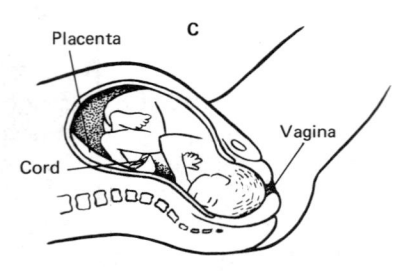

C

- Placenta
- Cord
- Vagina

The first stage of labor usually lasts several hours and is hard work. The mother needs to relax, rest, and be reassured. Give her water and fruit juices. In this picture the second stage of labor is well along. It is shorter than the first stage and the mother will now be pushing down with each contraction, helping to force the baby into the world.

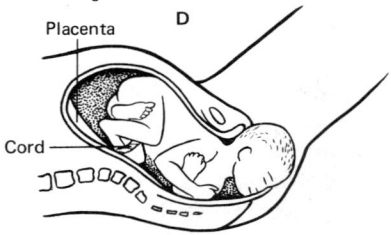

D

- Placenta
- Cord

The head of the baby has been partially born. This shows the usual position with the face down and the back of the head up. The bag of waters in which the baby is enclosed throughout the pregnancy may have broken at the beginning of labor, before or during the first stage. It may break now, or have to be torn with the fingers.

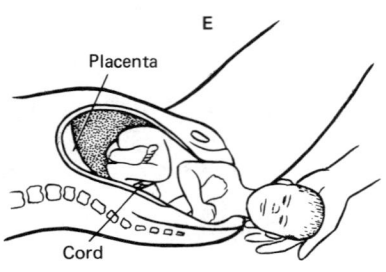

E

- Placenta
- Cord

Here you see the baby's head turned to the right as is usual. The shoulders are about to be born. The head must turn so that the baby's body can fit into the birth canal and come through more easily. After the birth of the baby there will be further uterine contractions and the placenta will be separated from the uterine wall and expelled.

FIGURE 15.2   The stages of childbirth.

7 What protection should be given an appendicitis victim? In the case of appendicitis, what should a first-aider not do?
8 How should the victim of the epileptic seizure be protected during and after the attack?
9 What is the explanation for the unconscious state, fainting? How can the victim be protected?
10 If intoxication is suspected, what additional checks should be made? What is the relationship, if any, between intoxication and diabetic coma, and insulin shock? How can a person help the victim of intoxication become sober?

SELECTED REFERENCES

AMERICAN MEDICAL ASSOCIATION, *Today's Health Guide*. Chicago: AMA, 1965.

AMERICAN NATIONAL RED CROSS, *Standard First Aid and Personal Safety*. New York: Doubleday, 1973.

BERLAND, THEODORE, "Appendicitis, the Forgotten Killer," *Today's Health*. Chicago: AMA, May, 1964.

COLE, WARREN H., and PUESTOW, CHARLES B., *First Aid: Diagnosis and Management*. New York: Appleton-Century-Crofts, 1965.

EPILEPSY ASSOCIATION OF AMERICA, *Facts*. Washington, D.C.: The Association, 1968.

HAFEN, BRENT Q., and KARREN, KEITH J., *First Aid and Emergency Care Workbook*. Denver, Colo.: Morton Publishing Co., 1977.

HENDERSON, JOHN, *Emergency Medical Guide*, 4th ed. New York: McGraw-Hill, 1978.

POTTHOFF, CARL J., "First Aid—Convulsions," *Today's Health*, March, 1969.

POTTHOFF, CARL J., "First Aid—Fainting," *Today's Health*, September, 1962.

POTTHOFF, CARL J., "First Aid—Unconsciousness," *Today's Health*, November, 1962.

SOFFER, ALFRED, "What You Should Know About Strokes," *Today's Health*, August, 1968.

16. DISASTER PREPAREDNESS

A program which has received great emphasis in this country in the past generation is Civil Defense. Recently, to broaden the concept of preparedness or protection, the name has been changed from *Civil Defense* to *Defense Civil Preparedness Agency*. The national program is administered by the Department of Defense.

Preparedness against nuclear attack is protection also against other disasters as the tornado, flood, hurricane, and earthquake. There is a great need for organization and leadership in the different disaster programs. If this leadership and organization for each program is not available, it would seem better that they be combined more or less into one.

This work of disaster preparedness is done mostly by volunteers. They need to be constantly recruited and trained. Communication and information are very important here and the workers should be kept informed and up to date. Safe places need to be located and maintained; emergency care training must be provided and kept up to date; food and other necessities must be provided.

It is recognized today by the leadership of the federal government and the states individually that disaster problems are not the same for all and that each area must plan for such differences. The Midwest most frequently experiences tornados—the most violent and destructive of all storms. The eastern and southern states are hit by the greatest number of hurricanes. The West is more familiar with the earthquake and its violence; while most areas of the country have experienced violent floods from the great rivers. These problems, together with the fires, winter storms, pollution disasters, heat waves, oil spills, and chemical accidents, create a great variety of disasters. Some of these problems are man-made; however, most of them are acts of nature which cannot be prevented. People must learn to cope with them.

The Defense Civil Preparedness Agency (DCPA) program in the United States is a national program designed to aid our population in times of disaster, regardless of whether the cause is natural or man-made. There have been several great disasters in recent years and in each case it was Civil Defense, now DCPA, that functioned successfully and helped the area or community return to normal life. The great Alaskan earthquake, Gulf States hurricanes, numerous floods, and the Kansas tornado are examples of disasters in which Civil Defense played a major role.

The Defense Civil Preparedness Agency continues to emphasize the danger of atomic warfare and the need for fallout shelters, radioactive monitors, communications, and necessary supplies. Since several countries, Russia and China in particular, possess great nuclear devices and have or will have the capability of delivering them to all parts of the world, the United States must be ready to meet any and all emergencies.

The program of preparedness differs with the different states. All states are urged to prepare against the possibility of nuclear warfare. Also each state is expected to prepare for other emergencies which are most likely to come to them. Federal funds are available for administrative salaries, staff help, and communication, rescue, and other types of equipment.

If an enemy should threaten or attack the United States, the entire nation would be mobilized to repulse the attack, destroy the enemy, and prevent or reduce the loss of life. Much assistance would be available to individuals from the local, state, and federal governments, and the U.S. armed forces. Should there be an attack, many lives would be saved through effective emergency preparedness and action. Some of the elements of an effective disaster preparedness programs are the disaster shelter and volunteer, emergency care training, radiological monitors, and the disaster supplies and warning signals.

THE DISASTER SHELTER

There are many buildings, tunnels, subways, mines, caves, and other areas with protection factors sufficient to protect our population from radioactive fallout. The minimum protection factor required is 40. This means that an individual within the designated shelter would be 40 times safer than on the outside. Many existing buildings and other areas possess protection factors of 100, 200, or more. These areas need to be found and made ready for shelter use.

The goal in recent years has been to find sufficient shelter areas or spaces for our population, to have the areas surveyed by a licensed architect, and to sign a license agreement with each owner. It is then important that the area be officially marked as a fallout shelter and that supplies be placed within it.

Personnel must be recruited and trained to operate the shelter. This is the most important and most difficult part of the shelter program as

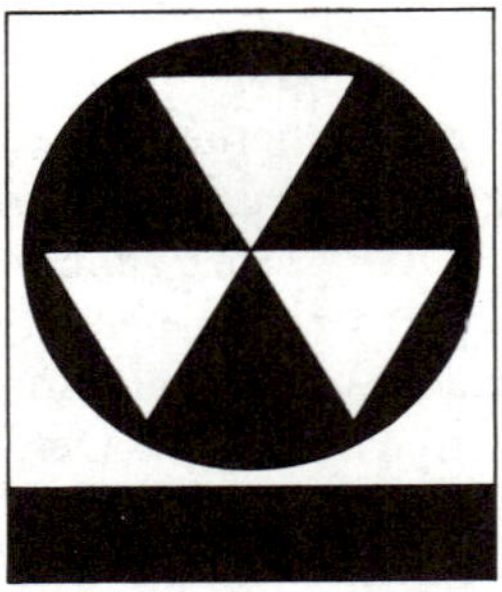

[256]   Disaster Preparedness

FIGURE 16.1   Public disaster shelter sign.

training must be continuous and meaningful. Otherwise it will fail. Keeping the shelter staff interested, up to date, and active is imperative. To be effective, the shelter must have managers, radioactive fallout monitors, communication personnel and equipment, and emergency care personnel and equipment to handle all health problems.

Priority must be given to shelter planning for our homes, schools, industries, and communities. Farmers must give some serious thinking about shelters to protect their family and livestock.

The three key factors for protection against radioactive fallout are time, distance, and mass. The shelter can best provide the factor of mass which will give the protection factor of 40 or more. Shelters can also provide the factor of distance from the bomb or burst but this factor is not too predictable.

THE DISASTER VOLUNTEER

Disaster workers, including Defense Civil Preparedness Agency (DCPA), have been volunteers from the beginning. In the past few persons, including Civil Defense, were paid for participation in disaster activities. Our government has spent billions of dollars on defense preparedness while at the same time it has spent very few dollars in comparison on disaster preparation for our citizens in the home communities and at their jobs.

These questions and others arise concerning the civilian population and the military. Is there too much or too little spending on the military? Is there too little spending for protection on the home front? Is the home front as important as the military? Can the disaster preparation program be left to the individual, small group, school, or community, or should the federal and state governments assume a greater responsibility?

Presently in the Defense Civil Preparedness Agency program in cooperation with the different states, the greater dependence for help is upon the volunteer. However, federal funds together with state funds pay up to 50 percent of the salaries of the city or county administrator. Salaries of secretaries and other staff personnel are fully funded. Also funds are available for the purchase of certain supplies and equipment. Indeed this is helpful for the development of a program at the local or county level. It still remains that without the volunteers (the key persons) in disaster planning and action, the program could not exist.

EMERGENCY CARE TRAINING

The Medical Self-Help program of emergency care, the Civil Defense program of a few years ago, has been terminated. This program had been funded by the Department of Health, Education and Welfare (HEW) but the funding stopped. This was an excellent program and had been designed to go along with the Red Cross First Aid program. It included the materials of the Red Cross program and in addition materials on emergency child-birth, radioactive fallout and shelter, healthful living in emergencies, nursing care of the sick and injured, and infant care. Since the termination of this program, the Defense Civil Preparedness Agency (DCPA) and others now look to the American Red Cross and their Standard and Advanced courses to train the personnel in emergency care procedures for the sick and injured. The Red Cross has expanded their course content to cover or include other areas needed in disaster preparation.

The Trauma Program has grown nationally during the past few years. The Trauma Center, usually a hospital, is well located geographically to serve an area and is well equipped to handle emergencies from the standpoint of both personnel and equipment.

The Trauma Program has had a great impact upon emergency care training and the securing of necessary equipment for handling emergencies. Many persons throughout the country have taken the Emergency Medical Technician (EMT) course. This training exceeds the normal first-aid training. It requires some 80 hours of study and practice. The EMT course gets specific in the areas of cardiovascular and respiratory problems, transportation of the injured, and extraction of the injured. The EMT course also includes much practice in the use of sophisticated equipment.

Following closely after the Trauma Program is the Ambulance Program. Many cities, counties, rural areas, and small communities have secured ambulances and have developed an Ambulance Program. Usually the ambulance has been purchased and equipped with matching funds from the state and federal governments. The ambulance attendants for

[258] Disaster Preparedness

the most part are persons who have had similar experiences in the military, or have had first-aid training and the EMT course. They are skilled attendants doing a very fine and much needed job.

The Ambulance Program has become an important and necessary service in this country. Even though the cost may be high, the service is necessary, and it is expected and appreciated by most. Along with the Trauma Center and the Ambulance Program, the newest development is the Heliocopter Program. Heliocopters are available in many locations to move accident victims to other locations where their needs can be better met. This is a fast and most efficient method of transportation, and many hospitals now have landing pads on their buildings or very close by their buildings.

RADIOLOGICAL MONITORS

The need for radiological monitors will continue as long as the danger of radiation from the atomic bomb exists. There will be a continued need for the shelter program for the same duration, and this may be a very long time.

Trained persons are needed to man the detector equipment and to keep our citizenry informed as to the level of radiation. During such times it will be necessary to know how much exposure each person has had, and how safe the food, water, and other necessities are for use.

Monitor courses will continue to be offered by units of the Defense Civil Preparedness Agency throughout the country. Interested persons will need to be recruited regularly and trained so as to assure the supply of trained persons to meet the needs of this very important phase of defense preparedness.

DISASTER SUPPLIES

A first-aid kit containing bandages, antiseptics, and other supplies is always useful. It can be stored in the shelter area, along with a first-aid handbook. Any specific medicines used by members of a family should be included. In addition, some member or members of a household should be trained in emergency care. Suggested items for a shelter are listed as (1) emergency care items and (2) useful shelter equipment.

Emergency Care Items

adhesive compresses—(Band-Aids) assorted sizes
adhesive tape

alcohol—70%
ammonia inhalant
antiseptic solution
sterile, cotton tipped applicators
aspirin or bufferin
bandage—2 inches wide
bandages—2 or 3 triangular
cotton—1 box, sterile
cough medicine
diarrhea medicine
ear drops
first-aid handbook
laxative
medication—any specifically indicated
motion sickness tablets
nose drops
petrolatum
safety pins
salt
scissors
splint, several sizes
thermometer
tweezers
water purification tablets

Useful Shelter Equipment

battery-type radio
flashlight with extra batteries
cooking and eating utensils
bottle and can opener
matches and candles
lantern
tools—wrenches, screwdriver, pliers, hammer, crowbar, saw, axe, broom, and shovel
sanitary supplies
rope—1 inch, 25 feet long
cots and blankets
card table and chairs
games for children
pencils and crayons
books and magazines
card games
clock—winding type

[260] Disaster Preparedness

DISASTER WARNING SIGNALS

The two standard signals of the Defense Civil Preparedness Agency which have been adopted in most communities are the attack warning signal and the attention or alert signal.

Attack Warning Signals

This signal will be sounded only in case of enemy attack. The signal itself is a three to five minute wavering sound on the siren, or a series of short blasts on whistles, horns, or other devices, repeated as is deemed necessary. The Attack Warning Signal means that an actual enemy attack against the United States has been detected and that protective action should be taken immediately. This signal has no other meaning and will be used for no other purpose (except for the monthly practice or drill).

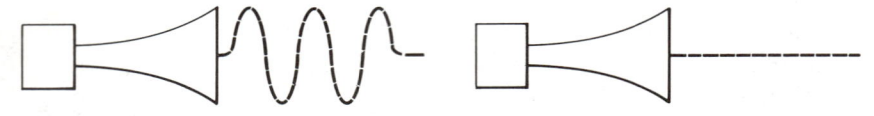

FIGURE 16.2 Attack warning signal.

Attention or Alert Signal

This signal is used by some local governments to get the attention of the citizens in a time of threatening or impending natural disaster or some other peacetime emergency. The signal itself is a three to five minute steady blast on sirens, whistles, horns, or other devices. In most places, the Attention or Alert Signal means that the local government wants to broadcast important information on the radio or television concerning a peacetime emergency or possible disaster.

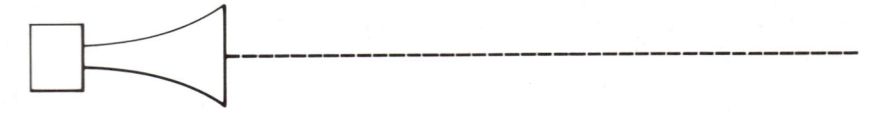

FIGURE 16.3 Attention or alert signal.

ACTIVITIES

1. Visit the fallout shelters in the community and get information about their stored supplies.
2. Volunteer as a Defense Civil Preparedness Agency worker and take

training in radiological monitoring, communications, or first aid. Report to your class and give an evaluation of your experiences.
3   Visit the local or area Trauma Center and discuss its program with the personnel. Report or prepare a paper on the findings.
4   Visit the Mutual Aid Coordinator for the Defense Civil Preparedness Agency and review the area program needs and progress. Get materials from the coordinator that can be meaningful and helpful to your classmates.
5   Write a paper concerning the need for the Shelter Program of the Defense Civil Preparedness Agency in the United States.

QUESTIONS TO ANSWER

1   How does the program of first aid differ from the EMT program?
2   How can the population of this country best be protected from radioactive fallout? What is meant by the protection factor?
3   What is the Defense Civil Preparedness Agency's shelter program? Defend or refute this program.
4   What supplies are needed in the fallout shelter? Presently who pays for them? How long will they remain useful?
5   What is the most difficult obstacle in our national disaster effort? How can it best be surmounted?
6   What persons are needed in a shelter situation to properly and adequately manage the shelter?
7   Is it possible to maintain safe sanitary conditions in a shelter? How?
8   Visit the Ambulance Program headquarters in your community. Inspect the ambulances and equipment, and discuss with the personnel its program, training, and charges.
9   What are the national Defense Civil Preparedness Agency signals? Inquire of 25 or more persons at random and find out the percent of those who know and understand the signals.
10 Visit your local or county Defense Civil Preparedness Agency headquarters. Examine the communications equipment. Inquire about the training programs and the need for volunteers.

SELECTED REFERENCES

AMERICAN NATIONAL RED CROSS, *Advanced First Aid and Emergency Care*. New York: Doubleday, 1973.
AMERICAN NATIONAL RED CROSS, *Standard First Aid and Personal Safety*. New York: Doubleday, 1973.
COLE, WARREN H., and PUESTOW, CHARLES B., *First Aid Diagnosis and Management*. New York: Appleton-Century-Crofts, 1965.

HENDERSON, JOHN, *Emergency Medical Guide*, 4th ed. New York: McGraw-Hill, 1978.
OFFICE OF DEFENSE CIVIL PREPAREDNESS AGENCY, *Annual Statistical Report*. Washington, D.C.: Department of Defense, 1973.
OFFICE OF DEFENSE CIVIL PREPAREDNESS AGENCY, *Protection in the Nuclear Age*. Washington, D.C.: Department of Defense, February, 1977.
OFFICE OF DEFENSE CIVIL PREPAREDNESS AGENCY, *Responsibilities and Authorities*. Washington, D.C.: Department of Defense, 1977.
OFFICE OF DEFENSE CIVIL PREPAREDNESS AGENCY, *Your Chance to Live*. San Francisco: Far West Laboratories for Educational Research and Development, 1972.
STATE OF ILLINOIS EMERGENCY SERVICES and DISASTER AGENCY, *Hazard Analysis*. Springfield: The Agency, 1976.
STATE OF ILLINOIS OFFICE OF PUBLIC INSTRUCTION, *School Emergency Planning Guide*. Springfield: The Agency, 1976.

PART IV
TYPES OF EMERGENCY CARE VICTIMS

This part of the book discusses the persons and types of injuries that are involved most frequently in accidents. These are the victims that the first-aider should be prepared to work with when providing first-aid protection. To assist the first-aid person, the most common types of injuries sustained are identified.

The following chapters are included in Part IV:

17 Traffic Accident Victims
18 Home Accident Victims
19 Public Accident Victims
20 Industrial Accident Victims
21 School Accident Victims

17. TRAFFIC ACCIDENT VICTIMS

One of the crucial problems of modern society is the growing motor-vehicle traffic. The number of vehicles is increasing throughout the world. However, the United States maintains a substantial lead in the total number of vehicles and highway users. Man has attempted to cope with the conditions and problems created by the traffic explosion, but to date the solution continues to elude traffic experts as the number of traffic accident victims continues to rise annually. More and more people are critically injured and meet death as a result of traffic collisions.

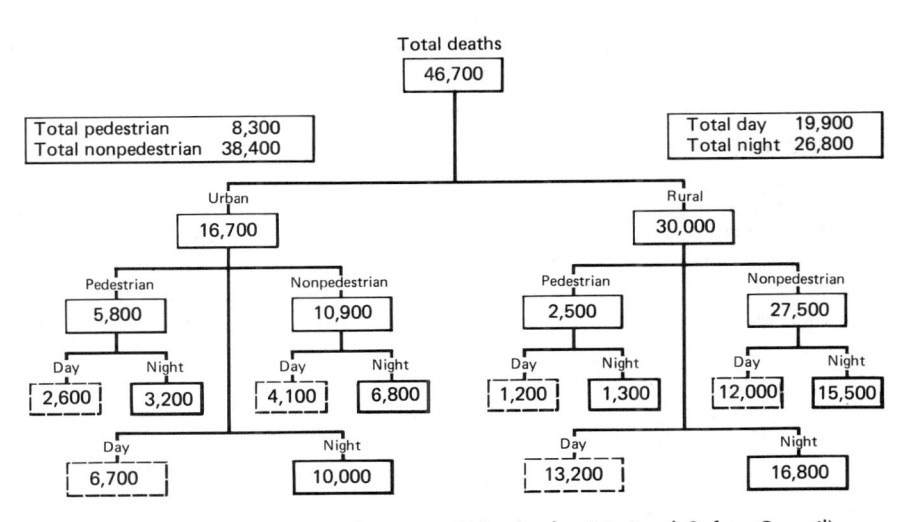

```
                          Total deaths
                            46,700

Total pedestrian    8,300                    Total day     19,900
Total nonpedestrian 38,400                   Total night   26,800

             Urban                                  Rural
            16,700                                 30,000

    Pedestrian      Nonpedestrian          Pedestrian      Nonpedestrian
      5,800            10,900                2,500            27,500

   Day    Night     Day    Night         Day    Night     Day     Night
  2,600   3,200    4,100   6,800        1,200   1,300   12,000   15,500

     Day       Night                       Day             Night
    6,700     10,000                     13,200           16,800
```

FIGURE 17.1 Principal classes of motor vehicle deaths. (National Safety Council)

[265]

[266]   Traffic Accident Victims

In a recent year more than 46,700 Americans died on the nation's highways in some 40,000 separate traffic collisions. Another tragic aspect of the traffic accident problem is that over 2 million persons were injured to the extent that they were disabled beyond the day of the accident. About 200,000 of these victims were permanently disabled for life. In urban areas some two fifths of the victims were pedestrians, and in rural areas the victims were principally occupants of motor vehicles. Approximately one half of the deaths occurred at night, with the proportion a bit higher in urban areas as opposed to a rural traffic environment.

Traffic collisions are traumatic accidents that can cause severe damage to all body parts. The first-aider should become familiar with the nature and scope of this problem in order to deal effectively with traffic victims.

TYPES OF TRAFFIC COLLISIONS

The following sections outline briefly how people met death in traffic collisions on the country's highways. The accident data presented are based upon the National Safety Council's annual publication *Accident Facts*.[1]

Total Motor-vehicle Accidents

As discussed in Chapter 1 motor-vehicle death victims totaled in excess of 46,700 in a recent year. About two fifths of the collisions were in an urban area while the remainder happened on rural highways, including state and interstate. The total analysis of the traffic accident problem includes deaths resulting from mechanically or electrically powered highway-transport vehicles in motion both on and off the highway.

Pedestrian Accidents

About 8,300 pedestrians die in motor-vehicle collisions each year. The greatest number of these occur on urban streets. Most of the victims were injured or killed while crossing or entering streets. Usually the crossing is between intersections, with the ratio of such incidence varying for individuals of different ages. Drivers must remember that pedestrians have the right of way at intersections.

Collisions Between Motor Vehicles

The greatest number of traffic victims meet death in this type of collision. Over 20,000 of the total motor-vehicle deaths that occurred in a recent year were in this category. These include deaths from collisions

[1] National Safety Council, *Accident Facts*. Chicago: The Council, 1977.

FIGURE 17.2 DEATHS AND INJURIES OF PEDESTRIANS IN THE UNITED STATES, 1976

	All Ages		Age of Persons Killed and Injured						
Actions	No.	%	0-4	5-9	10-14	15-19	20-24	25-44	45-64	65 and Over
Crossing or entering	67,000	61.9	71.2	77.8	63.5	47.2	45.3	48.2	61.8	75.0
—at intersection	24,700	22.8	8.0	19.2	23.4	20.4	20.1	21.7	30.1	41.5
—between intersections	42,300	39.1	63.2	58.6	40.1	26.8	25.2	26.5	31.7	33.5
Walking in roadway	8,600	7.9	2.2	2.4	8.6	15.0	12.2	9.5	8.7	6.7
—with traffic	6,200	5.7	1.3	1.3	6.0	11.1	10.2	7.5	5.6	4.2
—against traffic	2,400	2.2	0.9	1.1	2.6	3.9	2.0	2.0	3.1	2.5
Standing in roadway	4,600	4.2	1.2	0.4	2.1	7.1	8.9	7.6	5.7	2.1
Pushing or working on vehicle				0.1	0.5	3.3	4.5	4.9	2.5	1.3
in roadway	2,300	2.1	*	0.8	0.5	0.8	2.4	3.3	1.5	0.4
Other working in roadway	1,500	1.4	1.3	8.6	6.2	1.6	0.2	0.3	0.2	0.5
Playing in roadway	4,200	3.9	11.3	6.4	10.9	11.5	11.8	10.5	7.7	4.7
Other in roadway	9,400	8.7	6.3	3.5	7.7	13.5	14.7	15.7	11.9	9.3
Not in roadway	10,700	9.9	6.5							

Source: National Safety Council.

[267]

[268]   Traffic Accident Victims

usually of two or more motorcars. Scooters, motorized bicycles, farm tractors, trolley buses, and road machinery are a part of the problem because each of these is classified as a motor vehicle. The development of proper visual habits will help motorists avoid collisions with other vehicles.

It should be noted that the highest death rate from traffic collisions between motor vehicles is in the over-75- and 15–24-year-old age ranges. All other age ranges have a death rate slightly lower than these two.

Noncollision, Overturning, Running Off Roadway

The second highest incidence of traffic accidents occur in this area. About 13,000 traffic victims were claimed in this category in a current analysis of accident data. Most of these incidences happened on highways outside of urban areas. Such accidents are classified according to the first event. For example, if a car runs off the highway and then hits a tree, death is classified as a run-off-the-road accident. Fatigue, lack of sleep, and alcohol are the reasons for many of these accidents.

Drivers between the ages of 15 and 24 have the highest death rate in this category. The 24- to 44-year-old driver has the next greatest death rate.

Usually these tend to be dramatic-type collisions with numerous serious injuries occurring. The first-aider should become acquainted with the common injuries sustained in such occurrences and be prepared to cope with such. Figures 17.3 and 17.4 identify the parts of the body most frequently injured. Therefore, a part of the first-aid class should be devoted to the care and protection of these common injuries.

Collisions with Railroad Trains

Collisions with trains account for about 1,200 deaths each year. Although this does not seem to be a significant number, these deaths are senseless occurrences. For example, some deaths occur when a driver runs into a train already moving across the crossing. Other collisions happen when the motorist has stopped his car on the tracks and the vehicle becomes stalled. It appears that these two types of collisions generally could be avoided. It seems reasonable to expect that any person could see something as large as a train (except perhaps in dense fog, etc.). In most cases persons can get out of a car stalled on the railroad tracks so that no deaths would be involved in the collision.

Collision with Bicycles

About 900 lives are lost each year in vehicle-bicycle collisions. Most of these involve 5- to 14-year-old children. The proportion between rural and urban incidences is about even.

Types of Traffic Collisions [269]

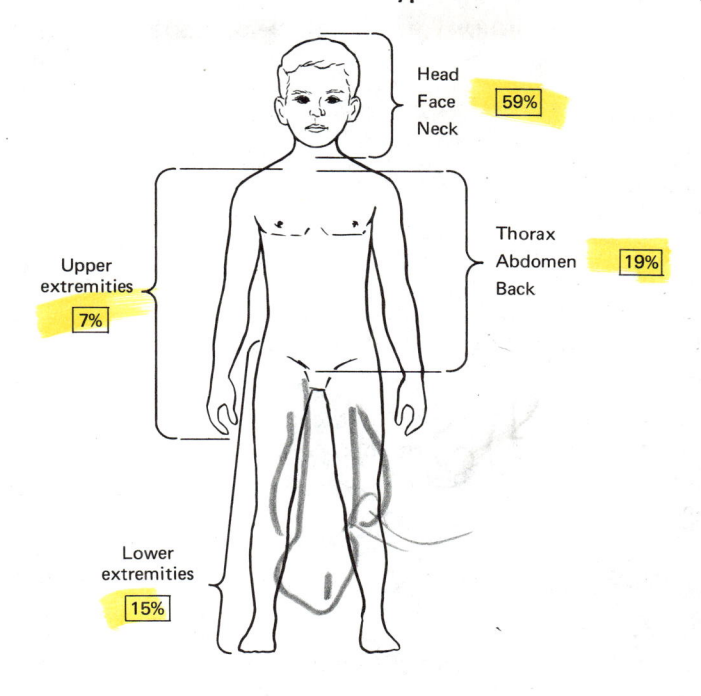

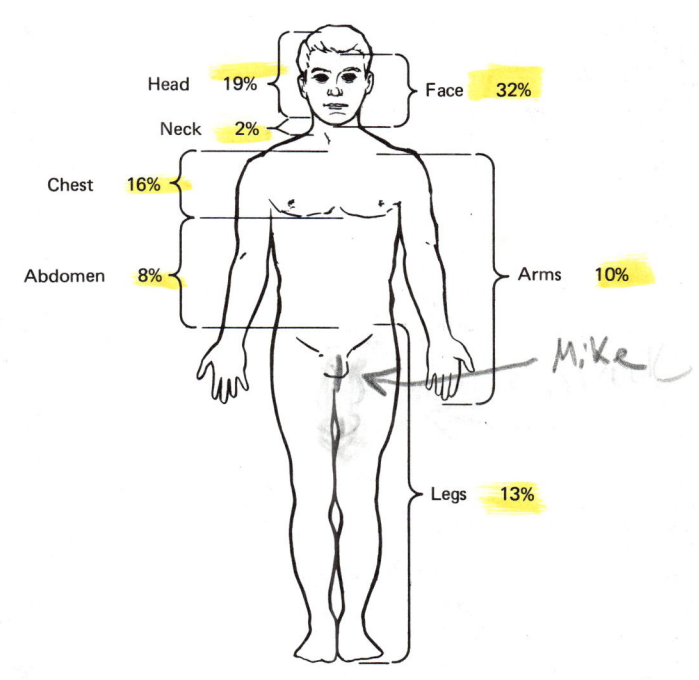

FIGURE 17.3 Distribution of injuries to children (above) and adults (below). (Alan M. Nahum, *Stapp Car Crash Conference.* Society of Automotive Engineers, 1968)

Traffic Accident Victims

FIGURE 17.4 DISTRIBUTION OF SKELETAL AND TISSUE/ORGAN INJURIES TO CHILDREN IN MOTOR VEHICLE ACCIDENTS

Injury Location	Skeletal Injuries (% of total)	Tissue/Organ Injuries (% of total)
Whole body	21	79
Head, face, neck	17	brain, 16; other, 67
Thorax, abdomen, back	19	81
Upper extremities	20	80
Lower extremities	38	62

Source: Alan M. Nahum, *Stapp Car Crash Conference*. Society of Automotive Engineers, 1968.

Caution should be exercised by the motorists because of the unexpected actions of the youngster on the bike. Extensive implementation of bicycle safety programs in the nation's elementary schools could do much to eliminate this problem.

Collisions with Fixed Objects

Deaths in this area occur at the rate of about 3,200 per year. Such incidents involve collisions with fixed objects such as walls, bridges, and abutments where the collision took place while all the vehicle wheels were still on the highway. The death rates are highest in the 15- to 44-year-old age ranges.

This is usually a very serious collision because of the great impact between the moving vehicle and a fixed object. Among the causes of these accidents is loss of vehicle control due to excessive speed, alcohol, or fatigue.

Other Collisions

There are some traffic collisions that occur infrequently. These include motor-vehicle collisions with animals, animal-drawn vehicles, and street-cars. The potential of vehicle-animal collisions is greatest during the hunting season. Motorists should be aware of this collision possibility and take caution on those highways known to be in heavily populated deer areas.

Motorcycle Accidents

The number of motorcycles in use in the United States has increased about 270 percent in the past ten years. The general trend has been for the number of motorcycle rider deaths to increase also. About 3,000 such deaths are recorded annually. The use of helmets by riders and passengers, developing educational programs, and better cycle design are helping to

Age of Drivers   [271]

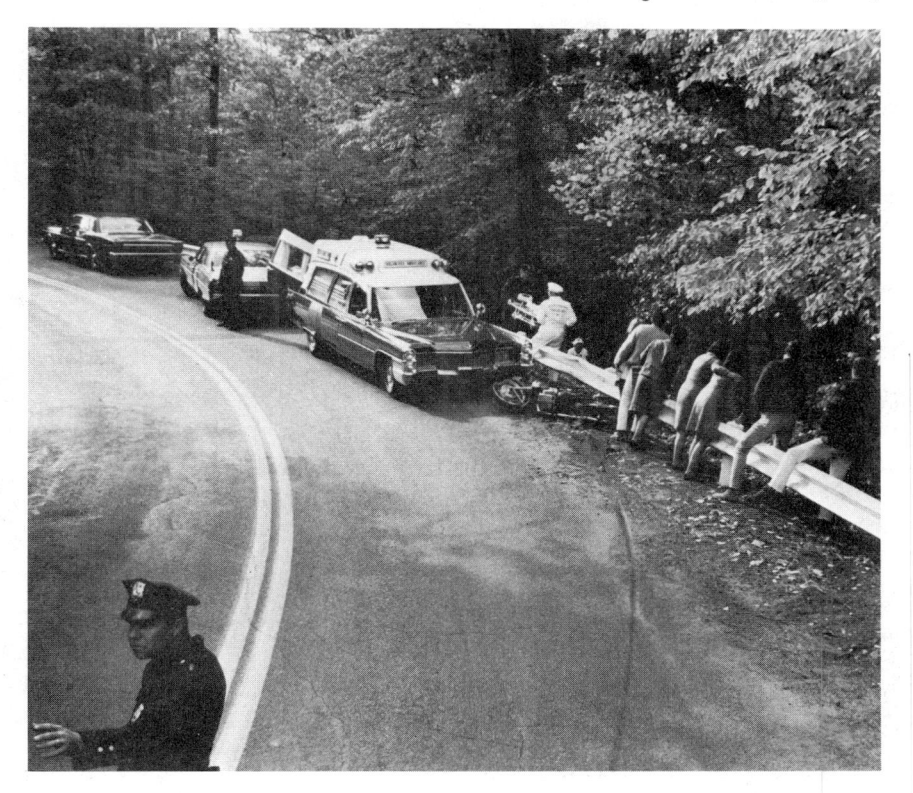

FIGURE 17.5 Motorcycle accidents have become more frequent occurrences. (Metropolitan Life Insurance Company)

reduce the number of cycle deaths. With the helmet requirements of the Highway Safety Act of 1966 rescinded, the cycle death rate in all probability will continue at a high level.

AGE OF DRIVERS

The number of drivers in the United States is fast approaching 134 million. An analysis of the number of drivers in each age group is shown in Figure 17.7. Upon examination of the information in this figure, it is obvious that the great majority of our drivers are under 50 years of age. There is a significant concentration of drivers in the under-30 age range.

It is estimated that in the early 1980's approximately 4 million new drivers will be added each year. By the later 1980's it is probable that close to 40 percent of our driving population will be under 25 years of age. This is an important consideration for the first-aider in that this is the age where the greatest incidence of traffic collisions occur.

FIGURE 17.6 MOTORCYCLE * AND TOTAL MOTOR-VEHICLE DATA, 1960–1976

| | Vehicles |||| | Deaths ||||
| | Motorcycles || Total Mot. Veh. || Motorcycle Riders || All Mot. Veh. Occupants ||
Year	No.	Yearly % Change	No.	Yearly % Change	No.	Yearly % Change	No.	Yearly % Change
1960	575,497		74,500,000		731		29,750	
1961	595,669	+ 3.5	76,400,000	+2.6	697	− 4.7	29,850	+ 0.3
1962	660,400	+10.9	79,700,000	+4.3	759	+ 8.9	32,300	+ 8.2
1963	786,318	+19.1	83,500,000	+4.8	882	+16.2	34,700	+ 7.4
1964	984,763	+25.2	87,300,000	+4.6	1,118	+26.8	37,900	+ 9.2
1965	1,381,956	+40.3	91,800,000	+5.2	1,515	+35.5	39,450	+ 4.1
1966	1,752,801	+26.8	95,900,000	+4.5	2,043	+34.9	42,800	+ 8.5
1967	1,953,022	+11.4	98,900,000	+3.1	1,971	− 3.5	42,700	− 0.2
1968	2,100,547	+ 7.6	103,100,000	+4.2	1,900	− 3.6	44,100	+ 3.3
1969	2,315,916	+10.3	107,700,000	+4.5	1,960	+ 3.2	45,200	+ 2.5
1970	2,814,730	+21.5	111,200,000	+3.2	2,330	+18.9	43,500	− 3.8
1971	3,345,179	+18.8	116,300,000	+4.6	2,410	+ 3.4	43,200	− 0.7
1972	3,801,932	+13.7	122,300,000	+5.2	2,700	+12.0	44,700	+ 3.5
1973	4,353,502	+14.5	129,800,000	+6.1	3,130	+15.9	44,050	− 1.5
1974	4,966,132	+14.1	134,900,000	+3.9	3,160	+ 1.0	36,400	−17.4
1975	4,966,844	+ **	138,000,000	+2.3	2,800	−11.4	36,300	− 0.3
1976	5,110,000	+ 2.9	142,400,000	+3.2	3,000	+ 7.1	37,400	+ 3.0

Source: Vehicles—Federal Highway Administration; motorcycle rider deaths, 1960–1967—National Center for Health Statistics; motorcycle rider deaths, 1968–1976, and motor-vehicle occupant deaths—National Safety Council.

* Includes motor scooter, motorized bicycle, and motorized tricycle.

** Less than 0.05 per cent.

FIGURE 17.7 AGE OF DRIVERS—TOTAL NUMBER AND NUMBER IN ACCIDENTS

| | All Drivers | | Drivers in Accidents | | | | Per No. of Drivers | |
| | | | Fatal | | All | | | |
Age Group	Number	%	Number	%	Number	%	Fatal *	All **
Total	133,800,000	100.0%	59,000	100.0%	28,400,000	100.0%	44	21
Under 20	13,600,000	10.2	9,800	16.6	5,100,000	18.0	72	38
20–24	15,700,000	11.7	12,300	20.9	5,600,000	19.7	78	36
25–29	16,100,000	12.0	7,400	12.5	3,800,000	13.4	50	24
30–34	14,300,000	10.7	6,300	10.7	3,000,000	10.6	44	21
35–39	12,000,000	9.0	3,900	6.6	2,000,000	7.0	33	17
40–44	11,300,000	8.4	3,900	6.6	1,700,000	6.0	35	15
45–49	11,800,000	8.8	3,500	5.9	1,700,000	6.0	30	14
50–54	11,200,000	8.4	2,800	4.8	1,400,000	4.9	25	13
55–59	9,000,000	6.7	2,400	4.1	1,300,000	4.6	27	14
60–64	6,800,000	5.1	2,100	3.5	1,000,000	3.5	31	15
65–69	5,700,000	4.3	1,600	2.7	900,000	3.2	28	16
70–74	3,700,000	2.8	1,200	2.0	300,000	1.0	32	8
75 and over	2,600,000	1.9	1,800	3.1	600,000	2.1	69	23

Source: Drivers in accidents based on reports from 25 state traffic authorities. Number of drivers by age are National Safety Council estimates based on reports from state traffic authorities and research groups.
* Drivers in Fatal Accidents per 100,000 drivers in each age group.
** Drivers in All Accidents per 100 drivers in each age group.

[274] Traffic Accident Victims

CAUSES OF TRAFFIC COLLISIONS

Figure 17.8 depicts the various causes reported for traffic collisions. In general these causes are related to driver failure, highway failure, or vehicle failure.

Traffic Violations

Traffic violations are related to traffic collisions. Speed too fast for conditions, failure to yield the right of way, following too closely, and improper overtaking are the most common violations reported by police officers. It has been estimated that traffic violations were committed in seven of ten traffic collisions.

Alcohol

Alcohol is the most common factor relating to traffic accident causes. "Drinking is indicated to be a factor in at least half of fatal motor vehicle accidents, according to resident studies." [2]

This fact needs to be recognized by the first-aider because the true extent of a traffic accident victim's condition may be difficult to determine if the person is under the influence of alcohol.

BODY PART INJURED

In traffic collisions the human body is injured to a severe or lesser degree depending upon the type of collision, the speed and condition of the vehicle, and the evasive action performed by the driver. Usually the head, face, chest, and lower extremities are the parts of the body most frequently injured.

Children

When children are involved in traffic collisions the head, face, and neck area are damaged in about 60 percent of all accidents. The abdomen, back, and thorax sustain about 19 percent of the total number of injuries, and the lower extremities account for about 15 percent. Upper extremities receive injuries in about 7 percent of all traffic collisions. Children are injured mostly because restraining devices are not used. During sudden changes of vehicle speed or during impact, a child's body moves forward quickly. Usually when the child is in the rear seat, fewer and less severe injuries are received. Figure 17.4 depicts the distribution of skeletal injuries of tissue-organ injuries in children.

[2] Ibid., p. 52.

Body Part Injured [275]

FIGURE 17.8 FACTORS IN TRAFFIC DEATHS AND INJURIES

The precrash phase
I. Human
  A. Age and sex
  B. Driving skill
    1. training
    2. licensing
  C. Medical considerations
    1. alcohol
    2. drugs
    3. other medical factors
      (a) physiological
      (b) psychological
      (c) pathological

II. Car
  A. Sensory inputs
  B. Vehicle condition
  C. Maneuverability
  D. Human engineering; accessibility of controls
  E. Brakes
  F. Tires

III. Environment
  A. Roadway
  B. Roadside, shoulders, obstructions
  C. Intersections and other discontinuities
  D. Weather
  E. Communications, signals
  F. Operational control
  G. Speed, speed control

The crash phase
I. Human
II. Car
  A. Impact phenomena
  B. Occupant protection
    1. structural factors
    2. interior design
    3. restraints
  C. Pedestrian protection
III. Motorcyclist
IV. Highway
  A. Median design
  B. Protected abutments
  C. Breakaway materials for roadside objects, light poles, etc.

The postcrash phase
I. Car
  A. Gas spillage, fire
  B. Design factors, access for rescuers, easy egress for occupant
II. Ambulance services
III. Emergency facilities
IV. Definitive care
V. Rehabilitation

Source: "The Physician's Role in Highway Safety," *Modern Medicine*.

Adults

In comparing adult injuries with those sustained by children, the following have been observed: About 32 percent of the adult injuries are to the face; the head is involved in 19 percent and the neck in 2 percent. The next most frequent area of the adult body injured is that of the chest and abdomen; about 16 percent of the total injuries are to the chest and 8 percent to the abdomen. These usually result from impact with the car's steering wheel and column. Legs are involved in about 13 percent of the total, and the arms are injured about 10 percent of the time.

The differences in the distribution of injuries sustained by adults as opposed to children are probably due to the differences in their relative positions inside a car and the stability of each due to size and weight.

[276] Traffic Accident Victims

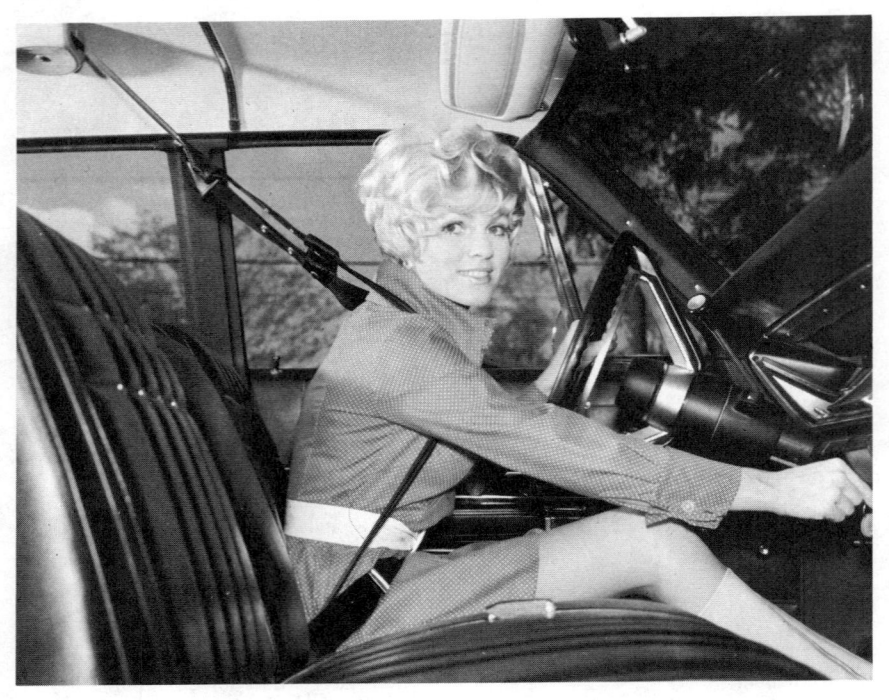

FIGURE 17.9 Inertia reel harness helps to lessen severity of traffic collisions. (American Seating Company, Grand Rapids, Michigan)

ACTIVITIES

1. Develop a paper on the use of occupant restraining devices used by children.
2. Visit a local hospital and determine the number of emergency victims admitted as a result of traffic collisions.
3. Organize a panel discussion with two classmates on the subject "Trends in Motorcycle Deaths and Injuries."
4. Write a term paper on the topic "Youth Versus Age as Prerequisites for Judicious Driving."
5. Draw a human figure and identify the areas most frequently injured in children and adults as a result of a traffic collision.

QUESTIONS TO ANSWER

1. Approximately how many Americans are killed in traffic accidents each year?
2. What is the most common type of motor-vehicle collision?

3 Approximately how many drivers will enter our driving population in the early 1980s?
4 Identify the most common types of injuries sustained by children involved in traffic collisions.
5 What is the most frequent factor associated with traffic accident causes?
6 During the past decade what percentage increase in motorcycle usage has the United States experienced?
7 What was suggested that might help lessen the number of bicycle collisions?
8 What part of the adult body is most frequently injured in traffic collisions?
9 Where do most of the noncollision traffic accidents occur?
10 In what location do pedestrians most often become accident victims?

SELECTED REFERENCES

AARON, J., and STRASSER, M., *Driver and Traffic Safety Education*. New York: Macmillan, 1977.

CHAYET, NEIL, *Legal Implications of Emergency Care*. New York: Appleton-Century-Crofts, 1969.

COLE, WARREN H., and PUESTOW, CHARLES B., *First Aid: Diagnosis and Management*. New York: Appleton-Century-Crofts, 1965.

KULOWSKI, J., *Crash Injuries*. Springfield, Ill.: Charles C Thomas, 1960.

NATIONAL SAFETY COUNCIL, *Accident Facts*. Chicago: The Council, 1977.

SELZER, M., GIKUS, P., and HUELKER, D. (eds.), *The Prevention of Highway Injuries*. Highway Safety Research Institute, Ann Arbor, Mich.: The University of Michigan, 1967.

SOCIETY OF AUTOMOTIVE ENGINEERS, *Twelfth Stapp Car Crash Conference*. New York: The Society, 1968.

STRASSER, M. K., et al., *Fundamentals of Safety Education*. New York: Macmillan, 1973.

U.S. DEPARTMENT OF TRANSPORTATION, *First Annual Report to Congress—Highway Safety Act of 1966*. Washington, D.C.: U.S. Government Printing Office, 1968.

U.S. DEPARTMENT OF HEALTH, EDUCATION, AND WELFARE, *Motor Vehicle Injury Prevention Program*. Washington, D.C.: The Department, 1966.

18. HOME ACCIDENT VICTIMS

Most Americans regard the home as a place where they can escape the highway, relax from pressures of work, and enjoy the security such an environment provides. Usually the home is thought of as a friendly, safe place to be. The facts, however, do not bear this out.

Home accidents are the most common cause of personal injury. About one third of all nonfatal accidental injuries and more than one fourth of all fatal injuries happen in and around the home. This is grim evidence that our homes are not as safe as they are thought to be.

Medical attention is required by about 15 million individuals who are injured annually in home accidents. In home accidents during a recent year some 24,000 persons were fatally injured, and about 100,000 injuries resulted in some permanent impairment.[1] Further, the nation suffers an annual loss of some 14.4 million workdays due to home injuries sustained among the nation's work force. This loss of productivity exceeds the loss resulting from on-the-job accidents.

The National Safety Council states that home accidents cost the nation about $6.3 billion each year, exclusive of property damage. Obviously there is a drain upon our human and economic resources.

With the expanding population and the introduction of new hazards around the home, it is expected that home injuries will continue to occur in significant numbers. The knowledge of these facts should cause all persons to become concerned. Further, it would be wise for one person in each family to become a trained first-aider. When one member of a family is trained in first aid, the other members generally tend to have a greater knowledge of first aid. Also the entire family tends to become safety conscious and avoids more accidents than the family without a

[1] National Safety Council, *Accident Facts*. Chicago: The Council, 1977.

Types of Home Accidents   [279]

first-aid-trained person. With a first-aider around, the seriousness of many home injuries could be lessened and the possibility of permanent impairment thwarted.

TYPES OF HOME ACCIDENTS

It is apparent that home accidents represent a serious problem in every community and need to be given more attention. The curtailment of home injuries should be the object of nationwide accident prevention efforts. The principal types of home accidents are falls, fire burns, suffocation, poisoning, firearm injuries, and poisoning by gases.

Falls

Falls are the most frequent cause of accidental death in the home. Approximately 7,700 such deaths are recorded each year. This is about twice as many deaths as from any other single cause. In the age group over 65, falls account for the greatest number of fatal home accidents. Usually, persons fall from one level to another. Common examples are falling down stairs, on floors, and off ladders.

Fire Burns

Fire is a serious threat to the lives of all family members. In a current report, deaths as a result of fires, burns, smoke asphyxiation, and falling objects amounted to about 5,100 persons. Although these deaths occurred in all age ranges, the majority were concentrated in the under-4 and over-65 age group. In addition to the known deaths there are in excess of 500,000 persons who are seriously injured due to fire.

Suffocation

During a typical year about 2,300 persons die in suffocation accidents. Ingested objects cause about 1,600 of these deaths, while suffocation-mechanical accidents account for some 700 deaths. Most of these fatalities occur in children under 4 years of age. By far the largest majority involved infants under one year. The inhalation or ingestion of objects or food plus smothering in bedclothes or thin plastic were the most frequent causes reported for these deaths.

Poisoning

About 3,400 individuals die each year from accidental ingestions of solids and liquid substances. It is estimated that about 500,000 such ingestions happen annually. Aspirin and other household product such as paints,

[280] Home Accident Victims

pesticides, cosmetics, and plants account for a significant percentage of these poisonings.

Firearms

A great many persons are injured through the misuse of firearms in the home. The National Safety Council reports that about 1,200 persons are fatally injured each year. Most of these deaths are due to carelessness on the part of family members. Gun-cleaning incidents, playing with guns, and the "unloaded" gun take many lives yearly. The greatest number of these fatalities are in the 15- to 24-year-old age range with the 5 to 14 age group a close second. Usually firearm accidents involve men and boys.

Poisoning by Gases

Accidental gas poisoning accounts for approximately 900 deaths each year. About one fourth of these are due to carbon monoxide involving cooking stoves, heating equipment, and standing motor vehicles. Persons in the 45 to 64 and 25 to 44 age groups seem to be the most frequent victims of gas poisoning.

Other Home Accidents

Those accidents not classified in the preceding sections include drowning, burns from hot substances, electric current, and blows sustained from falling objects. There are about 3,400 deaths related to these types of accidents. Drownings account for about 850 of these deaths and seem to be rising. Perhaps this increase is due partially to the growing number of home swimming pools. A recent study reveals that there are over 500,000 permanent home pools, 2 million portable pools, and more than 10 million plastic wading pools used by over 25 million persons in the United States today.

CAUSES OF HOME ACCIDENTS

Home accidents usually are the result of multiple causes and effect people in various ways. Primary factors in home accidents relate to both human and environmental sources.

Human factors, which are difficult to identify or understand, usually relate to emotional, physical, and mental characteristics of the individual. Fear, worry, fatigue, inadequate knowledge, and generally poor health are potential hazards to a person's safety.

Environmental hazards most often related to home accidents are faulty home design, poor housekeeping, and defective equipment and appliances. Such hazards are to be found outside the house as well as within.

ACCIDENTS AMONG CHILDREN

It is estimated that there are over 20 million persons injured in home accidents each year. Of this number about half are children under 15 years of age. Approximately two thirds of the fatal accidents to children under 5 happen at home, and home injuries account for about 60 percent of all injuries to children. Annually some 4.3 million days of school time are lost due to home accidents involving elementary and secondary students.

As already mentioned, the leading causes of accidental deaths among children under 5 are suffocation, inhalation and ingestion of objects, fires, poisoning, and drownings. Falls are the primary cause of nonfatal injuries to children in this age bracket.

The high incidence of home accidents which involve children are due in large measure to insufficient knowledge, lack of experience, and their inability to recognize hazards. Also the lack of parental supervision is a factor in the involvement of children in home accidents.

ACCIDENTS AMONG ADULTS

Home accidents involve an unusually large number of aged adults. About half of all accidental home deaths are in persons over 65 years of age. Among the basic factors that account for this high susceptibility to accidents are impaired vision and hearing, degeneration of the nervous system, and the common cell and tissue impairments related to old age.

Fractures of the hip, neck, and femur are common in this group. The general brittleness of bones and osteoporosis are conditions that predispose this age range to home injuries.

In an effort to eliminate accidents among older persons, there must be two basic steps. One is to provide our senior citizens with hazard-free environments. This includes homes and other places they might visit from time to time. The second step is to assist older persons in realizing their physical limitations and in appreciating the need to practice prudent safety measures.

FARM HOME ACCIDENTS

The home of the farm family today is comparable to the home of the urban family. Therefore, most of the same hazards exist in each environment. Hazards such as defective heating equipment and appliances, unsafe stairs and floors are the causes for numerous deaths and injuries among the members of farm families. The rural family performs chores and

Home Accident Victims

other light farm duties that are unique to them and subject them to type of hazards different from those of the urban family.

On the average there are about 1,000 deaths in farm-home-related activities each year and 170,000 disabling injuries. The number of injuries is estimated to be much higher than quoted because of the lack of adequate data on farm accidents. The farm home is a place where a trained first-aid person would be quite valuable owing to the frequency of home injuries.

ACTIVITIES

1. Develop a 20-item home hazard questionnaire. Make a copy available to all class members. Have each member evaluate his own home. Spend about 15 minutes of class time discussing their findings.
2. Contact the local Red Cross office. Determine the number of persons completing the Red Cross Standard and Advanced First-Aid Courses during the past year. Try to ascertain the number of families who would now have a trained first-aider in the home to provide emergency care to family members. Report to the class your findings.
3. Contact the local farm extension office to make an appointment. Interview the program director and determine the extent of the farm accident problem in the area.
4. Obtain the most recent edition of *Accident Facts* (National Safety Council publication). Analyze the section on home accidents. Develop a brief report on the subject "Home Accidents a Major Cause of Death in the United States."
5. Keep a scrapbook of newspaper stories that report the home accidents occurring in the local area. Determine the cause of each accident, how each could have been prevented, and the first-aid protection required for each type of injury suspected and identified.

QUESTIONS TO ANSWER

1. What hazards are found in the farm home that are not in the urban home?
2. What type of fractures are most common among adult home accident victims?
3. Identify the leading causes of death for children under 5 years of age.
4. About how many persons are killed and injured in home accidents annually?
5. What age group has the most frequent victims of home accidents?
6. What reasons are given for stating that home accidents may continue to occur in significant numbers?

7 What might account for the rising number of drownings around the home each year?
8 What environmental hazards most often relate to home accidents?
9 What are the most common causes of death by suffocation?
10 Identify the two basic factors related to home accidental deaths and injuries.

SELECTED REFERENCES

AMERICAN NATIONAL RED CROSS, *Standard First Aid and Personal Safety*. New York: Doubleday, 1973.

COLE, WARREN H., and PUESTOW, CHARLES B., *First Aid: Diagnosis and Management*. New York: Appleton-Century-Crofts, 1965.

GREEN, MARTIN I., *A Sigh of Relief—The First-Aid Handbook for Childhood Emergencies*. New York: Bantam Books, 1977.

HALSEY, MAXWELL (editorial consultant), *Accident Prevention*. New York: McGraw-Hill, 1961.

HENDERSON, JOHN, *Emergency Medical Guide*, 4th ed. New York: McGraw-Hill, 1978.

KLOTZ, S. D., *Guide to Modern Medical Care*. New York: Scribner, 1967.

NATIONAL SAFETY COUNCIL, *Accident Facts*. Chicago: The Council, 1977.

RUSLINK, DORIS, *Family Health and Home Nursing*. New York: Macmillan, 1967.

STRASSER, M. K., et al., *Fundamentals of Safety Education*. New York: Macmillan, 1973.

U.S. DEPARTMENT OF HEALTH, EDUCATION, AND WELFARE, *Family Guide Emergency Health Care*. Washington, D.C.: The Department, 1967.

19. PUBLIC ACCIDENT VICTIMS

Public accidents include those incidents related to recreation, transportation (except motor vehicle), and public buildings. These types of accidents have been rising in recent years because of the increase in the amount of leisure time that people have to devote to off-the-job activity. Safety experts have become concerned about the rise in deaths and injuries related to recreational and outdoor education activities. A basic question that must be answered is "How can people safely participate in leisure-time activities?" It would seem that a good part of the answer is related to planning, acquiring basic skills and knowledge, and the procurement of safe equipment. Physical condition must also be a primary consideration for all participants.

TYPES OF PUBLIC-RECREATIONAL ACCIDENTS

Today there are in excess of 100 million swimmers, 52 million boat users, 6 million water skiers, 30 million golfers, and 20 million hunters in the United States. Noncommercial flying is more popular than ever, with some 115,000 small aircraft in use. Most of these are owned by individuals and certainly add to the problem of public accidents.

All Public Accidents

Annually there are more than 21,500 public accidental deaths reported throughout the nation. This is a death rate of about 10.1 per 100,000 persons. These include deaths in public places or places used in a public way. Most sports and recreation deaths are a part of this total.

Types of Public-Recreational Accidents [285]

Although deaths are reported in each age range, the 65 and over, 15 to 24, and 45 to 65 have a significant number of public deaths each year. The number of disabling injuries is estimated to be approximately 2.7 million annually. However, this number is reported to be conservative due to the lack of an adequate system to collect and report such data.

Falls

Deaths as a result of falls in public places reach about 4,600 each year. The 65 and over age group is involved in more than four fifths of the total. The remaining deaths are scattered throughout all other age ranges. Most deaths of this type involve males more frequently than females.

The number of injuries sustained are unknown due to the lack of a satisfactory system for the collection of such information. But obviously the number of injuries would be in the thousands.

Drownings

Drownings account for about one fourth of all public accidental deaths. This seems to be an alarming number in view of the significant efforts that have been made to teach swimming and water survival techniques during recent years. But studies indicate that most of the general public would be rated as fair or poor swimmers. Perhaps this is a partial answer to the fact that there were some 4,500 persons who drowned in a recent year. This number does not include those persons drowned when a boat was involved.

Most drownings occur in the 15 to 24 age range with the 25 to 44 group a close second. Also there is a high incidence of drownings among the 5 to 14 and the under-4 age groups. Due to the high percentage of male swimmers, they are the most frequent victims of drownings.

Firearms

The number of persons using firearms for recreation has increased about 25 percent in the past decade. This is the largest increase of participants in any leisure-time activity.

The National Rifle Association has attempted to make firearm use a safe activity through the organization of clubs and the sponsorship of training classes. No doubt these efforts have been fruitful. But the fact remains that about 900 persons are killed each year in firearms accidents. Some 600 to 800 of these are hunting deaths. For each fatality there are about six nonfatal hunting injuries. This number does not include those mentioned in Chapter 18 related to the home accident problem.

FIGURE 19.1 SCOPE OF THE BOATING ACCIDENT PROBLEM IN THE UNITED STATES. ACCIDENT DATA BY STATE

	NUMBER OF ACCIDENTS				NUMBER OF VESSELS INVOLVED IN ACCIDENTS				NUMBER OF PERSONS		AMOUNT OF DAMAGE (DOLLARS)
	Total	Fatal	Non-Fatal Injury	Property Damage Only	Total	Fatal	Non-Fatal Injury	Property Damage Only	Killed	Injured Non-Fatally	
Total	6308	1170	1401	3737	8002	1178	1485	5339	1466	2136	$10,352,100
Alabama	121	33	30	58	146	34	31	81	40	44	144,500
Alaska	69	13	7	49	76	13	7	56	15	11	179,600
Arizona	115	7	28	80	141	8	28	105	8	42	204,400
Arkansas	41	21	7	13	47	21	7	19	26	10	29,900
California	898	97	174	627	1,227	95	186	946	125	263	1,586,400
Colorado	26	6	4	16	32	6	5	21	6	6	13,700
Connecticut	88	22	18	48	111	22	18	71	24	24	113,500
Delaware	18	6		12	21	6		15	7	1	30,500
District of Columbia	13	3	2	8	17	3	2	12	4	7	32,600
Florida	620	60	125	435	737	60	128	549	70	168	1,970,700
Georgia	98	20	22	56	128	20	22	86	26	37	97,300
Hawaii	62	4	10	48	74	4	10	60	4	13	228,200
Idaho	41	7	11	23	47	7	13	27	10	19	41,400
Illinois	121	35	30	56	159	35	32	92	55	56	118,600
Indiana	99	19	30	50	133	19	32	82	22	41	91,700
Iowa	66	11	13	42	84	11	15	58	11	26	67,100
Kansas	44	11	13	20	56	12	13	31	14	16	36,600
Kentucky	72	32	14	26	83	34	15	34	42	24	139,700
Louisiana	139	40	32	67	162	41	33	88	54	56	141,300
Maine	52	10	13	29	64	10	13	41	13	19	65,700

[286]

Maryland	173	17	35	121	237	17	36	184	18	49	587,200
Massachusetts	112	27	19	66	158	27	19	112	43	25	120,300
Michigan	369	58	170	141	454	59	178	217	70	227	399,100
Minnesota	121	40	34	47	168	40	37	91	49	52	66,400
Mississippi	54	17	7	30	66	17	9	40	26	15	40,500
Missouri	189	16	47	126	224	17	50	157	18	73	196,600
Montana	15	9	2	4	17	9	2	6	13	4	2,000
Nebraska	36	2	15	19	55	2	16	37	3	18	32,100
Nevada	67	4	10	53	78	4	10	64	4	16	104,200
New Hampshire	7	5		2	8	5		3	7		4,300
New Jersey	229	25	43	161	302	25	44	233	31	69	423,300
New Mexico	26	6	7	13	31	6	7	18	8	11	43,600
New York	368	65	75	228	481	66	79	336	83	129	510,100
North Carolina	184	46	41	97	222	46	42	134	53	54	350,400
North Dakota	5		3	2	8		3	5		3	4,000
Ohio	101	31	13	57	127	31	14	82	40	29	120,800
Oklahoma	59	17	15	27	73	17	17	39	23	21	49,200
Oregon	125	32	22	71	147	32	24	91	36	38	198,600
Pennsylvania	81	30	24	27	99	30	25	44	41	37	70,300
Rhode Island	41	2	5	34	57	2	7	48	2	8	132,500
South Carolina	144	46	27	71	177	46	32	99	54	46	159,400
South Dakota	6	1	1	4	8	1	1	6	1	5	9,000
Tennessee	94	30	20	44	119	30	22	67	32	34	55,400
Texas	328	56	63	209	424	56	76	292	71	111	380,700
Utah	47	9	12	26	60	10	12	38	14	25	105,200
Vermont	14	5	3	6	17	5	3	9	8	6	19,600
Virginia	122	31	30	61	147	31	31	85	42	43	199,500
Washington	212	36	23	153	279	36	23	220	42	30	330,100
West Virginia	15	8	2	5	16	8	2	6	9	4	32,100
Wisconsin	137	31	47	59	171	31	51	89	35	68	97,500
Wyoming	13	7	2	4	14	7	2	5	8		8,000
Guam	1			1	1			1		2	300
Puerto Rico	9	3	1	5	11	3	1	7	4	1	166,300
Virgin Islands	1	1			1	1			2		100

Source: United States Coast Guard.

[287]

[288] Public Accident Victims

Fire Burns

There are about 6,000 lives lost each year in accidents occurring in public places that are caused by fires and falling objects. This number includes deaths from fires, burns, asphyxiation, and falls. The need for rigid building and fire codes in order to eliminate such accidental deaths is obvious. Most cities are working toward the establishment and enforcement of such codes.

Flying

Flying as a recreational sport has increased significantly in recent years. It is reported that presently some 65 percent of all aircraft in use are classified for noncommercial general aviation purposes. The modern airplane is a very safe vehicle. About 1,000 deaths were reported in a recent year, which represents a death rate close to 66 per 100,000,000 miles of travel. When compared to the death rates for other types of human activity, the air transport rate is about the lowest.

Water Transport

Boating is the most rapidly expanding recreational activity in the United States today. Figure 19.1 depicts the scope of the boating accident problem as reported by the United States Coast Guard. The 1,200 deaths reported by the National Safety Council represents a figure that has tended to become stabilized in recent years. It is observed that in 90 percent of the cases a lifesaving device was not used. Yet in 61 percent of these cases a lifesaving device was available in the boat. As a result of the increase in the number of boat users, accidental deaths in this category could increase.

Education programs in boat safety should be increased to assure that those using such vehicles know how best to handle these craft. In view of the serious hazard to life via drowning, it would be wise for all boat users to complete a first-aid course in order to be able to handle water emergencies.

Railroad

There are about 400 public deaths each year related to locomotives. This number represents about a 60 percent decrease in train-related deaths during the past ten years. Today the number of railroad deaths is less than 1 percent of the total public accidental deaths recorded annually. With fewer trains in use, as highway and railroad grade crossings are eliminated, and as public safety programs educate the general populace, this type of accidental death should virtually be eliminated.

Other Transport

Each year there are about 200 deaths involving streetcars, bicycles, and animal-drawn vehicles. Because of the phasing out of streetcar use and animal drawn vehicles, this number has decreased significantly in the past two decades. It should be mentioned that this number does not include scooters, tricycles, subways, and trolley buses. These are reported under a different traffic accident classification and do occur in serious numbers each year.

All Other Public

Those accidents not classified previously include deaths from lightning, excessive heat or cold. There are about 8,100 public accident deaths reported each year in this category.

Camping

The camping movement has grown beyond all expectations in the past twenty years. This type of leisure-time activity has captured the interest of people from all walks of life. It is estimated that there are now approximately 16 million camping families in the nation. Overall the number of persons involved in camping is approaching 20 million.

Accidents have also accompanied the expanding interest in camping. Most states and in some instances federal agencies have established rules and regulations for the use of parks and other camp facilities in an effort to curb accidents. Facts are not available concerning injuries and deaths in this type of activity.

A SPECIAL PROBLEM: EPILEPSY

All types of people participate in recreational activities. These include persons with some type of physical impairment or condition of the nervous system. One special problem is that of epilepsy. The subject of epilepsy and seizures is treated in Chapter 15. The discussion that follows relates the problem to swimming, a common activity for persons subject to seizures.

The following information is based upon an article appearing in the *National News*, a publication of the Epilepsy Foundation of America.[1]

The first and most important thing to do for a child having a grand mal seizure while swimming is to get him out of the pool, according to

---

[1] Epilepsy Foundation of America, *National News*. Washington, D.C.: The Foundation, Vol. 1 No. 2 (April–May, 1968).

Kenneth Israel, M.D., psychiatric consultant for the Michigan Epilepsy Center in Detroit. Breathing stops temporarily during the seizure so the swimmer is not likely to inhale much water initially. But as he emerges from the seizure, muscles relax and the danger of drowning increases.

Specialists in the field of epilepsy say there is no standard answer as to whether or not limitations should be placed upon an epileptic person who swims. If a child is known to have seizures, it might be wise to keep him in shallow water to simplify rescue.

Persons involved with an epileptic child who wishes to swim should balance the good and danger to the child as well as the good and danger to the group. The child with infrequent seizures probably should be allowed to swim if his condition is known to the instructor and if the instructor is aware of simple first-aid techniques to employ in the event of a seizure.

The swimming instructor should rely upon the child's parents and/or physician for answers to these questions: What type of epilepsy does the child have? Are seizures completely controlled by medication? If not, are the seizures frequent or do they occur only rarely?

Although the child with frequent seizures also would benefit physically and psychologically from swimming lessons and would be reasonably safe under the watchful eyes of informed instructors, he might require the full-time attention of those instructors, thus possibly endangering other children should they need assistance.

Following are some of the questions most frequently asked by instructors and by parents of epileptic children.

> *Question:* Does physical activity, such as swimming, increase the possibility of seizures?
>
> *Answer:* On the contrary, physical activity and generally keeping the body in good physical shape tend to ward off seizures.
>
> *Question:* Is it possible to support a child in shallow water during a seizure?
>
> *Answer:* It's possible if his head can be kept above water without tightly restricting his movements. By the time he is removed from the water, he might be coming out of the seizure anyway.
>
> *Question:* If there is nothing soft at poolside on which to place a child having a grand mal seizure, is head damage from the convulsing movements possible?
>
> *Answer:* Yes, but severe damage is not likely. A couple of towels folded under the child's head would take care of the problem.
>
> *Question:* Should oxygen be given to a swimmer to bring him out of a seizure?
>
> *Answer:* Generally, no. Research indicates administration of oxygen merely prolongs a grand mal seizure. The only time oxygen is useful is if the child becomes cyanotic (turns blue, indicating serious lack of oxygen in the blood).

CAUSES OF PUBLIC ACCIDENTS

Public accidental deaths and injuries are caused by a variety of factors. Usually the primary causes relate to the violation of the basic principles of safe living and are concerned with unsafe behavior and an unsafe environment.

Undoubtedly the human element is responsible for a great many recreational accidents. The boat user, hunter, swimmer, or fisherman gets into difficulty because of some unsafe act that has been committed or some careless chances that have been taken. A poor attitude toward the safety of self and others is the basic reason for most accidents of this type.

A great many accidents occur because the person chooses a poor piece of equipment or machinery and lacks the skill for safe performance. Also he may permit the environmental conditions to become so unsafe that hazards exist all about. Good equipment and safe conditions are essential to safety in all leisure-time activities.

Many public accidents occur because there is a lack of supervision. Parents and others responsible for children, groups, or visitors should supervise the activities in which they participate. Unsupervised swimming, boating, hunting, or camping events can lead to disaster. Make certain that each of these activities is supervised and a skilled first-aider with proper first-aid equipment is a part of each such excursion.

Accidents can be the result of a lack of knowledge. Information related to each activity participated in is a must for each person. A lack of knowledge usually causes a person to perform in an unsafe and haphazard manner. Therefore individuals should educate themselves if formal education programs are not available. The American National Red Cross, National Rifle Association, State Conservation Departments, and others have training programs available. It is suggested that these be explored by all persons desiring to increase their knowledge of recreational activities.

ACTIVITIES

1 Contact the local Red Cross chapter. Discuss with the director the content of the Red Cross swimming program. Develop a report to be given orally to your class or group.
2 Write to the State Conservation Department, or other appropriate agency, requesting information on the number of boats, hunters, and fishermen in your state. Make a series of posters for display in class depicting these facts. Be prepared to discuss each.
3 Develop a research paper on the subject "Attitudes Cause a Disproportionate Share of Public Accidents."
4 Keep a scrapbook of recreational accidents reported in local news

[292] Public Accident Victims

media. Determine the cause of each accident and suggest how each could have been prevented.
5 Contact five public or private campgrounds. Determine the various safety practices and measures that have been established in each. Summarize these for a ten-minute class presentation.

QUESTIONS TO ANSWER

1 What accidents are included in the public accident category for reporting purposes and in the discussion of this chapter?
2 How does the death rate for flying accidents compare to the death rate of all public accidents?
3 Identify five factors to keep in mind in dealing with a swimmer who is subject to epileptic seizures.
4 The 65 and over age group account for what fraction of the total number of deaths resulting from falls in public places?
5 What is the most rapidly expanding leisure-time activity in the United States?
6 In what percentage of the fatal drownings reported was a lifesaving device used?
7 How does environment relate to the causing of public accidents?
8 What organization is attempting to train individuals in the use of firearms?
9 Is knowledge important in the prevention of recreational accidents? Briefly discuss.
10 Based upon recent studies, how are most swimmers rated—good, fair, poor? What might be done to improve this situation?

SELECTED REFERENCES

AMERICAN ASSOCIATION FOR HEALTH, Physical Education and Recreation, *Journal of AAHPER*. Washington, D.C.: The Association, monthly publication.
AMERICAN NATIONAL RED CROSS, *Standard First Aid and Personal Safety*. New York: Doubleday & Co., 1973.
HENDERSON, JOHN, *Emergency Medical Guide*, 4th ed. New York: McGraw-Hill, 1978.
NATIONAL SAFETY COUNCIL, *Accident Facts*. Chicago: The Council, 1977.
NATIONAL SAFETY COUNCIL, *Family Camping*. Chicago: The Council, 1968.
NATIONAL SAFETY COUNCIL, *Family Safety*. Chicago: The Council, bi-monthly publication.
NEW YORK UNIVERSITY, *Family Recreation and Safety*. New York: Center for Safety Education, 1961.

SEATON, D. C., et al., *Administration and Supervision of Safety Education.* New York: Macmillan, 1969.

STRASSER, M. K., et al., *Fundamentals of Safety Education.* New York: Macmillan, 1973.

U. S. COAST GUARD, Boating Statistics—1975. Washington, D.C.: Department of Transportation, 1976.

20. INDUSTRIAL ACCIDENT VICTIMS

Accidental deaths involving industrial workers have been reduced 71 percent in the past 64 years. An estimated 18,000 to 21,000 lives were taken in 1912 in on-the-job accidents, whereas in 1976, with a work force triple in size and producing about eight times as much, industrial accidents claimed but 12,500 work deaths. The death rate for all industrial accidents was 14 for each 100,000 workers during a recent year.

Disabling injuries totaled approximately 2.2 million during a recent year, a number that has been somewhat constant in spite of the increase

FIGURE 20.1 SCOPE OF THE WORK ACCIDENT PROBLEM

Industry Group	Workers (000)	Deaths 1976	Change from 1975	Death Rates 1976	1966	% Change	Disabling Injuries 1976
All INDUSTRIES	87,800	12,500	−500	14	20	−30%	2,200,000
Trade	20,300	1,300	0	6	8	−25%	400,000
Manufacturing	19,000	1,700	+100	9	10	−10%	470,000
Service	20,800	1,800	−100	9	13	−31%	400,000
Government	14,900	1,700	0	11	13	−15%	320,000
Transportation and public utilities	4,800	1,500	−100	31	40	−23%	180,000
Agriculture	3,500	1,900	−200	54	69	−23%	200,000
Construction	3,700	2,100	−200	57	74	−23%	200,000
Mining, quarrying	800	500	0	63	108	−42%	40,000

Source: National Safety Council.

Falls [295]

in the number of industrial workers. The reduction in work deaths and injuries has no doubt been the result of the accident prevention and education programs pioneered in industry. OSHA requirements also have influenced the lowering of industrial accidents.

Industrial safety has been a major concern of the nation since the beginning of the present century. The loss of our human resources in work accidents has been the subject of much legislation at both the state and national levels. Such legislation has placed legal and moral responsibilities upon the employer for the safety of his employees.

The various industrial safety programs implemented have significantly reduced the incidence of on-the-job accidents. The problem currently facing the employer is how to keep the worker safe while off the job. Generally speaking, the ability of industry to operate at a profit in the future will be related to the number of off-the-job accidents eliminated.

WHERE ACCIDENTS OCCUR

Of the 12,500 workers killed in 1976, about 1,300 lives were lost in the trade industries. There also were 49,000 disabling injuries reported for this type of industry. The manufacturing industries accounted for 1,700 deaths and 470,000 major injuries, whereas in service industries deaths were 1,800 accompanied by 340,000 disabling injuries. Government-related industries experienced some 1,700 deaths and 32,000 injuries, and transportation and public utilities accounted for 1,500 deaths and 180,000 disabling injuries. Agriculture, one of the nation's leading industries, had 1,900 work deaths and 19,000 injuries reported; the construction industry had 2,100 deaths among workers along with 200,000 serious reportable injuries. The lowest number of work deaths was recorded in the mining industry. There were 500 deaths and only 40,000 disabling injuries experienced in a recent year.

FALLS

Next to traffic collisions there are more people killed by falls than by any other type of accidental occurrence. For example, falls kill about 3,000 on-the-job employees each year. Moreover, approximately one fourth of all work injuries are caused by falls.

People on the job fall off ladders or fall as a result of spilled liquids or poor housekeeping conditions. It should be pointed out that a person does not have to fall off something high in order to be hurt. Falls on the same level are among the most frequent type of accident reported.

[296]   Industrial Accident Victims

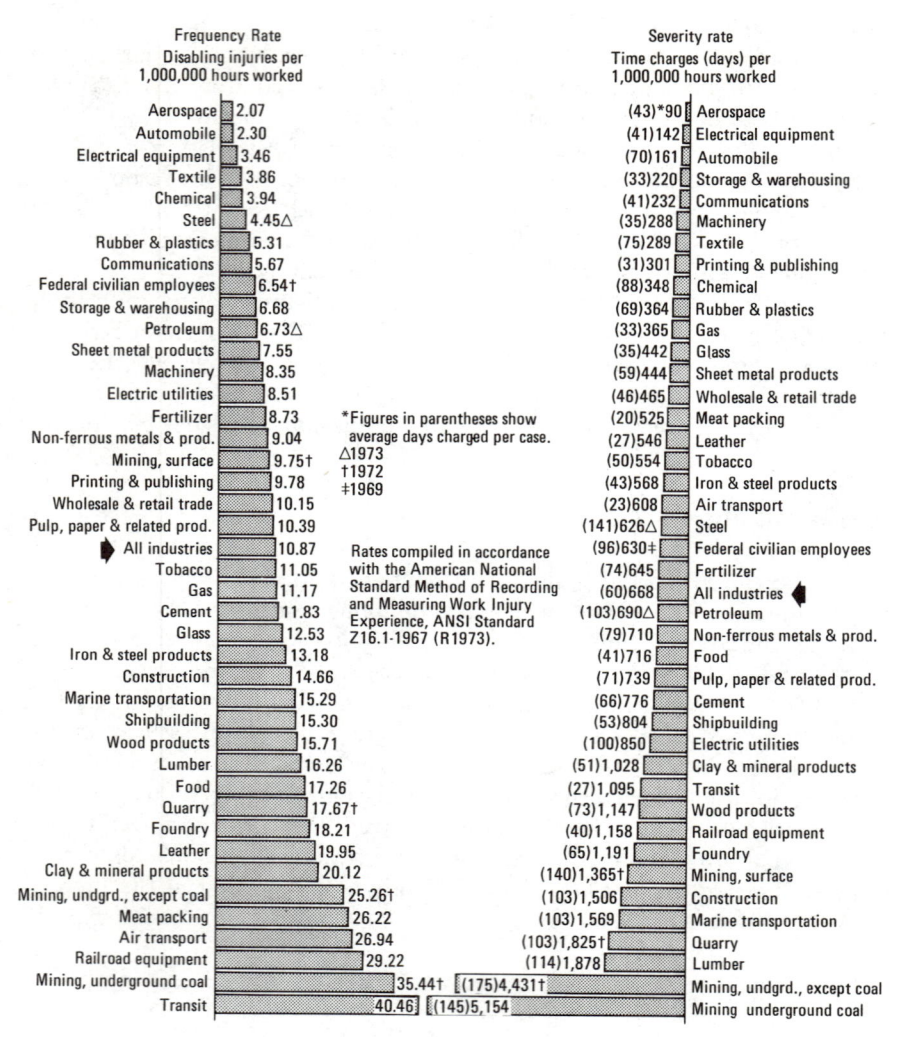

Frequency Rate Disabling injuries per 1,000,000 hours worked		Severity rate Time charges (days) per 1,000,000 hours worked	
Aerospace	2.07	(43)*90	Aerospace
Automobile	2.30	(41)142	Electrical equipment
Electrical equipment	3.46	(70)161	Automobile
Textile	3.86	(33)220	Storage & warehousing
Chemical	3.94	(41)232	Communications
Steel	4.45△	(35)288	Machinery
Rubber & plastics	5.31	(75)289	Textile
Communications	5.67	(31)301	Printing & publishing
Federal civilian employees	6.54†	(88)348	Chemical
Storage & warehousing	6.68	(69)364	Rubber & plastics
Petroleum	6.73△	(33)365	Gas
Sheet metal products	7.55	(35)442	Glass
Machinery	8.35	(59)444	Sheet metal products
Electric utilities	8.51	(46)465	Wholesale & retail trade
Fertilizer	8.73	(20)525	Meat packing
Non-ferrous metals & prod.	9.04	(27)546	Leather
Mining, surface	9.75†	(50)554	Tobacco
Printing & publishing	9.78	(43)568	Iron & steel products
Wholesale & retail trade	10.15	(23)608	Air transport
Pulp, paper & related prod.	10.39	(141)626△	Steel
All industries	10.87	(96)630‡	Federal civilian employees
Tobacco	11.05	(74)645	Fertilizer
Gas	11.17	(60)668	All industries
Cement	11.83	(103)690△	Petroleum
Glass	12.53	(79)710	Non-ferrous metals & prod.
Iron & steel products	13.18	(41)716	Food
Construction	14.66	(71)739	Pulp, paper & related prod.
Marine transportation	15.29	(66)776	Cement
Shipbuilding	15.30	(53)804	Shipbuilding
Wood products	15.71	(100)850	Electric utilities
Lumber	16.26	(51)1,028	Clay & mineral products
Food	17.26	(27)1,095	Transit
Quarry	17.67†	(73)1,147	Wood products
Foundry	18.21	(40)1,158	Railroad equipment
Leather	19.95	(65)1,191	Foundry
Clay & mineral products	20.12	(140)1,365†	Mining, surface
Mining, undgrd., except coal	25.26†	(103)1,506	Construction
Meat packing	26.22	(103)1,569	Marine transportation
Air transport	26.94	(103)1,825†	Quarry
Railroad equipment	29.22	(114)1,878	Lumber
Mining, underground coal	35.44†	(175)4,431†	Mining, undgrd., except coal
Transit	40.46	(145)5,154	Mining underground coal

*Figures in parentheses show average days charged per case.
△1973
†1972
‡1969

Rates compiled in accordance with the American National Standard Method of Recording and Measuring Work Injury Experience, ANSI Standard Z16.1-1967 (R1973).

FIGURE 20.2   Work accident injury rates by industry. (National Safety Council)

OFFICE ACCIDENTS

Individuals who work in offices usually have the false impression that accidents do not occur in this type of work environment. The National Safety Council reports a .71 accident frequency rate and a 107 severity rate for office accidents when compared to other type work accidents.

Office Accidents [297]

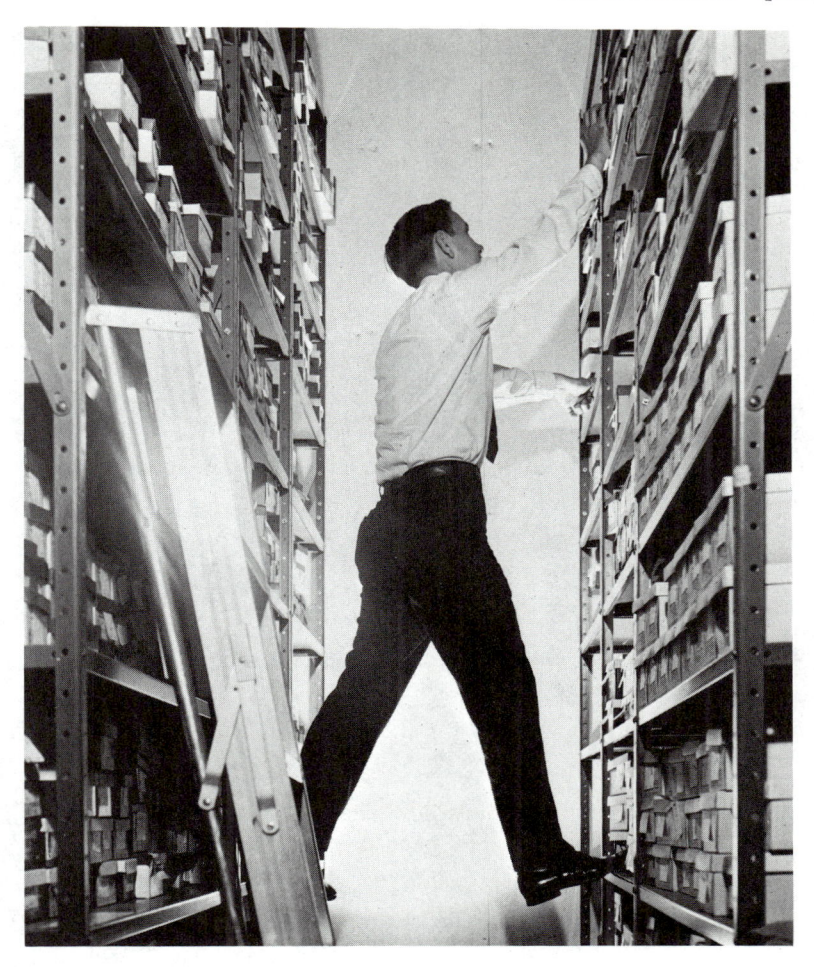

FIGURE 20.3 Falls from ladders are common industrial accidents. (AEtna Life & Casualty)

Often these are falls on stairs or caused by coffee spills, paper clips, or telephone cords. High heels, certain dress fashions, loose jewelry, thumbtacks, razor blades, sharp pencils, and paper cutters are also potential sources of office accidents.

Improper lifting is the cause of injuries in the office as well as in the performance of job tasks in other places. Figure 20.5 shows the proper way to lift articles, light or heavy.

[298]   Industrial Accident Victims

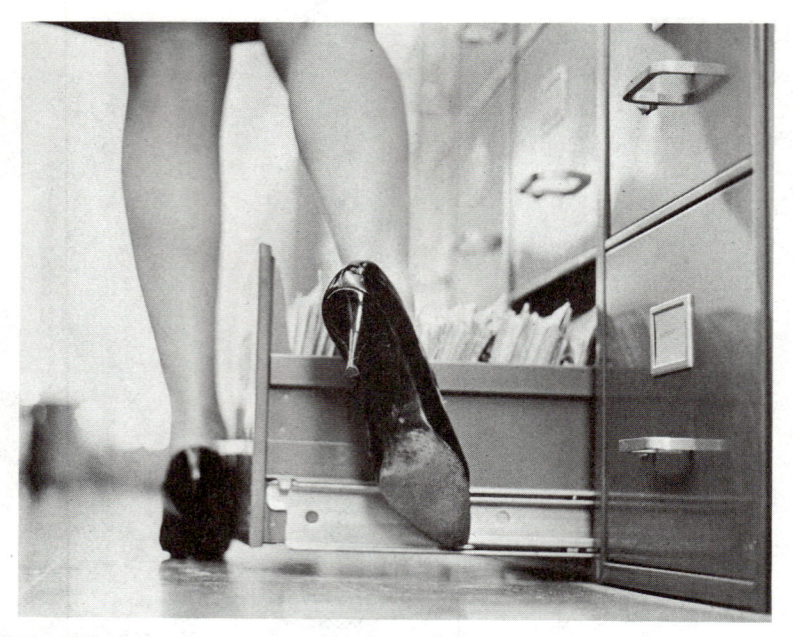

FIGURE 20.4   Open file cabinets can cause office accidents. (AEtna Fire & Casualty)

LIFTING

As mentioned, improper lifting is the source of injuries in the office as well as in industrial jobs. The back is usually strained because

1. The size of the job that the back has to do.
2. The amount of strength the back has to do that job.
3. The way a man goes about his job, bending or twisting in awkward positions; hurrying, quick, rough motions; or a "never-say-die" attitude of not giving up when tired.[1]

The subject of strain is discussed more thoroughly in Chapter 11, for first-aid protection refer to that chapter. However, as a summary of the problem relative to back strain and lifting the following are listed:

1. Most back strains result from making the back do more than it has the strength to do.
2. The majority of back strains heal when restraining the back is avoided.
3. As the swayed-in position of the lower back is its weakest, to avoid strain means to avoid increasing the curve in the lower back at all times.
4. When doing anything that requires standing, one foot is placed on some-

[1] William K. Ishmael and Howard B. Shorbe, *Care of the Back—Industrial Edition*. Philadelphia: Lippincott, 1962.

Lifting [299]

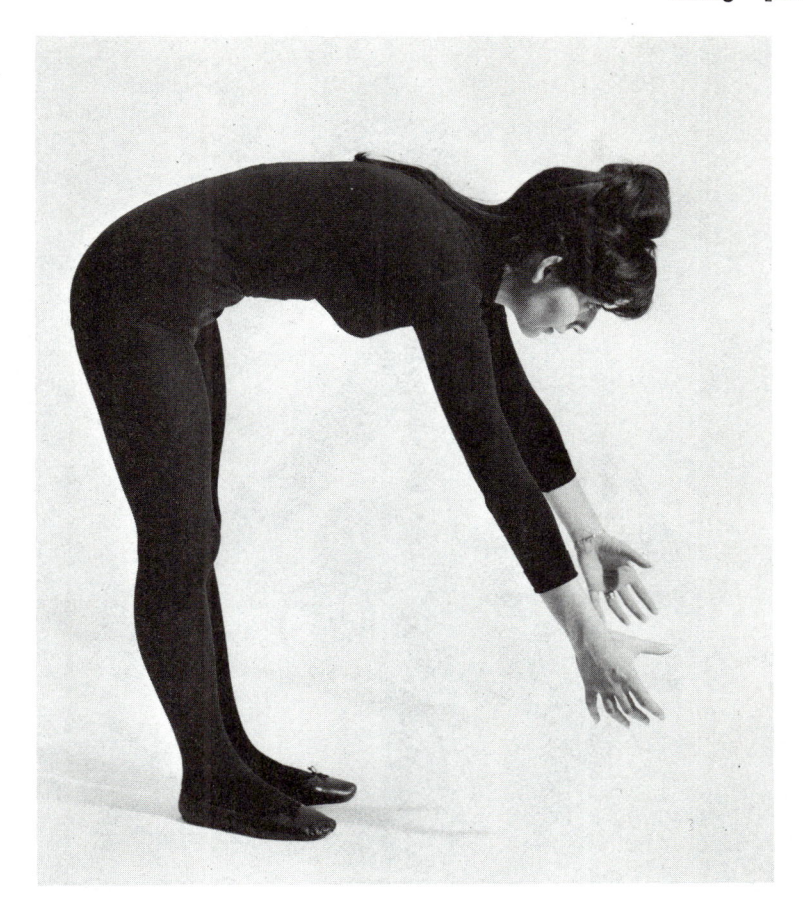

FIGURE 20.5A Improper method of lifting. (AEtna Life & Casualty)

thing that will bend the knee and hip and flatten the lower back, to lessen strain.

5. When sitting, one or both knees are kept higher than the hips. The legs are crossed or the feet are placed on a stool, keeping the knees bent. When driving a car, the seat is kept close to the pedals to elevate the knees to relieve strain.

6. As a measure to correct low back sway, bending exercises to strengthen the abdominal muscles are helpful. These exercises also stretch the contracted low back muscles.

7. It is usually necessary to consult a physician to detect and correct deficiencies or diseases that weaken the back structures.

8. A person is not to lose sleep or go beyond his endurance. He should rest before he gets too tired, but sufficient general exercise is necessary to prevent weakness from lack of use.

[300]   Industrial Accident Victims

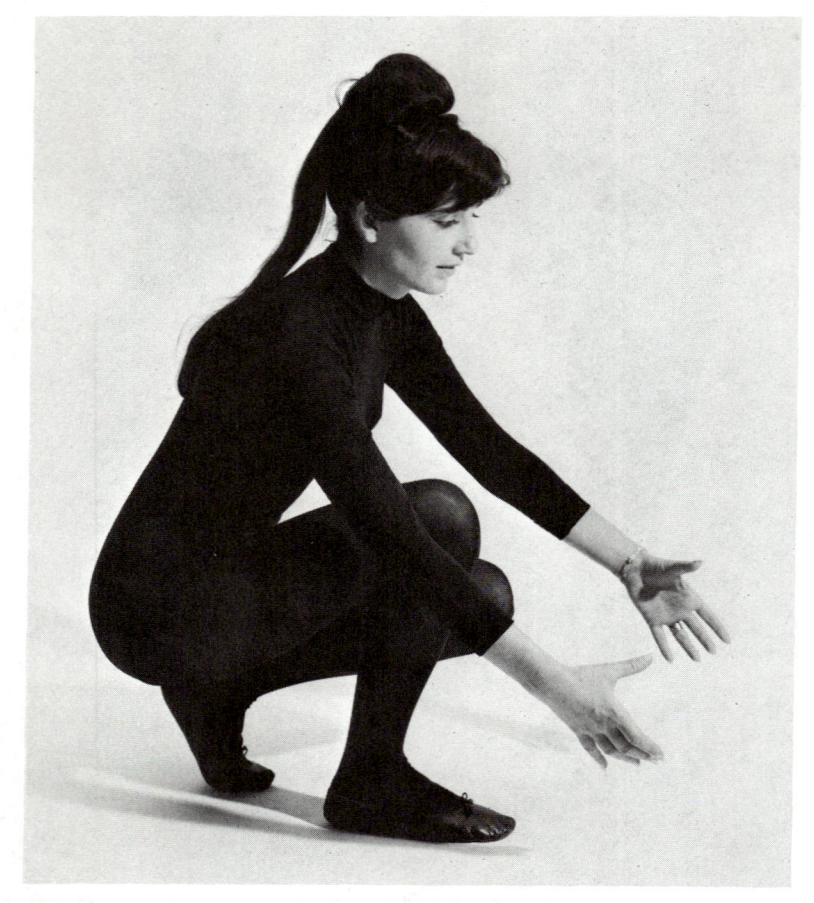

FIGURE 20.5B   Proper method of lifting. (Aetna Life & Casualty)

9   If a person has more than an average amount of low back sway, or if his back is strained, special remedial exercises must be done before excessive general exercise is attempted.
10   A person is to control his weight. The smaller the waistline, the less strain on the back.[2]

COST OF WORK ACCIDENTS

The total cost of work accidents in 1976 was in excess of $17.8 billion. This amount included $7.9 billion for visible costs (wage losses, insurance and medical costs) and $7.9 billion for other costs (money value of worker-lost-time and time required to investigate and handle each acci-

[2] Ibid., p. 22.

Cost of Work Accidents [301]

dent). Also there were $2 billion in fire losses reported. On the average it cost industry about $200 for each work accident.

The losses mentioned are the losses computed for lack of development of comprehensive on- and off-the-job accident prevention programs by all industries. In addition the need for first aid and industrial hygiene staff and facilities is evident. With such personnel and facilities industry eliminates some of the work cost losses through prompt attention to all injuries.

Lost Time

It is significant to note that there were 245 million man-days of time lost due to industrial accidents during a recent year. This lost time interrupted production schedules and made it necessary for the industries involved to operate on a less efficient basis. Work accidents are a major blow to the nation's economy.

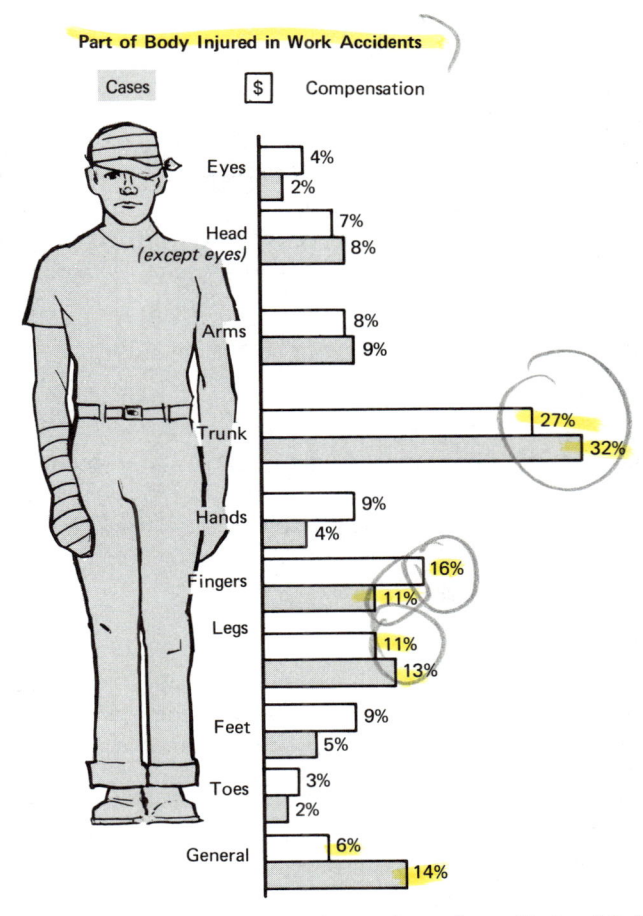

Part of Body Injured	Cases	Compensation
Eyes	4%	2%
Head (except eyes)	7%	8%
Arms	8%	9%
Trunk	27%	32%
Hands	9%	4%
Fingers	16%	11%
Legs	11%	13%
Feet	9%	5%
Toes	3%	2%
General	6%	14%

FIGURE 20.6 Body parts frequently injured in work accidents. (National Safety Council)

[302] Industrial Accident Victims

CAUSES OF INDUSTRIAL ACCIDENTS

Work accidents are due to a number of causes. However, upon examination of reports submitted by industries to the National Safety Council and other organizations, it is possible to conclude that most of these accidents are the result of (1) unsafe human acts or (2) an unsafe environment.

Unsafe Human Acts

Acting in an imprudent manner tends to cause industrial accidents. The person's behavior while performing work tasks will in large measure determine whether the work will be performed safely. Carelessness, horse play, using equipment improperly, and operating at unsafe speeds are among the primary unsafe acts that cause work deaths and injuries.

Unsafe Environment

Unsafe work conditions are the basis for numerous work accidents. Improper work layout, defective equipment, unsafe dress, poor housekeeping, and inadequate machine guarding are some of the main environmental factors relative to work accidents. Conditions must be hazard-free if the person is to work accident-free. First-aid protection is needed frequently in many plants because of injuries sustained from an unsafe work environment.

PART OF BODY INJURED

Disabling work injuries total about 2.2 million according to State Labor Department reports. Of this number 12,500 were fatal and 80,000 resulted in some degree of permanent impairment. Figure 20.6 depicts the distribution of body parts injured in work accidents.

Frequency of Injury

Injuries to the trunk were the most frequent, 27 percent, and thumb and finger injuries next, 16 percent. The legs were injured in 13 percent of the reported cases, the feet and hands 6 percent, and the arms in about 9 percent.

Injuries to the trunk also account for the greater number of fatal incidents, and head injuries are the second most frequent cause of fatal work accidents. Permanent injuries most frequently involve the thumb and fingers, with injuries to the head second.

The trunk is that part of the body most often involved in temporary disabilities, with the thumb and fingers the second most frequent source of temporary injuries. The foot and hand are next in frequency.

Severity of Injury

Approximately one out of 100 compensable injuries results in a fatality. About one fourth leave some type of permanent impairment. Severity to the different parts of the body varies. Some two out of 100 fatal injuries are to the head. While about one out of 100 injuries to the trunk is fatal. For other body parts the number of fatal injuries is very small. Usually other parts of the body are involved in permanent or temporary disabilities only.

OFF-THE-JOB INJURIES

There are more workers killed and injured off the job than on the job. Therefore, this is the most important problem facing industry management today. The National Safety Council reports some 38,200 off-the-job

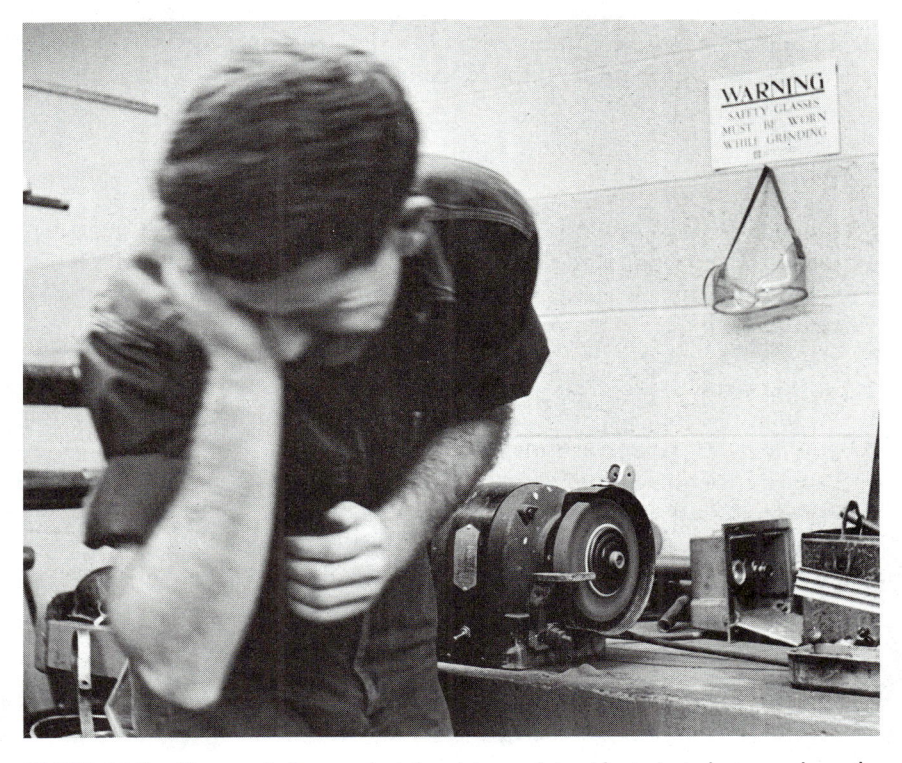

FIGURE 20.7 The eye is frequently injured in work accidents in industry and on the farm. (AEtna Life & Casualty)

[304]   Industrial Accident Victims

deaths as opposed to 12,500 on-the-job deaths. Injuries while off the job are about 3 million annually, compared to 2.2 million on the job. Industry is in business to make a profit, so that interest in off-the-job accidents is a national by-product of the profit motive. Because accidents are costly in production output and in the training of new workers, off-the-job safety programs emerged as the most dynamic influence in the industrial accident prevention movement of the 1960s. In the 1970s the Occupation Safety and Health Act has been an important deterrent to industrial accidents.

FARM ACCIDENTS

Farm-related occupations are among the most dangerous available to the nation's work force. The death rate for farm accidents ranks fourth when compared with other industries. There are approximately 1,700 deaths and 190,000 disabling injuries in agriculture-related accidents reported each year.

The lack of consistent supervision of farm workers on the job and insufficient educational programs perhaps account for the high incidence of farm accidents. Farm Bureau, 4-H Clubs, and other state agricultural organizations are developing programs of accident prevention for the farm population. These efforts should pay dividends in a lower frequency rate of accidents among the farm residents of the nation.

ACTIVITIES

1   Contact five local industries and request information concerning their accident frequency and severity ratings and first-aid facilities. Determine the adequacy of each of the industries' first-aid programs to take care of their accident problems.
2   Develop a first-aid program to take care of an industry with 500 workers. Include necessary facilities, staff, and equipment.
3   Write a research paper on the subject "The Influence of Off-the-Job Accidents in American Industry."
4   Back injuries are common among industrial workers. In cooperation with an industrial nurse develop a rehabilitation program to strengthen a back that has been severely strained in the lower lumbar region.
5   Develop a series of posters depicting five of the most common types of work accidents needing first-aid protection. Describe the first-aid protection required.

QUESTIONS TO ANSWER

1. What is the percentage reduction in the past 64 years of accidental deaths involving industrial workers?
2. What are the two factors responsible for work-related accidents?
3. Identify causes of office accidents.
4. Discuss briefly the causes of back strain.
5. How many persons are killed each year in occupational-type farm accidents?
6. Why are industries concerned about off-the-job accidents?
7. Define "visible" as opposed to "other" costs of occupational accidents.
8. When sitting, what can be done to avoid back strain?
9. How many man-days are lost yearly due to industrial accidents?
10. What role does an unsafe environment play in causing accidents?

SELECTED REFERENCES

AMERICAN NATIONAL RED CROSS, *Standard First Aid and Personal Safety*. New York: Doubleday, 1973.

BRENNAN, WILLIAM T., and LUDWIG, DONALD J., *Guide to Problems and Practices In First Aid and Emergency Care*. Dubuque, Ia.: Wm. C. Brown, 1976.

COLE, WILLIAM H., and PUESTOW, CHARLES B., *First Aid: Diagnosis and Management*. New York: Appleton-Century-Crofts, 1965.

HALSEY, MAXWELL (editorial consultant), *Accident Prevention*. New York: McGraw-Hill, 1961.

HENDERSON, JOHN, *Emergency Medical Guide*, 4th ed. New York: McGraw-Hill, 1978.

ISHMAEL, WILLIAM, and SHORBE, HOWARD, *Care of the Back—Industrial Edition*. Philadelphia: Lippincott, 1962.

NATIONAL SAFETY COUNCIL, *Accident Facts*. Chicago: The Council, 1977.

NATIONAL SAFETY COUNCIL, *Accident Prevention Manual for Industrial Operations*. Chicago: The Council, 1976.

National Safety Council Supervisors Safety Manual. Chicago: The Council, 1967.

STACK, HERBERT, and ELKOW, J. DUKE, *Education for Safe Living*. Englewood Cliffs, N.J.: Prentice-Hall, 1966.

21. SCHOOL ACCIDENT VICTIMS

Since 1920 the accidental death rate for elementary schoolchildren has decreased approximately 50 percent. During the same period of time the accidental death rate for secondary students declined, then stabilized, and in recent years has been on the increase. Outstanding jobs of implementing programs of education for safe living have no doubt accounted for the success in elementary schools. At the secondary and college levels there seems to be a lack of interest and desire to prevent accidents. As a result, accident prevention programs have not been developed to the same degree as on the elementary school level. But a need for such programs is evident, for the leading cause of death for all persons under 24 years of age is accidents.[1] Figure 21.1 portrays this fact.

The school has two basic responsibilities toward the development of safety education and accident prevention programs. One of these responsibilities is that of keeping the child safe while in school and, to the degree possible, to and from school. Secondly, the school has the task of educating the child in the modification of personal behavior and in the development of appropriate habits, knowledge, and skills essential for safe living. These responsibilities are either a legal or moral responsibility. A program that accomplishes appropriate results must be continuous and comprehensive in nature.

[1] National Safety Council, *Accidents Facts*. Chicago: The Council, 1977.

THE ELEMENTARY SCHOOL

Accidents account for approximately one third of all deaths involving preschool and elementary-age children. Thus, it is essential that they receive an early education in safety. The preschool child must be introduced to principles and practices of safe living by his parents. A program of safety education should be an integral part of a child's elementary school education and experiences. It is through the educational process that young children will learn to live safely in today's society. A primary objective of the elementary school should be to provide an instructional program that prepares youngsters to live, play, and work in a basically hostile environment. Unless this is accomplished elementary schoolchildren will continue to be involved in a great many accidents each year.

To care for students who are injured at school, a first-aid facility and a school nurse should be available at all times. The principles outlined in Chapter 3 and suggestions in Chapter 25 could be used as guides by elementary schools in the organization and development of such a program.

FIGURE 21.1 LEADING CAUSES OF DEATH IN UNITED STATES, AGES 1–24

Cause	Number of Deaths			Death Rates		
	Total	Male	Female	Total	Male	Female
1 to 14 Years: ALL CAUSES	22,539	13,537	9,002	44.6	52.5	36.4
Accidents	10,429	6,939	3,490	20.6	26.9	14.1
Motor-vehicle	4,607	2,936	1,671	9.1	11.4	6.7
Drowning	2,060	1,570	490	4.1	6.1	2.0
Fires, burns	1,197	657	540	2.4	2.5	2.2
Firearms	492	391	101	1.0	1.5	0.4
Cancer	2,518	1,418	1,100	5.0	5.5	4.4
Congenital anomalies	1,883	948	935	3.7	3.7	3.8
Pneumonia	837	419	418	1.7	1.6	1.7
Homicide	702	397	305	1.4	1.5	1.2
Heart disease	567	318	249	1.1	1.2	1.0
Stroke (cerebrovascular disease)	309	164	145	0.6	0.6	0.6
15 to 24 Years: ALL CAUSES	47,545	35,508	12,037	118.9	176.8	60.5
Accidents	24,121	19,416	4,705	60.3	96.7	23.7
Motor-vehicle	15,672	12,224	3,428	39.2	61.0	17.2
Drowning	2,520	2,280	240	6.3	11.4	1.2
Poison (solid, liquid)	1,332	1,048	284	3.3	5.2	1.4
Firearms	758	681	77	1.9	3.4	0.4
Homicide	5,493	4,258	1,235	13.7	21.2	6.2
Suicide	4,736	3,787	949	11.8	18.9	4.8
Cancer	2,701	1,626	1,075	6.8	8.1	5.4
Heart disease	1,045	631	414	2.6	3.1	2.1

Source: National Safety Council.

THE SECONDARY SCHOOL

The National Safety Council reports that the accident fatality rate for the 15- to 19-year-old group is about 2.6 times that of the 10- to 14-year-old age group. Overall the accident frequency rate for secondary school students is high. Perhaps this is due to the different activities of this age group as opposed to those activities of junior high school students. Also, the apparent lack of educational programs for safe living in secondary schools would suggest a lack of interest and concern for the prevention of accidents among high school students.

As mentioned previously, the accident frequency and severity rate involving high school youth has been on the increase in recent years. Increased accidents in motor vehicles, physical education classes, swimming, athletics, and recreational activities are being experienced.

The application of accident prevention principles should be a basic part of the educational experiences provided secondary school students. School administrators and teachers should be concerned over the development of sound programs of education for safe living among this age group. An understanding of the needs of the high school students would certainly include the problems of accidents that injure and kill thousands of these persons annually. It is required by law in many states that some phases of safety education be taught in the schools. Perhaps the requiring of a comprehensive safety education program is a good share of the answer in the quest to eliminate accidents at the high school level. However, teachers with a genuine interest in safe living should be employed to teach such courses. The teacher's attitude and teaching ability are very important if students are to incorporate safety into their activities. Good teaching in the driver education classes and active enthusiastic safety clubs could make students more safety conscious.

First-aid courses should be available in all schools. By having had such courses students could eliminate many hazards to life through the proper use of first-aid protective measures. If possible, a doctor should be present at interscholastic athletic activities.

COLLEGE AND UNIVERSITY ACCIDENTS

College and university students are involved in numerous accidents each year. One study states that of the 207,000 full-time students surveyed, 14,487 injuries were reported to student health services during the 1965–1966 academic year. Of this number approximately 1,247 were disabling injuries.

Male college students were victims of about three fourths of all injuries reported. Approximately 1 out of 8 males and 1 out of 12 females enrolled in colleges and universities were treated for injuries.

Types of Accidents [309]

The study further reports that 8 percent of all injuries were disabling beyond the day of the accident, with the males having a higher percentage of such accidents than the girls. Some one third of the reported incidents occurred off campus. The location of on-campus accidents is as follows: 52 percent, athletics or recreation; 20 percent, residence halls; 15 percent, school buildings; 11 percent, school grounds; 2 percent, motor vehicles. In contrast the location of off-campus accidents is as follows: 31 percent, recreation; 29 percent, residence; 25 percent, motor vehicle; 4 percent, work; 11 percent, other.[2]

In recent years there has been an expanded interest in campus safety. However, much yet remains to be accomplished in the development of educational and environmental safety programs for college students. Hazards involving laboratories, classrooms, dormitories, physical education classes, and fire are a constant threat to the safety of these students.

Improved health services also seem to be in order for many campuses. Classes in first aid should be available to all students desiring to obtain this instruction. Those students enrolled in teacher education curricula could benefit immensely from a first-aid course.

TYPES OF ACCIDENTS

Accidents involving elementary and secondary school students occur in a wide variety of activities and environments. Reports on school accidents collected by the National Safety Council and other agencies suggest that the amount of exposure and hazard related to each activity accounts for the frequency and severity of certain accident patterns. The following is a brief discussion of the types of accidents that relate to elementary and secondary school youth. Figures 21.2 and 21.3 outline the extent of the school accident problems.

Shops and Laboratories

Injuries occur most frequently among secondary school boys in industrial arts classes, whereas girls are injured more often in science and home economics classes. Because of the absence of shop and laboratory programs at the elementary level, injuries of this type are almost nonexistent.

Buildings—General

Both boys and girls sustain frequent injuries in the classroom at the high school level. Accidents in corridors and on stairs are the next most common type of accident inside the school building. The frequency of

[2] National Safety Council, *Accidents Facts*. Chicago: The Council, 1968, p. 89.

Grounds—Unorganized Activities

Accidents associated with playing on apparatus, ballplaying, and running are most common at the elementary level. The same pattern applies to junior high school boys. Senior high school youths seldom receive injuries sustained in these types of activities.

Grounds—Other

Accidents related to fences, walls, steps, and walks do occur, but the overall frequency is very low. First grade through the sixth are the grade levels involved most often. For such accidents the frequency rate for boys is about twice that for girls.

Physical Education

Studies indicate that approximately 50 percent of all school and college injuries occur in physical education, recreation, and athletic activities. The National Safety Council reports that about 67 percent involve boys and some 59 percent involve girls. Most activities associated with the foregoing areas are potentially dangerous. Therefore all students should be taught the proper safety skills associated with these activities in order to perform safely.

Touch football, basketball, softball, and apparatus are the activities where high school boys are most frequently injured, whereas basketball, volleyball, apparatus, and organized games are the common areas where secondary school girls are injured. At the elementary level, class games, softball, and other organized games seem to involve both boys and girls in about the same proportions.

The most common types of injuries occurring in physical education classes are sprains, fractures, contusions, strains, dislocations, lacerations, abrasions, concussions, and eye injuries. About 80 percent of the injuries are sprains, contusions, and fractures.

Those persons responsible for students engaged in the foregoing activities (teachers, coaches, recreation leaders) should recognize the hazard potential, teach to prevent injuries from occurring, and be skillful in rendering first-aid protection should an accident occur.

Intramural Sports

Football seems to be the sport having the greatest number of accidents among boys at the high school level. Injuries associated with basketball, baseball, and touch football are about equal in number in this age range.

Types of Accidents [311]

FIGURE 21.2 STUDENT ACCIDENT RATE BY SCHOOL GRADE—BOYS

Location and Type	TOTAL	Kgn.	1-3 Gr.	4-6 Gr.	7-9 Gr.	10-12 Gr.	Days Lost per Inj.
Enrollment Reported (000)	1,157	77	249	268	295	243	
TOTAL School Jurisdiction	9.94	5.73	6.39	8.95	13.63	12.29	1.03
Shops and labs	.73	0	.01	.05	1.31	1.70	.63
Homemaking	.01	0	—	—	.02	.01	1.09
Science	.06	0	—	.01	.16	.09	.50
Driving (practice)	—	0	0	0	.01	—	1.20
Vocational, ind. arts	.51	0	0	.01	.93	1.16	.59
Agricultural	.01	0	0	0	.01	.01	.58
Other labs	.03	0	—	.01	.06	.06	.73
Other shops	.11	0	.01	.02	.12	.37	1.04
Building—general	2.01	1.82	1.53	1.85	3.18	1.53	.88
Auditoriums and classrooms	.88	1.24	.79	.93	1.24	.51	.69
Lunchrooms	.10	.04	.09	.12	.15	.07	.87
Corridors	.50	.26	.25	.34	.95	.48	1.03
Lockers (room and corridor)	.07	0	.01	.02	.16	.10	1.02
Stairs and stairways (inside)	.20	.07	.09	.15	.40	.18	1.23
Toilets and washrooms	.10	.12	.16	.13	.06	.05	.96
Grounds—unorganized activities	1.98	2.48	3.39	3.76	.73	.21	1.00
Apparatus	.40	1.04	.95	.55	.07	.02	1.13
Ball playing	.44	.06	.37	1.20	.22	.07	.84
Running	.55	.61	1.12	.94	.17	.04	1.02
Grounds—miscellaneous	.36	.48	.40	.49	.29	.28	1.20
Fences and walls	.04	.06	.06	.07	.03	.01	1.61
Steps and walks (outside)	.12	.25	.13	.13	.11	.10	1.01
Physical education	3.27	.35	.69	2.29	6.09	4.64	1.04
Apparatus	.30	.04	.12	.22	.52	.38	1.05
Class games	.35	.07	.21	.42	.55	.29	.90
Baseball—hard ball	.03	0	—	.01	.08	.06	.96
Baseball—soft ball	.16	0	.02	.17	.31	.16	1.39
Football—regular	.11	0	—	.04	.20	.25	1.59
Football—touch	.24	0	0	.09	.49	.43	1.14
Basketball	.52	0	.01	.19	.99	1.02	1.06
Hockey	.03	0	—	.01	.04	.05	.65
Soccer	.19	0	.03	.16	.32	.31	1.18
Track and field events	.12	0	.01	.08	.26	.13	1.27
Volleyball and similar games	.14	.02	.01	.08	.21	.31	.72
Other organized games	.43	.04	.11	.40	.82	.45	.90
Swimming	.07	0	0	.02	.12	.17	.62
Showers and dressing rooms	.07	0	.01	.02	.19	.06	.60
Intra-mural sports	.16	0	0	.04	.32	.31	1.50
Baseball—hard ball	—	0	0	0	—	.01	1.83
Baseball—soft ball	.01	0	0	0	.02	.01	6.81
Football—regular	.07	0	0	0	.13	.15	1.42
Football—touch	.02	0	0	.01	.04	.02	.68
Basketball	.03	0	0	.01	.05	.08	1.27
Inter-scholastic sports	1.04	0	—	.05	1.23	3.36	.86
Baseball—hard ball	.02	0	0	0	.01	.09	.81
Baseball—soft ball	.01	0	0	—	.01	.02	.61
Football—regular	.66	0	0	.01	.74	2.17	.90
Basketball	.15	0	0	.01	.23	.42	.70
Track and field events	.07	0	—	.02	.10	.18	.81
Special activities	.06	.03	.04	.10	.06	.06	1.84
Trips or excursions	.03	.03	.03	.05	.04	.02	1.53
Student dramatics	—	0	—	0	—	.01	.13
Student concerts	0	0	0	0	0	0	0

[312]   School Accident Victims

FIGURE 21.2—Continued

Location and Type	TOTAL	Kgn.	1-3 Gr.	4-6 Gr.	7-9 Gr.	10-12 Gr.	Days Lost per Inj.
Going to and from school (MV)	.16	.34	.18	.14	.18	.12	3.95
School bus	.07	.07	.06	.06	.09	.04	.92
Public carrier (incl. bus)	.01	.09	.02	.01	.01	0	7.30
Motor scooter	.01	.01	0	0	—	.02	6.50
Other mot. veh.—pedestrian	.04	.12	.09	.04	.04	.01	6.71
Other mot. veh.—bicycle	.01	.02	0	.02	.02	—	8.24
Other mot. veh.—other type	.02	.03	.01	.01	.02	.05	2.45
Going to, from school (not MV)	.17	.23	.15	.18	.24	.08	1.63
Bicycle—not mot. veh.	.03	0	.01	.03	.05	.01	1.38
Other street and sidewalk	.09	.20	.10	.09	.10	.06	1.16

Source: National Safety Council.

FIGURE 21.3   STUDENT ACCIDENT RATES BY SCHOOL GRADE—GIRLS

Location and Type	TOTAL	Kgn.	1-3 Gr.	4-6 Gr.	7-9 Gr.	10-12 Gr.	Days Lost per Inj.
Enrollment Reported (000)	1,105	72	235	258	286	238	
TOTAL School Jurisdiction	5.72	4.01	4.35	6.24	7.99	4.73	.98
Shops and labs	.17	0	.01	.03	.39	.28	.45
Homemaking	.06	0	0	.01	.17	.08	.35
Science	.05	0	0	.01	.13	.06	.43
Driving (practice)	—	0	0	—	0	.01	0
Vocational, ind. arts	.03	0	0	.01	.05	.06	.45
Agricultural	—	0	0	0	—	0	0
Other labs	.02	0	—	—	.02	.05	.61
Other shops	.01	0	.01	—	.02	.02	1.04
Building—general	1.36	1.02	.88	1.28	2.25	1.04	.87
Auditoriums and classrooms	.58	.67	.50	.63	.85	.31	.73
Lunchrooms	.05	.02	.06	.05	.07	.04	1.03
Corridors	.31	.12	.11	.25	.65	.23	.76
Lockers (room and corridor)	.04	.01	.01	.02	.10	.05	.44
Stairs and stairways (inside)	.23	.05	.05	.16	.44	.28	1.38
Toilets and washrooms	.07	.12	.08	.09	.06	.05	.80
Grounds—unorganized activities	1.25	1.68	2.37	2.46	.26	.08	.94
Apparatus	.38	.99	.93	.57	.04	.01	1.20
Ball playing	.21	.02	.15	.66	.06	.01	.63
Running	.34	.31	.76	.57	.07	.02	.84
Grounds—miscellaneous	.21	.22	.28	.28	.17	.14	1.17
Fences and walls	.02	.03	.04	.04	.01	0	1.38
Steps and walks (outside)	.08	.09	.09	.11	.08	.06	1.07
Physical education	2.16	.40	.51	1.80	4.26	2.25	.94
Apparatus	.37	.11	.11	.27	.69	.44	1.01
Class games	.25	.09	.13	.39	.36	.14	.80
Baseball—hard ball	.01	0	0	—	.01	.01	.63
Baseball—soft ball	.10	0	.01	.09	.20	.12	.75
Football—regular	.01	0	0	.01	.01	.01	.83
Football—touch	.03	0	0	.02	.06	.04	.50

Types of Accidents [313]

Location and Type	TOTAL	Kgn.	1-3 Gr.	4-6 Gr.	7-9 Gr.	10-12 Gr.	Days Lost per Inj.
Basketball	.22	0	.01	.08	.52	.30	.88
Hockey	.04	0	0	.01	.07	.08	.81
Soccer	.08	0	.01	.11	.14	.07	.91
Track and field events	.10	0	.01	.08	.24	.07	1.37
Volleyball and similar games	.18	0	.01	.11	.34	.29	.98
Other organized games	.32	.09	.10	.32	.65	.25	.93
Swimming	.04	0	0	.01	.09	.07	.71
Showers and dressing rooms	.05	0	0	.01	.14	.04	.81
Intra-mural sports	.04	0	—	.05	.07	.05	.84
Baseball—hard ball	—	0	0	0	—	—	0
Baseball—soft ball	—	0	0	0	.01	0	1.00
Football—regular	—	0	0	—	0	0	.50
Football—touch	—	0	0	0	0	.01	.75
Basketball	.01	0	—	.01	.01	.02	.98
Inter-scholastic sports	.18	0	0	.02	.19	.56	.74
Baseball—hard ball	0	0	0	0	0	0	0
Baseball—soft ball	.01	0	0	—	.01	.04	.69
Football—regular	—	0	0	0	—	.01	0
Basketball	.07	0	0	.01	.08	.22	.62
Track and field events	.04	0	0	.01	.05	.09	1.10
Special activities	.07	.11	.03	.07	.08	.10	1.32
Trips or excursions	.04	.11	.03	.04	.04	.04	1.11
Student dramatics	—	0	0	—	0	—	.25
Student concerts	—	0	0	0	—	—	0
Going to and from school (MV)	.17	.36	.16	.11	.22	.14	1.91
School bus	.08	.09	.05	.05	.13	.05	1.00
Public carrier (incl. bus)	.01	.08	.01	.01	.02	—	2.75
Motor scooter	—	0	—	0	—	0	.33
Other mot. veh.—pedestrian	.05	.14	.07	.03	.05	.02	3.85
Other mot. veh.—bicycle	—	0	0	0	—	—	1.75
Other mot. veh.—other type	.03	.05	.03	.02	.02	.07	1.54
Going to, from school (not MV)	.11	.22	.11	.14	.10	.09	2.42
Bicycle—not mot. veh.	.01	0	—	.02	.01	0	1.14
Other street and sidewalk	.07	.17	.07	.09	.06	.07	1.32

Source: National Safety Council.

A few elementary boys are involved in these game injuries also. But rarely are girls, at either the elementary or secondary level, involved in accidents in intramural sports.

Interscholastic Sports

In junior and senior high schools, football is the sports activity in which most boys sustain injuries, whereas basketball, track, and baseball injuries are fewer. Junior high boys are involved in some sports accidents, principally in football and basketball. Because of the absence of interscholastic sports events involving girls, these accidents are no problem to them.

At the junior high school level, bruises make up about 38 percent of the injuries; sprains, 33 percent; fractures, 13 percent; abrasions and lacerations, each 7 percent; and dislocations, around 2 percent. Legs, knees, ankles, backs, and shoulders are the most frequent parts of the body injured.

Special Activities

At the elementary and secondary school levels, various field trips, dramatic and concert program trips, etc. are usually accident-free, but the hazard potential is great. The National Safety Council reports that most of the accidents experienced are on field trips. Teachers should plan such excursions with student safety as a primary consideration. A person with a first-aid background should accompany all such groups.

Going to and from School

Students of all ages are exposed to hazards as they go to and from school. Accidents involving motor vehicles—school bus, public carrier, motor scooter, pedestrian, and bicycle rider—are frequent types of incidents related to each age group.

At the elementary level pedestrian, school bus, and bicycle accidents are the most frequent types of accidents with resultant injuries, whereas at the secondary level motor vehicle, motor scooter, and pedestrian accidents rank high.

The accident problems discussed here are principally reported as school-jurisdiction accidents. Obviously elementary and secondary school students are involved in accidents around the home and community that are nonschool-jurisdiction accidents. These are referred to in other parts of the text, mainly in Chapters 17, 18, 19, and 20.

ACCIDENT REPORTING

The basis for knowing the extent of a school's accident problem is a sound accident reporting system. Such a system allows the school to identify the type, severity, frequency, location, and cause of school accidents. With this information, remedial programs can be organized to assist in the elimination of accidents involving elementary and high school students. Chapter 3 includes the organizational aspects of an accident reporting system.

ACTIVITIES

1 Obtain from the National Safety Council a copy of the publication *Student Accident Reporting Guidebook*. Using this as a basis, develop an accident reporting system program for a school.

2 Contact ten schools in the area and determine the extent of their accident problem. Write an analysis of each school with suggested recommendations for improvement.
3 Design a first-aid facility for a school with 1,000 students. Include all the equipment and supplies needed for such a facility.
4 Write to the state's coaches' association. Request materials that they have available related to safety in sports. Prepare a ten-minute presentation for the class.
5 Contact 15 elementary school teachers to determine the number that are qualified in first aid. Also ascertain the extent to which they use or would use such training in their schools.

QUESTIONS TO ANSWER

1 Over the past 50 years the accident rate involving elementary schoolchildren has decreased 50 percent. True or False? What may have contributed to this?
2 What intramural sport has the most accidents involving high school boys?
3 Identify three of the common types of accidents that involve elementary students going to and from school.
4 What are the two basic responsibilities of the school in the development of a safety education program?
5 Accidents account for what percentage of deaths involving preschool and elementary-age children?
6 At what age should children be taught safety?
7 Briefly summarize the college accident problem.
8 Based upon Figures 21.2 and 21.3, what types of shop accidents occur most frequently at the junior high school level?
9 What percentage of all school injuries occurs in physical education classes?
10 What type of information is obtained from a uniform accident reporting system?

SELECTED REFERENCES

AMERICAN NATIONAL RED CROSS, *Standard First Aid and Personal Safety.* New York: Doubleday, 1973.
BAKHAUS, DO CARMO, PAMELA and PATTERSON ANGELO TO, *First Aid Principles and Procedures.* Englewood Cliffs, N.J.: Prentice-Hall, 1976.
FLORIO, A. E., and STAFFORD, G. T., *Safety Education.* New York: McGraw-Hill, 1972.
HALSEY, MAXWELL (editorial consultant), *Accident Prevention.* New York: McGraw-Hill, 1961.

HENDERSON, JOHN, *Emergency Medical Guide*, 4th ed. New York: McGraw-Hill, 1978.
NATIONAL SAFETY COUNCIL, *Accident Facts*. Chicago: The Council, 1977.
NATIONAL SAFETY COUNCIL, *Student Accident Reporting Guidebook*. Chicago: The Council, 1966.
SEATON, DON C.; STACK, HERBERT J.; and LOFT, BERNARD I., *Administration and Supervision of Safety Education*. New York: Macmillan, 1969.
STACK, HERBERT J., and ELKOW, J. DUKE, *Education for Safe Living*. Englewood Cliffs, N.J.: Prentice-Hall, 1966.
STRASSER, M. K., et al., *Fundamentals of Safety Education*. New York: Macmillan, 1973.

PART V
PRACTICAL APPLICATIONS

In this final part of the book the practical aspects of first aid, such as the techniques of bandaging, transportation methods, and types of first-aid supplies, are discussed. The last chapter is concerned with organizing emergency care services.

Included in Part V are the following chapters:

22 Essential Techniques to Master: Bandaging and Splinting
23 Transportation for Protection
24 First-Aid Supplies
25 Organizing Emergency Care Services

22. ESSENTIAL TECHNIQUES TO MASTER: BANDAGING AND SPLINTING

First-aid and emergency care information is quite practical. The opportunity to apply this knowledge is common, as accidents continue to happen every few seconds. There is no part of the first-aid program so meaningful as the practical application. First aid is a "learning by doing" activity. If given the chance to evaluate, students in first-aid classes usually indicate that more time should be given to the techniques, the practical application. To learn properly to bandage, splint, transport, or give artificial respiration, it is necessary to practice under the supervision of a capable instructor. In first-aid training, theory must be put into actual practice with sufficient time provided in the first-aid course for demonstration work.

BANDAGING MATERIAL

The bandaging material is used to hold the sterile dressing in place or to support an injury. Some of the common materials used for bandaging are roller gauze, muslin strips, elastic, triangular cloths, cotton webbing (ankle wrap), and adhesive tape. These bandaging materials are commonly confused with dressings. However, it is the sterile dressing that is placed over the wound. Gauze squares, adhesive compresses (Band-Aids), bandage compress, and roller gauze are examples of dressings.

BANDAGING TECHNIQUES

The bandaging techniques presented are fundamental to emergency care. It is important that they be understood and practiced until the

[320] Essential Techniques to Master: Bandaging and Splinting

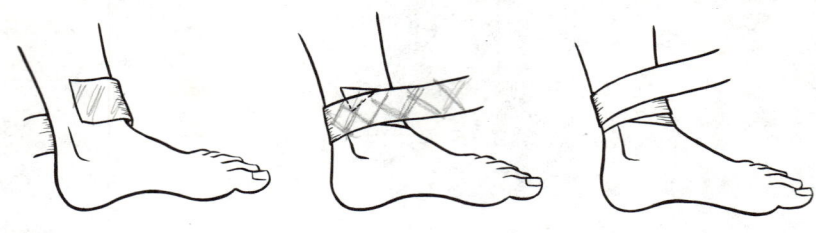

FIGURE 22.1 Steps in anchoring a roller bandage.

first-aider masters them. Once an emergency need arises it is too late for study and review; the application needs to be as automatic as possible.

The two most common bandaging errors are placing them either too tightly or too loosely. The purpose of bandaging is to secure the dressing over the injury, to protect, or to give support. If the bandage is too loose, it cannot adequately protect and it may come off. If it is too tight, circulation can be stopped.

Anchoring the Bandage

It is necessary that the bandage remain fixed in position, so it is suggested that the bandage, especially the roller-type bandage, be anchored. There are five steps in the anchoring procedure:

1. Circle the bandage around the arm or leg.

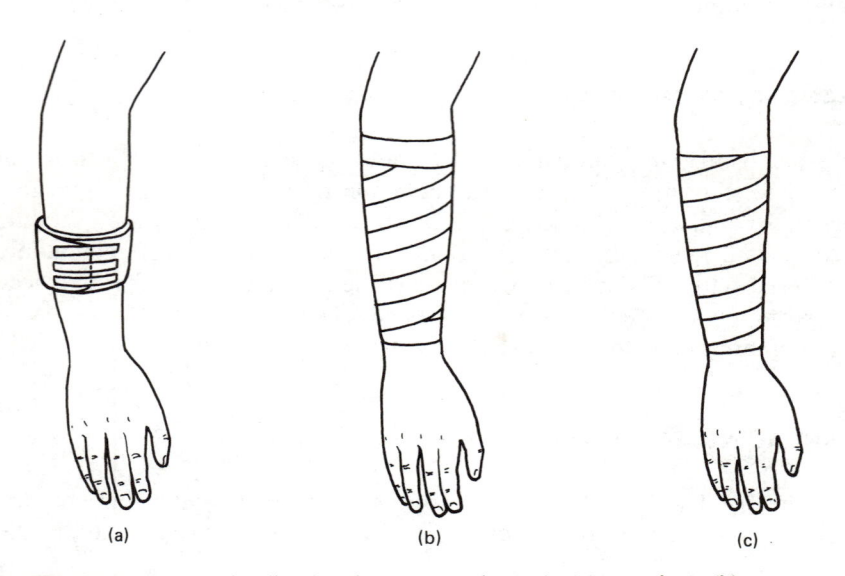

(a)   (b)   (c)

FIGURE 22.2 Types of roller bandaging (spiral turns): (a) complete, (b) open, and (c) closed.

2. Allow the end (beginning) of the bandage to project to one side, an inch or two.
3. Fold the projected end over the first turn of the bandage.
4. Cover the first turn with the second, securing the bandage.
5. Continue the circles upward on the arm or leg and apply each turn or circle as uniformly tight as possible.

Spiral Turns

Spiral turns are used on the fingers, arms, and legs. Such turns are made by going around the part, usually overlapping completely or partly each time the bandage encircles. Spiral turns can be described as complete, closed, or open, depending upon the degree that each turn of the bandage covers the previous turn. The open spiral does not overlap, whereas the closed spiral partially overlaps and the complete spiral entirely covers the previous lap or laps. The purpose of the spiral turns, usually done with a roller-type bandage, is to hold the dressing in place. When applying these three types of bandages, the first-aider should proceed as follows:

Complete Turn

1. Anchor the bandage.
2. Encircle the part, finger or arm, placing each turn completely over the previous turn.
3. Put enough turns in place to secure the dressing.
4. Secure the bandage by tying or with adhesive tape.

Open Turn

1. Anchor the bandage.
2. Place the second turn over the first turn.
3. Continue to encircle the part, but do not overlap. The open turn is used to secure a large dressing, as a burn dressing or when the supply of bandages is limited in amount.
4. Secure the bandage by tying or with adhesive strips.

Closed Spiral Turn

1. Anchor the bandage.
2. Cover the anchor the second turn while encircling over the first turn.
3. Continue to encircle and overlap each turn by one half so that the skin is completely covered. This method is used to secure a dressing when the supply of bandage material is adequate and the injured area is large.
4. Secure the bandage by tying or with adhesive tape strips. It is desirable to put adhesive strips in several places to make certain the bandage will remain in place.

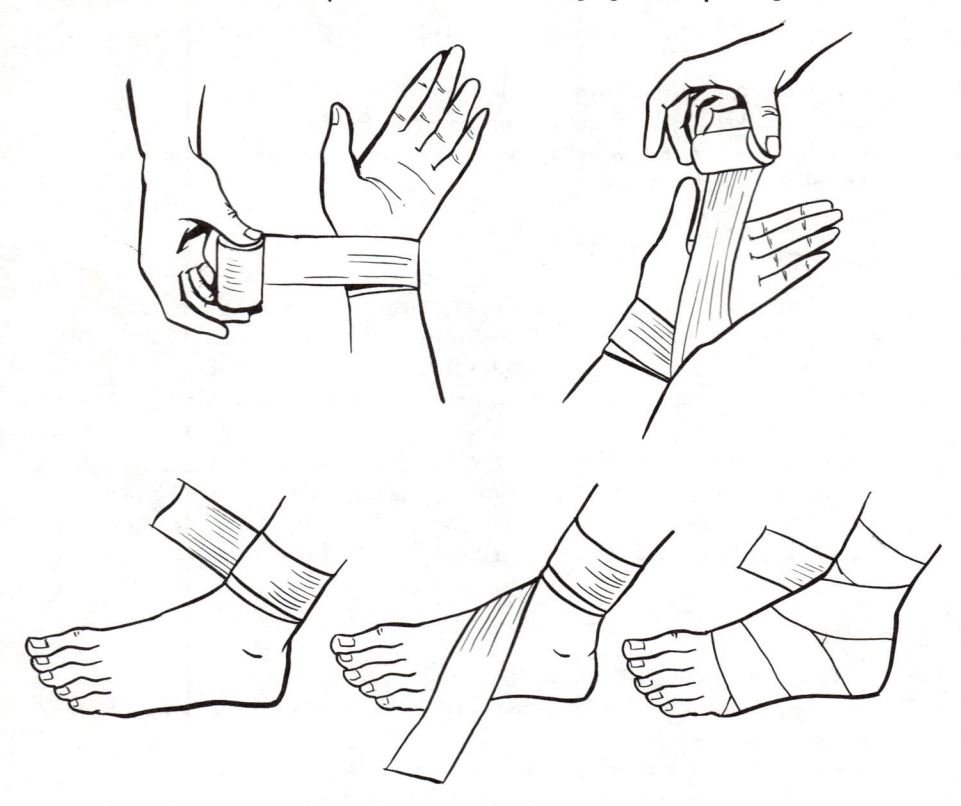

[322] Essential Techniques to Master: Bandaging and Splinting

FIGURE 22.3 Figure-of-eight bandage for hand and wrist, and for foot and ankle.

Figure-of-Eight

The figure-of-eight is a useful and helpful bandage. It can be used on most joints and the limbs, but it is especially desirable for supporting and protecting the finger, ankle, hand, and wrist. This bandage can be applied with roller gauze, muslin strips, ankle wraps, or elastic wraps. The most desirable materials for applying the figure-of-eight are the elastic wrap and the roller gauze. It is important that each turn be uniformly tight. If one turn is too tight, circulation will be stopped and the bandage will need to be removed and reapplied for comfort. When using the procedure for applying a figure-of-eight bandage, the first-aider should

1. Anchor the bandage around the wrist, finger, ankle, or other part.
2. Encircle the part again.
3. For the foot or wrist, encircle the hand or foot in the figure-of-eight manner, each turn being uniformly tight. Extra turns can be used on the foot, ankle, or wrist.
4. Continue the figure-of-eight, moving up and down the ankle or wrist and about the foot or hand and overlap each figure-of-eight pattern.

Bandaging Techniques [323]

5. Continue until the bandage is used up or until the part is sufficiently protected.
6. Secure with a strip of adhesive tape, applying the adhesive in the same figure-of-eight pattern.

Recurrent Turn for Finger

Bandaging an injured finger is a problem. It is difficult to bandage and to protect the finger, especially to keep the bandage secure. If the wound is large and if bleeding is severe, several layers of gauze or a compress may be needed to control the bleeding. The recurrent turn is a satisfactory method of bandaging for the fingers. To apply the recurrent turn bandage, the first-aider should

1. Fold the bandage (roller gauze) several times; the folds should be long enough to cover the finger from base to base on each side of finger.
2. Place the folded bandage over the finger. If this is a large wound or if bleeding is a problem, it is desirable to place a sterile compress (gauze square) beneath the folds of the roller gauze.
3. Take a spiral turn or two around the base of the finger to secure the bandage.
4. Fold the bandage over the entire finger another time or two.
5. Take additional spiral turns around the base of the finger to secure; then apply closed spiral turns over the entire finger and back to the base.

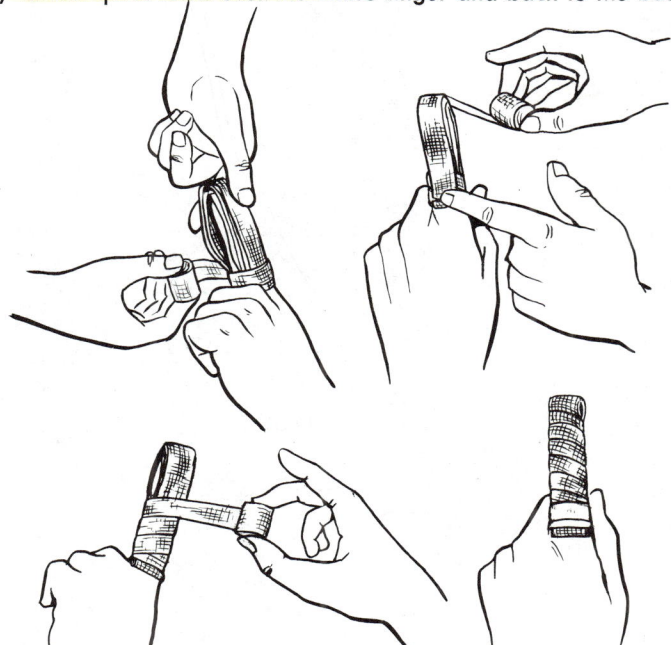

FIGURE 22.4 Finger bandaging, showing application of recurrent bandage by steps.

[324] Essential Techniques to Master: Bandaging and Splinting

6 Secure the bandage at the base of the finger by tying or with adhesive tape strips. To tie, cut down the middle of the bandage, knot, wrap in opposite directions, and tie.

Four-Tailed Bandage

The four-tailed bandage gets its name from its appearance. Strips of cloth, three to four inches wide and some three feet long, are ideal for this bandage. The strips are cut down the middle, leaving a portion midway in the strip of some five or six inches. This leaves four tails, hence the name. It is useful for giving support or for holding a dressing in place for the chin and nose in particular. Also it can be used on joints as the knee or elbow. The procedure for applying is as follows:

1   Place the bandage over the nose.
2   Keep the upper two tails low, going beneath the ears, and tie behind the head.
3   Keep the lower two tails high, crossing over the upper tails in front of the ears and tie on the back slope of the head.

Spiral Reverse

This bandage is most desirable for the body parts that taper, such as the arm or leg. The ankles and wrists are small, but the extremities get larger toward the body. The spiral reverse is a means of tightening the bandage as it progresses up the arm or leg. By reversing (turning the bandage over) it is secured. If the spiral reverse is not used on the lower

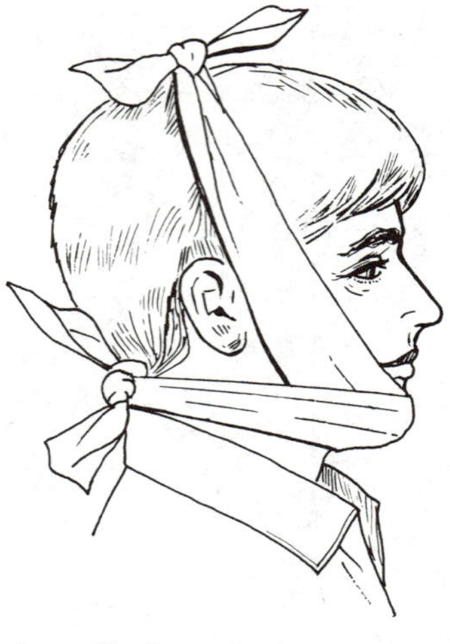

FIGURE 22.5   Four-tail bandage (for lower jaw).

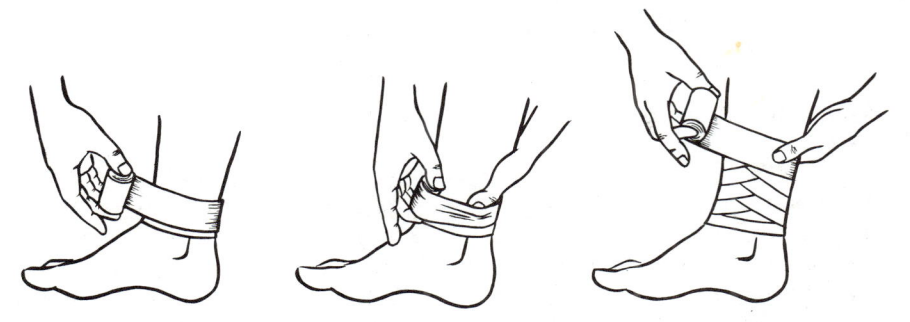

FIGURE 22.6 Spiral-reverse steps for tapering parts of the body (lower leg).

arm, the bandage tends to become loose and consequently is useless. This type of bandaging should be practiced by the first-aider until it is mastered. Holding the roll as illustrated will tend to prevent dropping it and will keep the bandage uniformly snug. To apply it, the first-aider should

1 Anchor the bandage at the wrist or ankle.
2 Continue up the arm or leg with the closed spiral turn.
3 When the arm or leg begins to taper, reverse (turn the bandage over) at each turn.

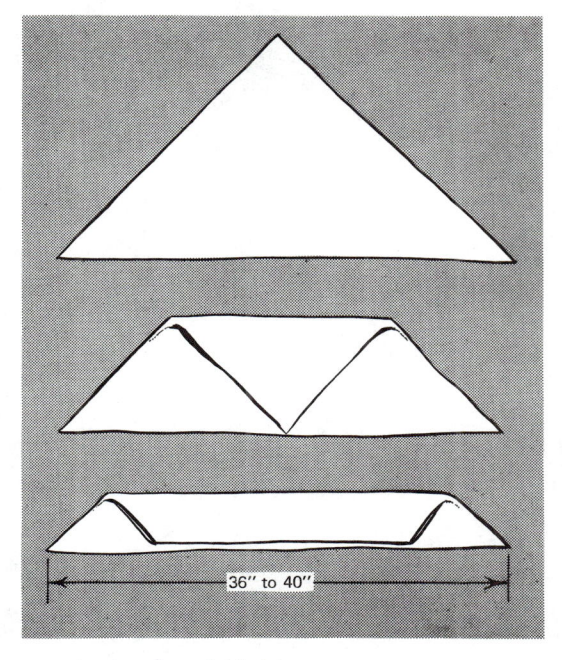

FIGURE 22.7 Triangular bandage folded into cravat.

[326] Essential Techniques to Master: Bandaging and Splinting

4   Continue up the arm or leg to just below the elbow or knee.
5   Secure by tying or preferably use several strips of adhesive tape.

TRIANGULAR BANDAGE

The triangular bandage is the most versatile in the first-aid kit. It is possible to protect the head, torso, shoulder, elbow, hand, hip, foot, and other areas by using the triangular bandage. This bandage can also be folded into a cravat and used to protect or support the foot, hand, neck, eye, throat, and head. It can also be used as a very desirable tourniquet and in applying splints to all parts of the body.

The triangular bandage can best be made from white muslin. An old sheet or tablecloth may also be used. It is helpful if several different sizes are available because of differences in physical makeup. A range of 40 to 50 inches across the base is best. A large bandage can be used on a small person, but the small bandage is useless on a large person. Triangular

FIGURE 22.8 Triangular bandage steps for protection of hand.

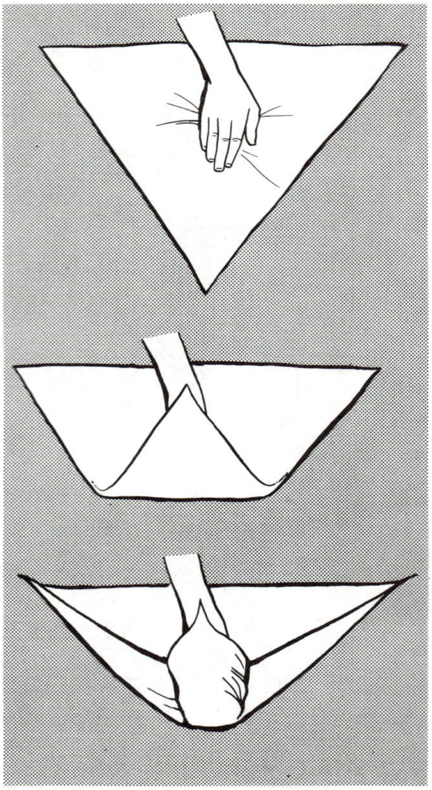

Triangular Bandage [327]

bandages can be easily made by taking a 40-inch square of muslin, folding it diagonally and then cutting along this folded line. If the edges are hemmed, the bandage will be stronger and it will serve for a longer period of time.

Hand and Foot

The entire hand or foot can be bandaged with one triangular bandage. If the hand is crushed, burned, or badly injured, it is possible to protect the part with this bandage. The sterile dressing should first be placed over the wound, then the triangular bandage used to secure the dressing in place. The person applying the triangular bandage on a hand and foot should

1. Place the open bandage on a flat surface; then put the hand or foot, six to eight inches from the base of bandage, in the center of the bandage.
2. Pull the point (right angle) up on the wrist or ankle.

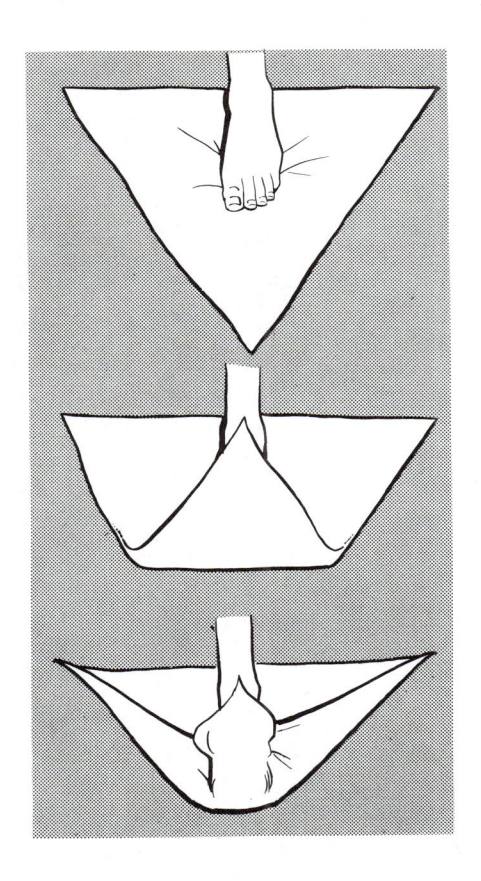

FIGURE 22.9 Triangular bandage steps for protection of foot.

[328] Essential Techniques to Master: Bandaging and Splinting

3   Bring the angle or point from the left, then from the right, over the front and around the ankle or wrist.
4   Tie the points in front of the ankle or wrist with a square knot.

Head

A triangular bandage can be used for covering the head. For example, the problem could be a burn or wound that must be protected. The procedure would be to

1   Place the bandage on a flat surface and fold the longest portion over about an inch, once or twice, depending upon the size of the bandage and the victim.
2   Place the bandage on the head so that the folded base rests on the forehead. If the flat portion of the forehead is not used, the bandage will slip and not hold securely.
3   Extend the angle (right angle) back over the head and down the back of the head and neck.
4   Bring the two folded ends completely around the head, just above the ears.
5   Secure in front with a square knot and tuck under the ends if they are long.

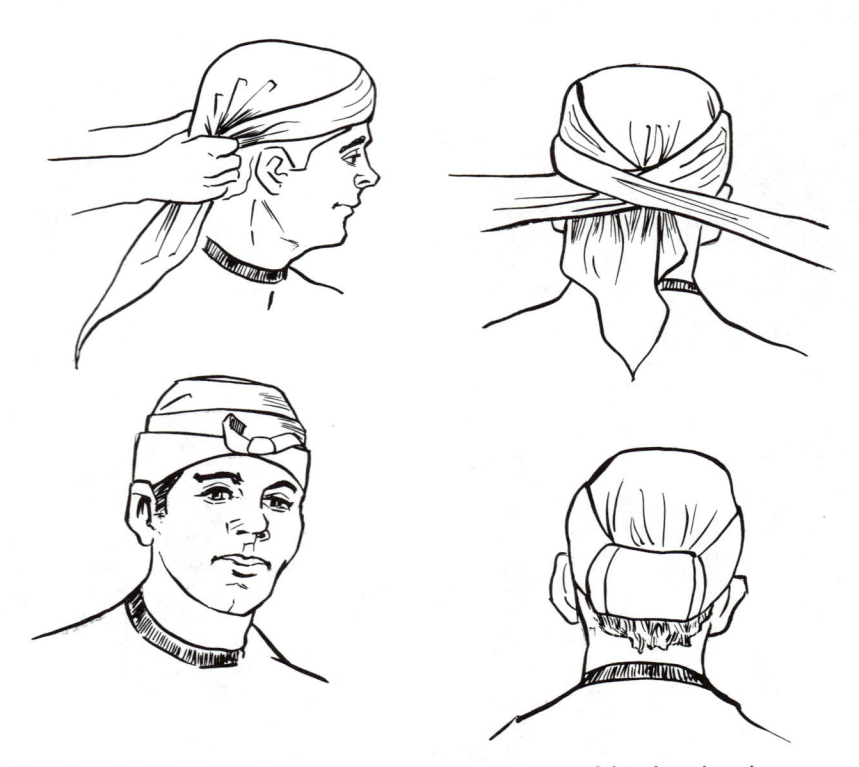

FIGURE 22.10   Triangular bandage steps for protection of head and scalp.

Triangular Bandage [329]

6 Tuck the part behind the head into and under the two circular turns about the head.

Torso—Chest and Back

One large trianguar bandage will cover the entire chest or back. This bandage is useful for large abrasions, burns, and other wounds. It can be used to secure a dressing and it affords reasonable protection. The procedure is to

1 Place the point (right angle) over the shoulder for either chest or back injuries.

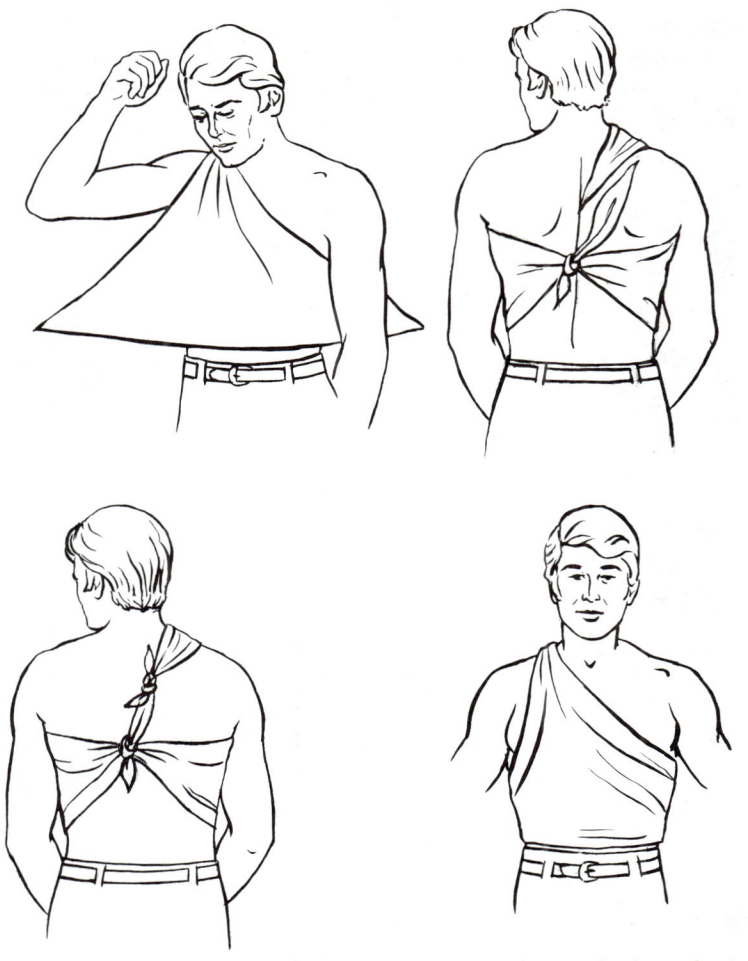

FIGURE 22.11   Triangular bandage steps for protection of torso (back or chest).

[330] Essential Techniques to Master: Bandaging and Splinting

2 Extend the two long ends around the body and tie with a square knot; this knot should be tied directly below the point (right angle).
3 With the 12 or 15 inches of bandage remaining, tie with the angle end above the shoulder, and with a square knot. If this remaining portion is not long enough to reach the shoulder and tie, then a strip of gauze or muslin will be needed to make this connection and to tie.

Hips and Shoulder

Two triangular bandages, one folded as a cravat and the other open, will effectively protect the hip or the shoulder. These two areas are very common sites for abrasions, and the injury can involve a large area. A dressing can be placed over the abrasion, burn, or laceration and the two bandages can effectively hold it in place. The procedure is to

1. Place one bandage flat on a table.
2. Fold the second bandage into a cravat, some three to four inches wide.
3. Roll the angle (right angle) of the first bandage around the cravat two or three times to fasten them together.

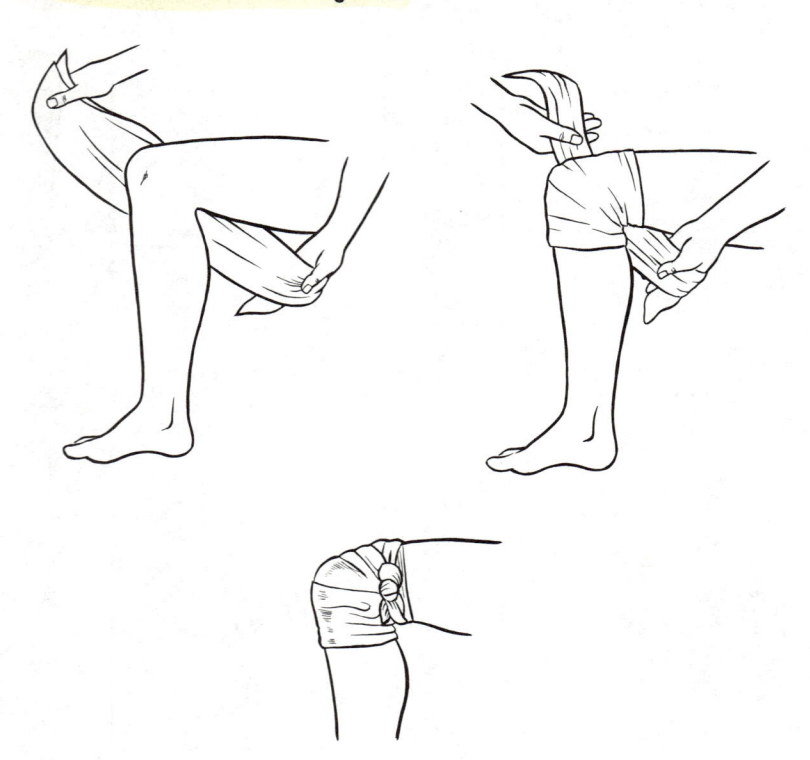

FIGURE 22.12 Triangular bandage steps for protection of elbow or knee.

Triangular Bandage [331]

4. Place the bandages on the injured shoulder or hip.
5. Extend the cravat around the neck and under the opposite armpit and tie with a square knot. The bandage being applied to the hip should be extended around the body and tied.
6. Extend the end of the second bandage around the arm, just above the elbow, then bring to the front and tie with a square knot. If it is the hip, the bandage should be extended around the leg, above the knee, and secured with a square knot.

Elbow and Knee

One triangular bandage folded as a cravat will cover either of these joints and give some protection to the area. The cravat should be folded wider than usual, some six to eight inches, as it will be covering a large area. It is also advisable to use a larger bandage if one is available. When using this procedure the first-aider should

1. Bend the elbow or knee unless there is an injury in the joint.
2. Place the bandage over the knee, extend the two ends around the leg, one end above and the other below, then cross the two ends and tie with a square knot.
3. For the elbow, place the bandage in the down position in the bend of the elbow joint, extend one end around the arm above the elbow, the other

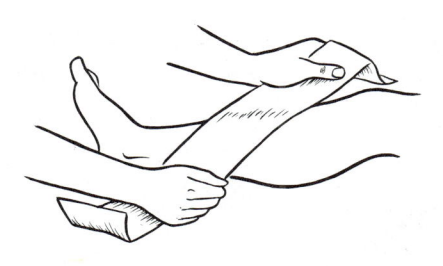

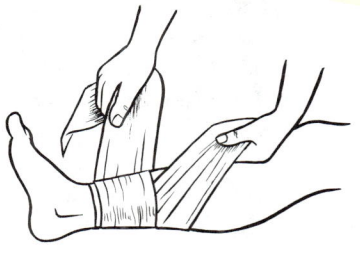

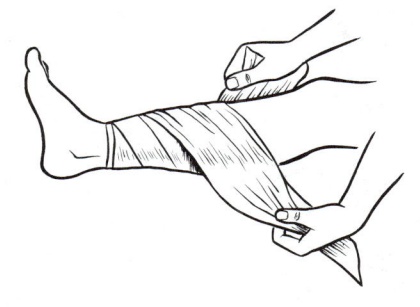

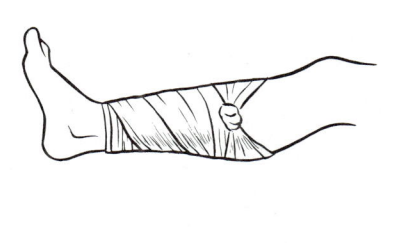

FIGURE 22.13 Use of triangular bandage for protection of lower leg.

[332]   Essential Techniques to Master: Bandaging and Splinting

around the arm below the elbow, then cross the two ends at the elbow joint in front and tie with a square knot.

Forearm

A single trianguar bandage, folded as a cravat, will protect or cover the lower arm. The procedure is to

1. Place one end of the bandage up the arm in a diagonal position.
2. Hold the bandage in this position, then with the longer end of the bandage, wrap it firmly around the forearm overlapping each time and going up the arm as far as possible.
3. Tie the two ends with a square knot to secure the bandage.

Ear and Chin

One triangular bandage will afford some protection to the ear, chin, or cheek. The procedure is as follows:

1. Fold the bandage into a cravat, some three to four inches wide.
2. Place a compress over the injury; then start with the cravat over the compress, then beneath the chin, across the flat portion of the head to prevent slipping.
3. Cross the two ends of the cravat just above and in front of the ear.
4. Extend the two ends of the cravat around the back of the head and across the forehead and tie on the opposite side of the head with a square knot.

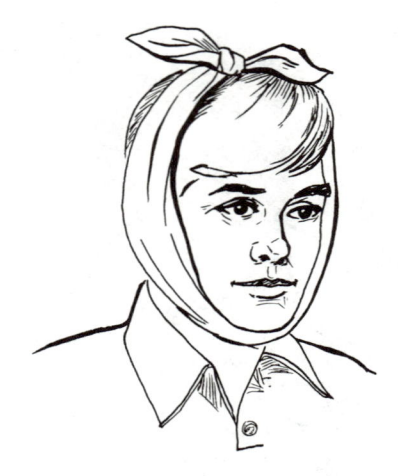

FIGURE 22.14   Triangular bandage as cravat for protection of lower jaw (ear and chin).

Triangular Bandage [333]

Arm Sling

Two triangular bandages are needed: preferably one that measures 50 inches or more across the base, and a second bandage, folded as a cravat, is desirable for holding the arm securely against the body and providing additional protection. When using this procedure the first-aider should

1. Place the bandage in position on the side away from the injury, one point over the shoulder with the base in a vertical position, the angle pointed toward the injury.
2. Move the injured arm across in a horizontal position, slightly elevated.
3. Bring the downward long point of the bandage up and over the injured shoulder, then around the neck.
4. Tie the two ends of the bandage with a square knot, on the side of the neck.
5. Leave the fingers on the injured hand exposed for observation.
6. Tie and tuck the point of the bandage, or pin with a safety pin.

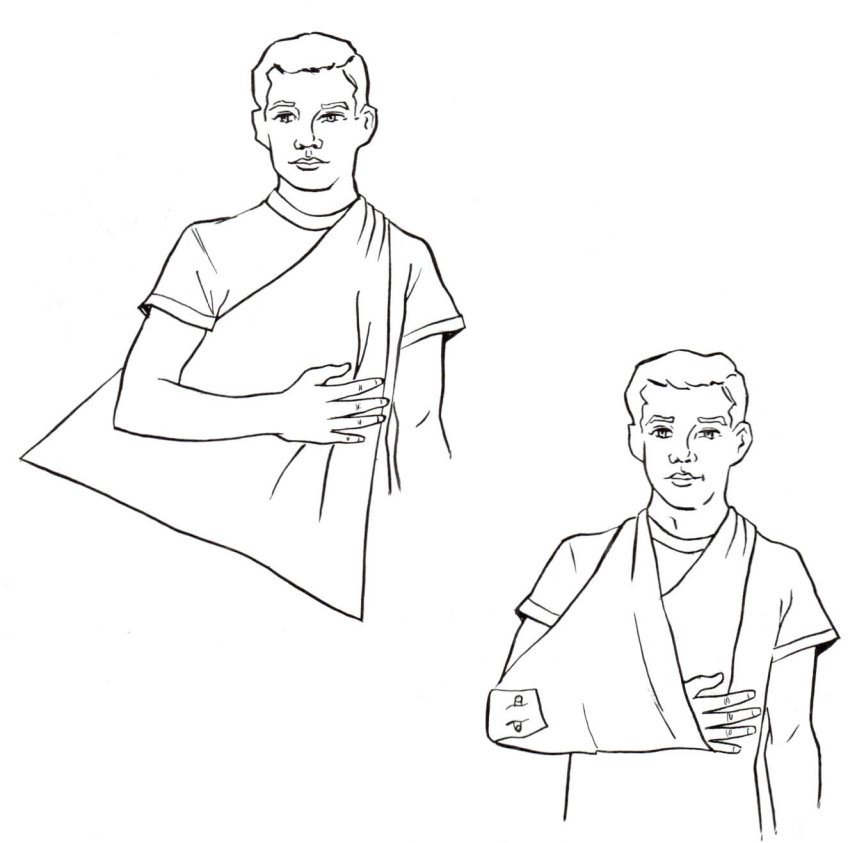

FIGURE 22.15 Triangular bandage—application of arm sling.

[334]   Essential Techniques to Master: Bandaging and Splinting

7) Use the second bandage, which has been folded as a cravat, to secure the injured arm to the body. Extend this bandage around the body, over the midpoint of the upper arm, and tie with a square knot on the opposite side of the body.

Pressure Bandage—Hand

This very important bandage has a dual responsibility. It is used for applying pressure to control bleeding from the palm and for putting the arm in traction. The splint is secured to the pressure bandage in traction splinting for the arm. The procedure is to

1. Have the victim hold a roll of gauze or a folded compress tightly in his hand.
2. Place the center of the folded bandage (cravat) over the wrist to the inside, which is held in an upward position.
3. Bring the other end of the bandage around and up and over the tightly clenched fist; then pull and hold this end securely.
4. Bring the other end (longer) around and up and over the fist and keep the bandage over the knuckles.

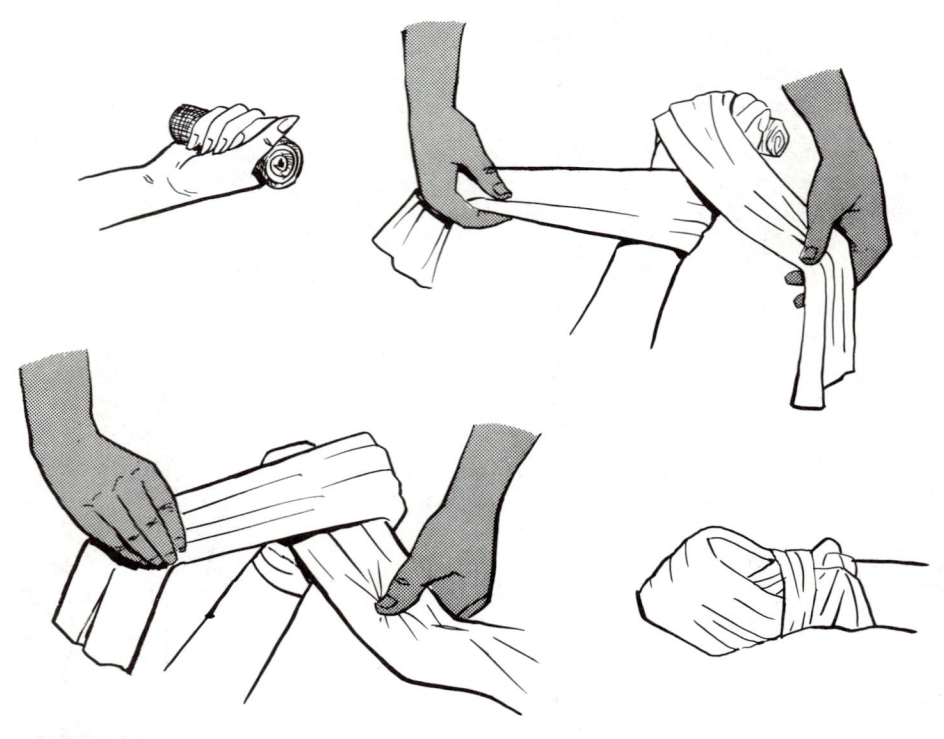

FIGURE 22.16   Triangular bandage as cravat for applying pressure bandage on the hand.

Triangular Bandage [335]

5. Cross the two ends of the bandage at the wrist, and then wrap the ends around the wrist securely in opposite directions and tie with a square knot. Tie well above the wrist; otherwise it may block the radial artery.

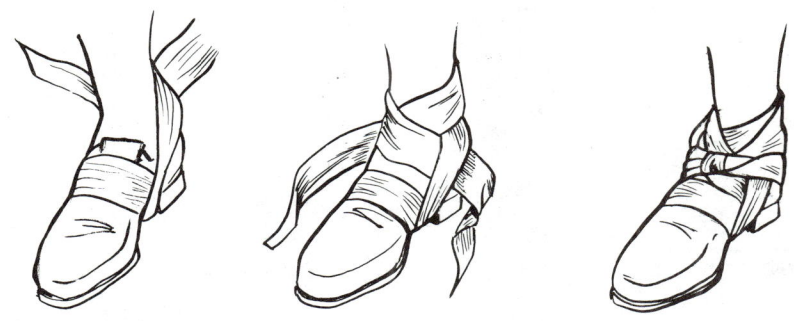

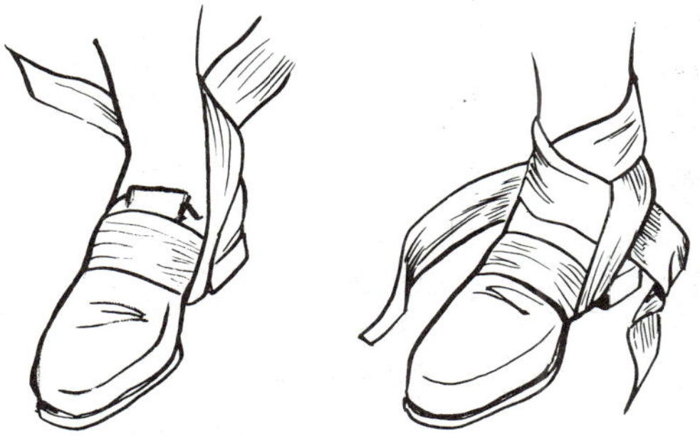

FIGURE 22.17 Triangular bandage as cravat for protecting and applying to ankle.

Ankle Wrap

This bandage has two important functions—to give support and protection to an injured ankle, and to place the leg in traction. The traction splint is fastened to the foot by means of the ankle wrap. This bandage must be put on the injured part securely if it is to serve its purpose. The procedure is to

1. Fold the triangular bandage into a three-inch cravat.
2. Take the shoe off, especially if a sprain is suspected.
3. Place the middle part of the cravat in the instep portion of the foot.
4. Cross the two ends of the cravat behind the heel.
5. Pull the ends in opposite directions and down, around and under the cravat.
6. Pull up on the cravat from each side to tighten and until the wrap is reasonably secure.
7. Tie on top or in front of the foot with a square knot.
8. Test to make certain that the bandage will not pull off over the foot. It must be secure.

Fracture of the Jaw

One triangular bandage will provide good support and protection to a fractured or dislocated jaw. In this situation the first-aider should

1. Fold the bandage as a cravat.
2. Place the middle portion of the cravat beneath the chin.
3. Bring the opposite ends over the flat portion of the head and tie with a square knot.
4. If the cravat is long enough, encircle the head again and tie.
5. Don't tie too tightly. The purpose is only to protect and to support.

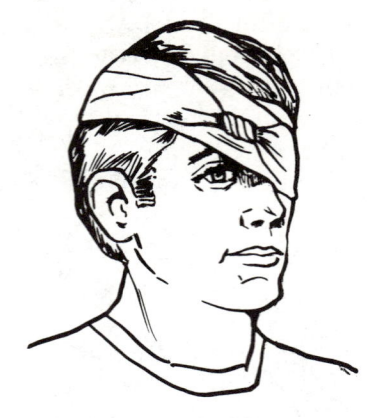

[336]   Essential Techniques to Master: Bandaging and Splinting

FIGURE 22.18   Triangular bandage as cravat for protecting eye.

Eye Injury

One triangular bandage folded as a cravat can afford protection to an injured eye, but if two cravats are available, even better protection can be obtained. The procedure is to

1   Place a sterile eye pad over the injured eye.
2   Fold the bandage as a cravat.
3   Place the cravat on an angle with the midportion covering the injured eye, continue around the head with the two ends of the cravat in opposite directions, tie with a square knot.
4   With two bandages, place one across the head with one extending downward and over the good eye.
5   With the second bandage, on an angle, tie around the head completely covering the injured eye with the cravat—the dressing will be over the eye and beneath the cravat.
6   Pull up with both ends of the first bandage to uncover the uninjured eye so that the victim can see. Tie the two ends of the cravat on top of the head with a square knot.

SPLINTING

There is a rule of long standing concerning broken bones, dislocations, and suspected fractures. "If there is any doubt, splint the victim before moving." Even if a wrong judgment is made, the splints will not harm the victim.

Frequently, individuals who intend to help will permit or assist the injured to his feet, then allow the victim to walk. If the injury is a fracture of the upper leg, pelvis, back, or smaller bones of the lower leg, the failure to splint can be dangerous.

Shock occurs to some degree in all body injuries, especially in fractures. The larger the bone, the more intense the shock. The way the victim is handled, including splinting or failure to splint and transportation, will influence the degree of shock. It is important that shock be protected first in fracture cases. First-aiders should act promptly to prevent or postpone it.

The first-aider should handle the suspected fracture carefully and avoid any unnecessary manipulation of the injured part. He should make every effort to determine the nature of the injury. If the injury is believed to be a fracture, it should be protected by splinting and suitable transportation should be provided to the hospital.

SPLINTING MATERIAL

Hopefully, splints will be available when needed. Splints can be purchased, self-made, or improvised from a variety of materials.

Purchased Splints

The most recent type of ready-made splint is the orally inflated plastic bandage-splint. Assorted sizes can be purchased to protect the hand, lower arm, elbow, ankle, knee, and lower leg. The splint is placed around the injured part and is easily and quickly inflated by mouth. The air pressure provides a comfortable cushion and also secures the position of the fracture. The plastic bandage-splints are simple and easy to apply quickly; they help combat shock, protect other tissues, and are washable and reusable. These splints are very desirable for use by rescue truck, ambulance, and playground attendants, school and industry personnel, and police.

The Thomas splint, sometimes called the half-ring, is the ideal splint for placing the upper arm or upper leg in traction. These splints should be readily available in schools and in industry where it is most likely that they will be needed. If the Thomas splint is not available, wooden improvised splints should be used for placing the leg or arm in traction.

Self-Made Splints

Preferably splints should be made from wood. The ideal material is plywood cut into different widths and lengths to fit the areas where they will be most needed. Two-ply plywood is satisfactory for making arm splints; however, four-ply should be used for making traction splints for the legs and arms. Four-ply plywood should also be used for making splints for pelvic fractures and knee fractures.

The plywood should be covered with white cloth or gauze, and strips of adhesive should be used to secure the cloth or gauze in place. Traction

[338]   Essential Techniques to Master: Bandaging and Splinting

splints for the leg and arm should be notched three or four inches deep at the two ends to help secure the bandages to the splints.

Suitable splints for the lower arm and wrist can be made from hardware cloth, a heavy square wire mesh. This wire can be cut into strips, four to five inches wide, and then folded into a compact package. The cut edges of the wire should be covered with adhesive tape strips.

Improvised Splints

If ready-made or self-made splints are not available, it is possible to improvise and provide some protection with materials at hand, such as newspapers, magazines, umbrellas, wooden strips such as rulers or tree limbs, folded heavy cardboard, or paper boxing. Improvised splints are most satisfactory on the wrist, lower arm, and lower leg. These areas are common fracture locations. Though fractures are serious and need protection, it is not necessary to hurry. It would be better to take sufficient time to prepare a splint than to do an unsatisfactory job and cause the victim added trouble and discomfort.

TYPES OF SPLINTING

There are two types of splinting, fixation and traction. In fixation splinting, the injured part is protected by fixing it in place. In traction splinting, the injured part is put into a state of stress or pull. The purpose is to apply enough traction or pull to compensate for the behavior of the muscles. Muscles tend to go into a state of contraction when a bone adjacent to the muscles is broken. This condition is especially dangerous in the upper leg because the muscles are heavy and strong. Also, there is only the one bone, the femur, in the upper leg. When the injured part is placed in traction, the muscle contraction is controlled and the bone is kept in position. The danger of overriding and the possibility of the simple fracture becoming compound are lessened and hopefully prevented. Traction splinting for the upper leg is most desirable. Much is made of traction splinting in hospitals for other body parts. The first-aider's concern is primarily with the arm and leg. The arm can also be put into traction to protect a broken humerus in the upper arm.

Fixation Splinting

This is fixing the broken bones in place by the use of wooden splints or improvised splints of magazines, newspapers, cardboard, and other materials. Fixation splinting will be discussed for several body locations.

Types of Splinting [339]

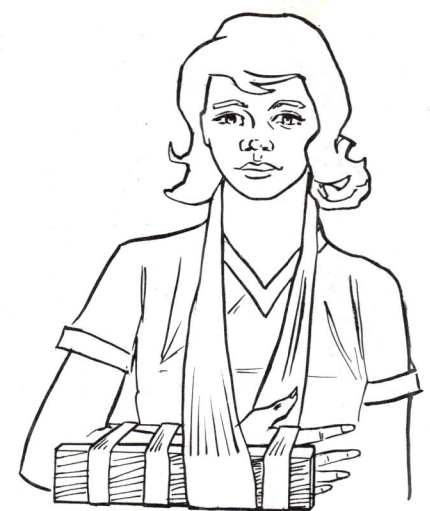

FIGURE 22.19 Fixation splinting for lower arm or wrist.

Lower Arm and Wrist The lower arm, including the wrist and hand, is a common area for fractures. There are two bones in the lower arm, the radius and the ulna. If a fracture is suspected in either one or both of these bones, the victim should be seated and the part protected by fixation. The following procedure should be used:

1. Two wooden padded splints are needed. These splints should be long enough to extend from the elbow down the arm and beyond the palm and fingertips for an arm fracture. The splints should extend from the middle of the lower arm and beyond the fingertips for a wrist injury, fracture, or sprain.
2. One splint should be on the palm side and the other splint opposite, so that the arm is centered between the splints.
3. The splints should be secured with roller gauze, elastic bandage, several neckties, or two or three triangular bandages folded as cravats. The fingertips should remain exposed at all times.
4. The injured arm should be placed in an arm sling with the fingertips exposed and the arm should be elevated.
5. Another triangular bandage should be folded as a cravat, and the injured area secured to the body. This bandage should surround the body from a midpoint in the upper arm.
6. The victim should remain quiet, sitting or reclining, until suitable transportation is provided.

[340] Essential Techniques to Master: Bandaging and Splinting

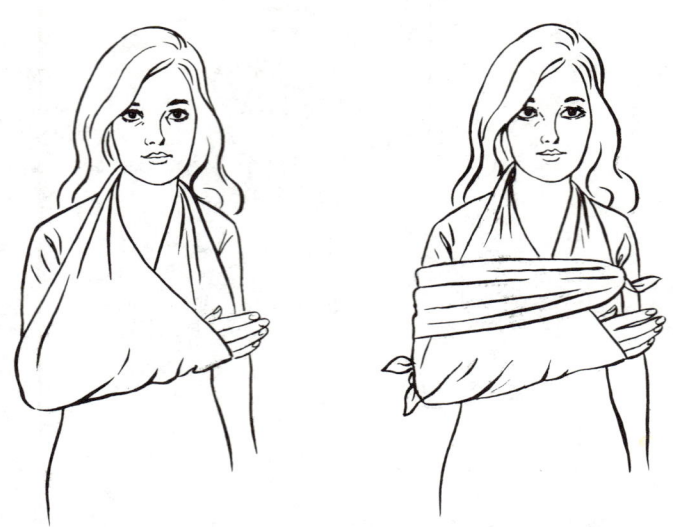

FIGURE 22.20 Triangular bandage—showing arm sling and use of cravat for protecting collar bone or shoulder separation.

Collarbone and Shoulder Fractures of the clavicle and separations and dislocations of the shoulder are common in contact sports, automobile accidents, and falls. All three injuries are protected by the first-aider in the same manner. The basic procedure is outlined as follows:

1. The victim should be placed in a sitting or semireclining position until transportation is provided.
2. The arm on the injured side should be placed in an arm sling, and the arm should be elevated reasonably.
3. A second triangular bandage should be folded as a cravat, and the injured arm should be secured to the body by placing the cravat around the arm, midway in the upper arm and tied reasonably tight on the opposite side of the body.

Upper Arm—Humerus This bone is not as commonly fractured as the lower arm bones or the wrist. Such a fracture would be indicated by pain from motion, swelling, and tenderness in the area. The following procedure should be used to protect the humerus:

1. The victim should be seated and quiet until transportation is provided.
2. Padded wooden splints should be placed on both sides of the arm, one from the armpit down the inside and past the elbow joint, the second from the shoulder down the outside of the arm and past the elbow joint.

Types of Splinting   **[341]**

3. The splints should be secured reasonably tight with triangular bandages folded as cravats, or with neckties or roller-type bandages.
4. The arm should be placed in an arm sling with the fingertips exposed and the arm reasonably elevated.
5. Two cravats should be used to secure the arm to the body, surrounding the body from a midpoint of the upper arm, then tying the cravat ends on the opposite side of the body.

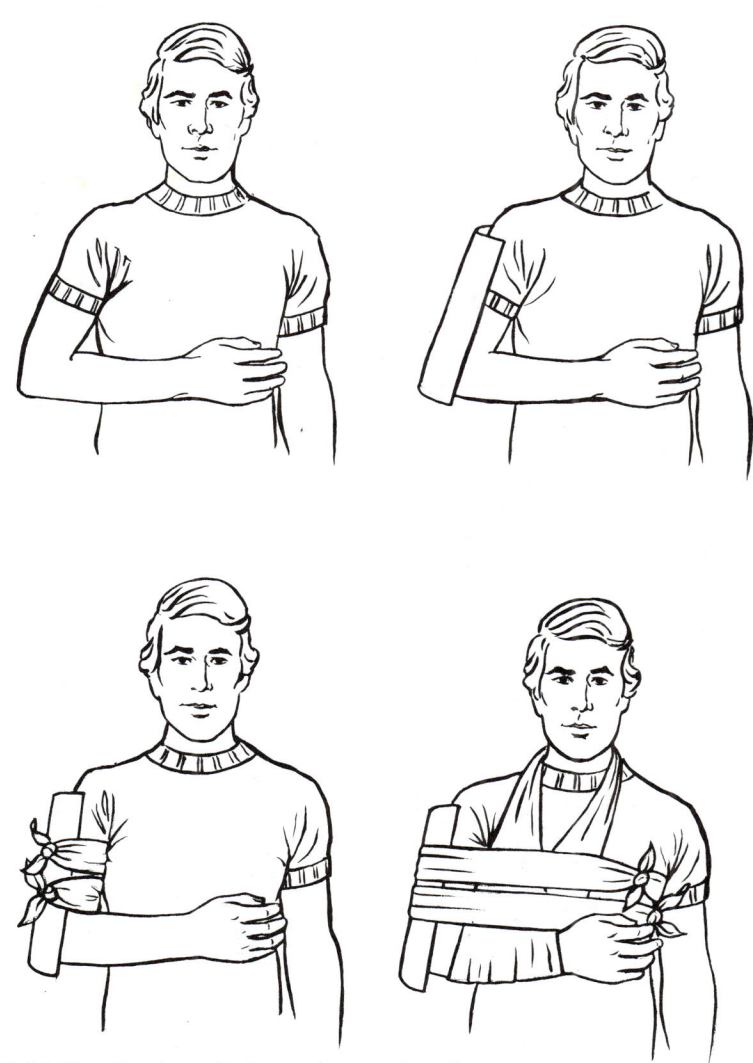

FIGURE 22.21   Fixation splinting and protection of upper arm.

[342] Essential Techniques to Master: Bandaging and Splinting

Elbow Joint This is a very important joint and protection should be given to prevent damage to the tissues that surround it. Henderson[1] states that such fractures may result in varying degrees of permanent disability. If the elbow is fractured, there may be discoloration, a false position of the part, pain, and shock. To give protection the first-aider should

1) Place the victim in a lying position to guard against shock.
2) The arm, including the elbow, should remain in the position it was found.
3) If the arm is straight, splint with a wooden splint from the armpit to and beyond the fingertips, placing the splint on the inside of the arm.
4) If the arm is bent, secure the arm to the body by means of an arm sling and by cravats to maintain the bent position.
5) Provide suitable transportation to medical help.
6) If the fracture is compound, cover the wound with a dressing; then apply the splints. The wound should be left for the physician to treat.

Finger Each of the four fingers has three bones, and the thumb two bones. The fracturing of a finger is rather common. When it occurs it is evident because there are pain, deformity, swelling, and inability to use the part. Finger injuries are common in physical activities, especially football, basketball, and baseball.

If the finger is injured, it could be a sprain, a dislocation, or a fracture. Only an x-ray can tell for certain the nature of the injury. In all three situations, splinting will protect. The procedure is to

1 Have the victim sit down and put his injured finger in an extended position.
2 Place a tongue blade, finger stall, or some firm material as a splint from the palm of the hand to beyond the fingertip on the underside.

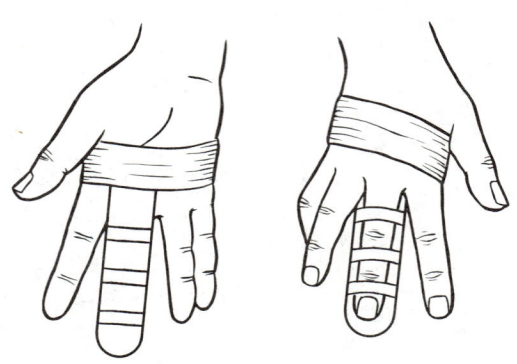

FIGURE 22.22 Fixation splinting for finger.

[1] John Henderson, *Emergency Medical Guide*, 4th ed. New York: McGraw-Hill, 1978, p. 198.

Types of Splinting [343]

3 Secure the splint with roller gauze or muslin strips.
4 Transport the victim to medical help for x-ray and treatment.
5 If it is evident that the finger is dislocated, place the hand in a downward position and exert a steady pull to position the finger.

Ankle The ankle is commonly fractured and sprained. There is no sure way for the first-aider to distinguish between a fracture and a severe sprain of the ankle. Injured persons need to be taken to the hospital and medical doctor for x-ray and protection. The first-aider should be given protection as follows:

1 The victim should get off the injured foot, then preferably remove his shoe.
2 The ankle should be elevated and ice packs should be used to control the swelling.
3 An elastic wrap or cotton webbing should be used to support and protect. This will also help to reduce swelling.
4 The victim should not be allowed to walk. He should be transported to the hospital and physician for x-ray and treatment.

Lower Leg—Tibia and Fibula The larger bone of the lower leg is the tibia, and if it is fractured it will be evident, as the victim will immediately cease to use the part. However, persons have been known to continue activity after a fracture of the small bone, the fibula. If the two bones are fractured, the victim will be disabled immediately. To protect fractures of the lower leg, the first-aider should

1 Place the victim in a reclining position.
2 Use ice packs or cold to limit swelling and bleeding.
3 Place the injured leg between two padded splints, one extending from the groin (between the legs), the second splint corresponding with the first in position but on the outside of the leg.
4 Secure the splints with four or five triangular bandages, folded as cravats but not tight enough to limit circulation.

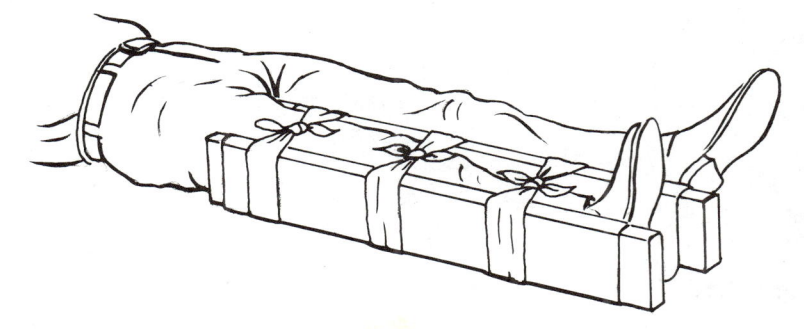

FIGURE 22.23 Fixation splinting for lower leg.

[344]   Essential Techniques to Master: Bandaging and Splinting

5. Place the victim on a litter and transport him to the hospital in a reclining position, preferably keeping the injured leg in an elevated position.

Kneecap—Knee or Patella   Henderson states

> The most common fracture of the knee occurs at the kneecap, as a result of a crushing blow. The great majority of such accidents are sustained in automobile accidents when the person riding next to the driver (suicide seat) is thrown forward against the dashboard.[2]

Knee fractures also result from athletic injuries and other crushing blows. The seat belt has proven to be the best device for preventing this type of accident in the automobile crash. Fractured kneecaps are indicated by swelling and pain in the joint. The victim will not attempt to straighten the knee, and it is frequently possible to feel the parts of the broken bone, the patella. To protect the knee and kneecap when it is injured

1. Place the victim in a lying-down position (supine) and protect against shock.
2. Apply cold compresses or ice packs to the injured area to limit swelling and bleeding.
3. Place a padded wooden splint, six inches wide and thick enough to support, from the buttocks to beyond the heel and on the underneath side of the leg.
4. Secure the extended leg which has been placed upon the splint with four or five triangular bandages, folded as cravats.
5. Place the splinted leg in an elevated position and wait for transportation.
6. Transport to a hospital and medical help in a lying position.

Upper Leg—Femur   The upper leg has only one bone, the femur. This bone supports the entire body weight when a person stands. If the shaft or main portion of the femur is fractured or broken, the individual will be immobilized at once. The upper end of the femur terminates into a round

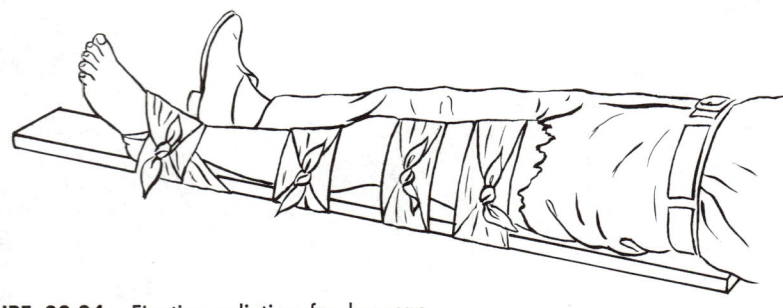

FIGURE 22.24   Fixation splinting for kneecap.

[2] Ibid., p. 120.

Types of Splinting [345]

ball-like part which fits into the pelvis to form a ball-and-socket joint, the hip joint. It is not uncommon for the head of the femur to be broken off, especially in older persons. Such injuries would be most difficult to ascertain without the x-ray. Fractures of the femur or upper leg can be protected by either fixation or traction splinting. For fixation splinting the first-aider should

1. Keep the victim down and protect for shock.
2. Straighten the leg as gently as possible.
3. Place a padded wooden splint from the armpit on the injured side to six to twelve inches beyond the feet.
4. Place a second padded wooden splint between the legs, from the groin to some six to twelve inches beyond the feet. Pad the area over the crest of the ileum to lessen pressure on the great trocanter of the femur.
5. Secure the two splints with six to eight triangular bandages folded as cravats. Place three or four of these cravats around the two splints and the injured leg, between the ankle and the groin; then with two or three additional cravats tie around the torso and the long splint.
6. Secure the two legs together, from hip to feet with two or three more triangular bandages as cravats.
7. Keep the victim down and comfortable until transportation is available to medical help.

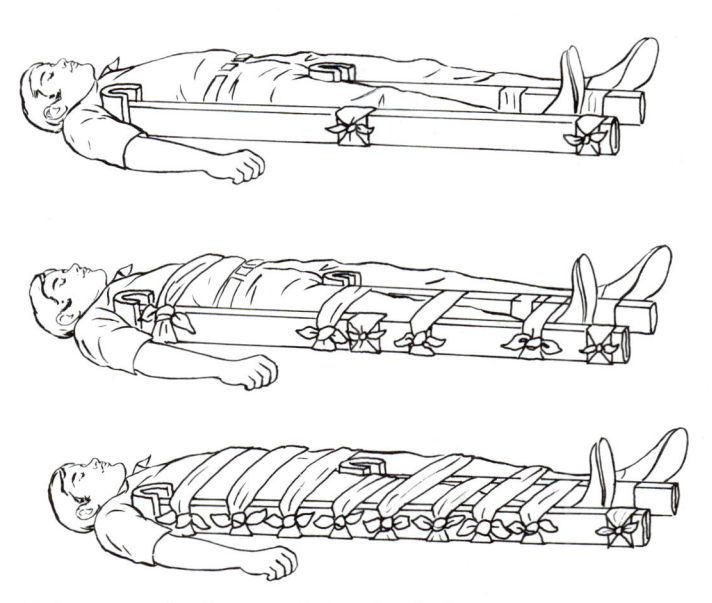

FIGURE 22.25 Steps for fixation splinting for thigh.

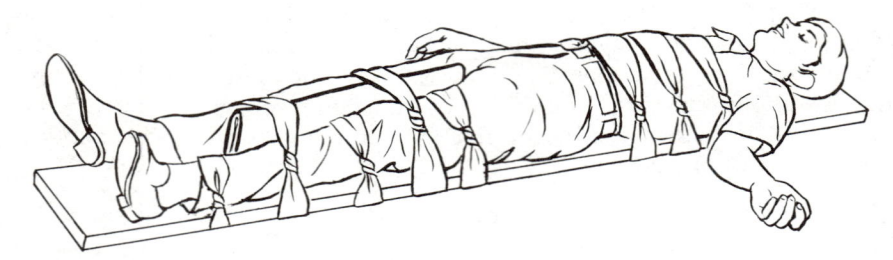

Essential Techniques to Master: Bandaging and Splinting

FIGURE 22.26 Improvised fixation splinting of a pelvic fracture.

Pelvis or Hip Fractures of the pelvis are most common in older people and usually result from falls. Fractures of the pelvis to persons of all ages are common in crushing-type injuries, such as result from automobile accidents. If there is any likelihood of a fracture to this area, the victim should not be permitted to get on his feet. It is dangerous because bone fragments could penetrate the bladder, reproductive organs, intestines, blood vessels, and nerves. Indications of a fractured pelvis are pain, inability to lift or move the leg, false position of the leg and/or foot, and a deep bruise. Frequently the leg and foot assume a turned-out position. The first-aid protection for a fracture of the pelvis is the use of fixation splinting. The first-aider should

1. Place the victim in a lying-down position (supine) and gently straighten the leg. The victim should be protected against shock.
2. Place a padded splint, a board six to twelve inches wide and at least an inch thick, beneath the victim on the injured side. The splint should extend several inches beyond the head and the feet.
3. Place a folded blanket or pad between the victim's legs.
4. With three triangular bandages folded as cravats, secure the leg to the splint, with three more cravats, secure the upper body or torso to the splint.
5. With two or three additional cravats, secure the two legs, going around the legs, splint, and folded blanket.
6. Transport the victim to the hospital in an ambulance or other suitable conveyance.

Neck and Back "The procedures for caring for a victim of a broken back are the same as those listed for one with a broken neck, with this important exception: The victim must be transported in the face-down position."[3]

Injuries to the back and neck should receive the utmost protection. Careless handling can injure the spinal cord and cause paralysis or death. First-aiders should not attempt to move the victim until sufficient help is available and a rigid platform is at hand for use as a litter. Planking is

[3] Ibid., p. 129.

Types of Splinting   [347]

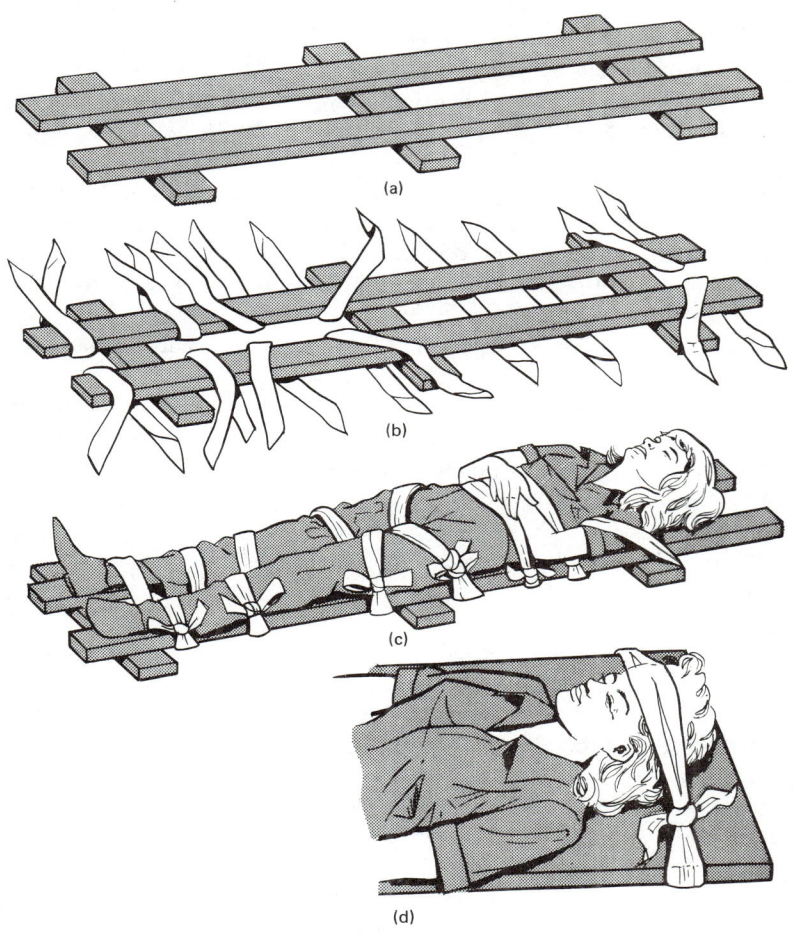

FIGURE 22.27 Protection for neck and back fracture: (a) rigid platform; (b) placement of cravats; (c) securing of patient to rigid platform with cravats; (d) securing the head and neck.

preferable because of the ease in securing the tringular bandages which are used as cravats. Such a platform can be made with a minimum of effort, or in an emergency a door can be used as the rigid-type litter. The first-aider can make several checks to determine where the back is injured. Back and neck injuries can be protected by the first-aider by applying fixation splinting:

1   Prepare a rigid platform from two boards longer than the victim's body and strong enough to support his weight without bending. Three or four cross boards, three or four inches wide, should be placed at the location where the feet, knees, hips, and shoulders of the victim will be. These boards

[348] Essential Techniques to Master: Bandaging and Splinting

should be nailed together, leaving a reasonable space between the two long boards for the cravats to secure the injured victim to the rigid litter.
2. If possible, pad the boards with a blanket.
3. Place the victim on the stretcher, face down for a back injury, face up for a neck injury. There should be sufficient people to easily lift the victim and to keep his head and body straight without any bending, twisting, or jarring. The lifters should carefully rehearse, one person should give the command, and then all should work as a unit. Special consideration should be given to the head and neck to prevent possible turning, twisting, or falling. It is advisable for one person to maintain the position of the head by applying a steady pull.
4. Secure the victim firmly by tying the legs, hips, torso, head, and neck. The arms can be folded across the body and secured at the wrists.
5. Pad on each side with pillows, paper, clothing, wrapped bricks, sand bags, etc., to keep the head in position. Nothing should be placed between the litter and the head. Place padding beneath the body curves.
6. Carefully place the victim in an ambulance on his rigid platform litter; transport slowly and carefully to the hospital and medical staff. If possible, the hospital should be advised that a back and neck injury victim is in transit.

Rib Injuries Fractured ribs are common. Such injuries result from sharp blows to the rib cage. A tender spot and short, painful, fast, and shallow breaths are indications of rib fractures. It is possible to protect the broken ribs and to lessen the danger by applying wide bandages or strips of

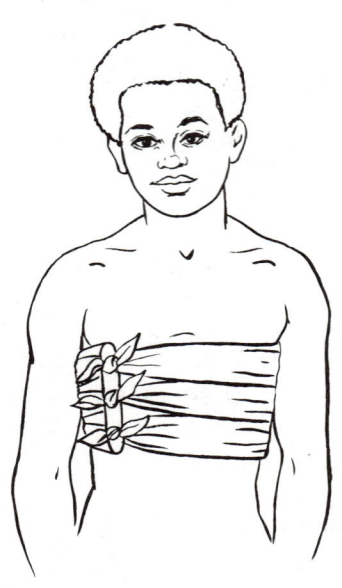

FIGURE 22.28 Triangular bandages as cravats—pressure bandage for broken ribs.

adhesive tape, two or three inches wide, around the rib cage and chest. "In cases where the ribs seem depressed because of injury, bandages should not be applied around the chest, lest the broken rib ends be driven deeper into the soft tissue."[4]

The first-aider can protect the fractured rib with fixation bandages. He should

1. Fold three triangular bandages into three-inch-wide cravats.
2. Place the first cravat around the body and cover the injured rib location. A pad or short padded splint should be placed on the opposite side for securing the knot.
3. Have the victim take a deep breath. As the victim exhales, the cravat should be tightened reasonably and secured with a square knot.
4. Place the second cravat just below the first cravat; tighten and secure with a square knot.
5. Place the third cravat above the first cravat; tighten and secure with a square knot.
6. Transport to the hospital, preferably in a reclining position. If the bandages cause pain, they should be removed.

Traction Splinting

Fractures of leg bones, especially the femur of the thigh, can be protected by traction splinting and using the Thomas splint or an improvised wooden splint. The Thomas splint consists of a metal ring large enough to encircle the upper leg. This ring is joined by a hinge and is connected to two metal rods long enough to extend beyond the toes.

The Thomas splint is a traction splint and it is recommended for use on the leg when traction is needed. The purpose of traction splinting is to immobilize the fractured bone ends by applying pull, thus helping to prevent tissue damage.

Leg—Thomas Splint The first-aider can apply traction to the leg by means of the Thomas splint. Two persons are needed for placing the arm or leg in traction—one for maintaining a steady pull on the leg during the process, and the other for doing the splinting. In applying the Thomas splint on the leg, the first-aider should

1. Place the victim in a back (supine) position and protect against shock.
2. Have the helper grasp the victim's foot on the injured leg, one hand on the toes, the other on the heel, and maintain a constant pull until the splinting is finished.
3. Fasten the Thomas splint into place, the short part toward the crotch and the longer part on the outside of the leg. The leg is centered in the splint and the buckle is secured. It should not be too tight.

[4] American National Red Cross, *Advanced First Aid and Emergency Care*. New York: Doubleday, 1973, p. 171.

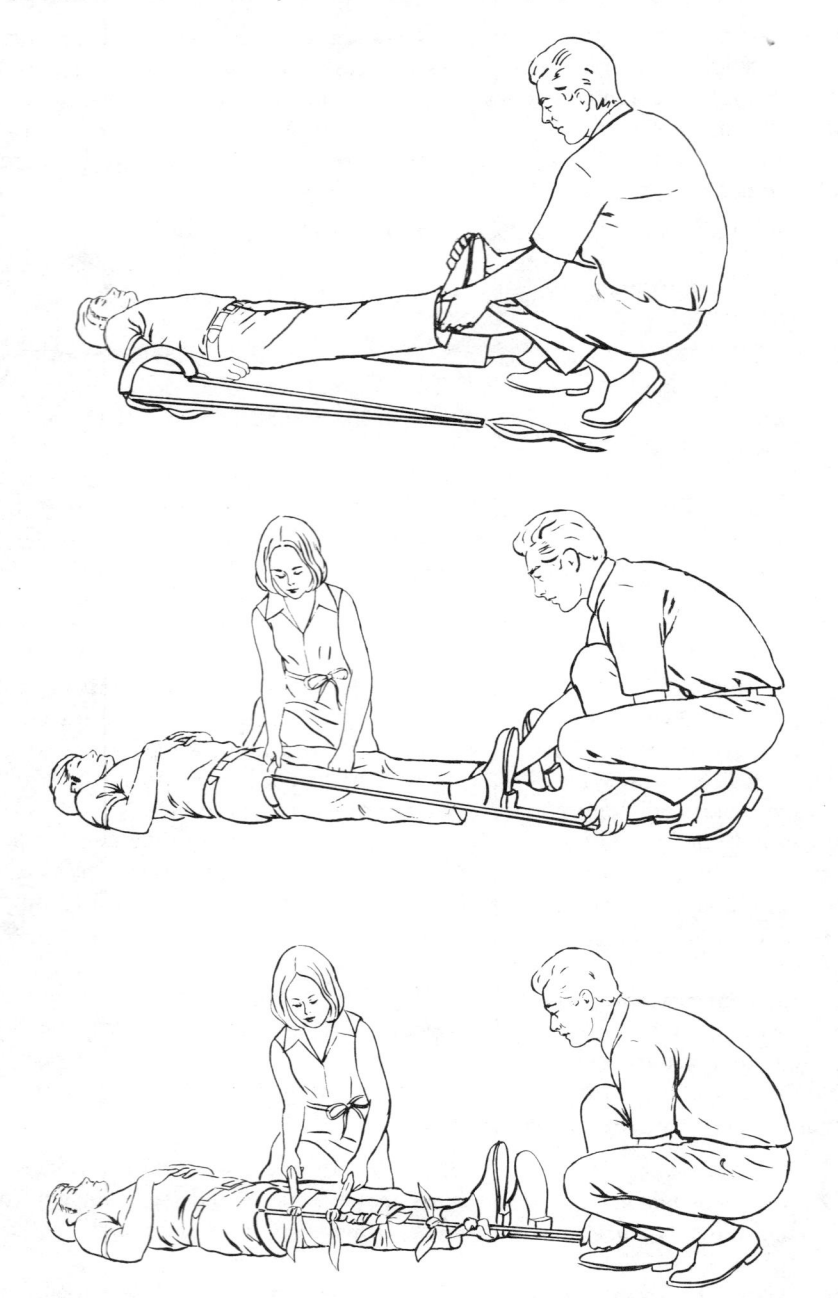

[350] Essential Techniques to Master: Bandaging and Splinting

FIGURE 22.29 Steps in applying Thomas splint for traction splinting of upper leg.

Types of Splinting [351]

4. With a triangular bandage folded as a cravat, apply an ankle wrap snugly on the foot.
5. With another triangular bandage folded as a cravat, fasten it to the foot end of the Thomas splint with a lock-hitch by making a loop over the splint end; go around the splint with the cravat, and press both ends through the loop to secure to the splint.
6. Pass the ends of the cravat that have been secured at the foot of the splint under the part of the ankle wrap that surrounds the victim's foot; then pull them toward the victim's foot to tighten, pass the end around the splint, and tie with a square knot in the center on top.
7. Insert a section of broom handle, strong piece of wood, or metal between the two ends of the cravat between the end of the splint and the foot, and twist. Sufficient traction or tension should be applied to compensate for the contraction of the leg muscles.
8. Support the leg in the splint with four to five triangular bandages as cravats, several neckties, or an elastic wrap. The leg can be cradled in the splint by passing neckties or cravats under the injured leg and across both sides of the splint, then reversing the directions and tying the cravats or neckties on top with a square knot.
9. Elevate the splinted leg a reasonable distance from the floor and allow the victim to rest.
10. Transport the victim to the hospital in a reclining position when suitable transportation is available.

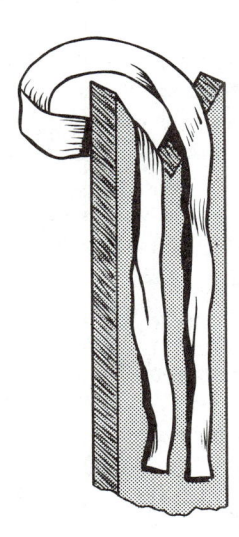

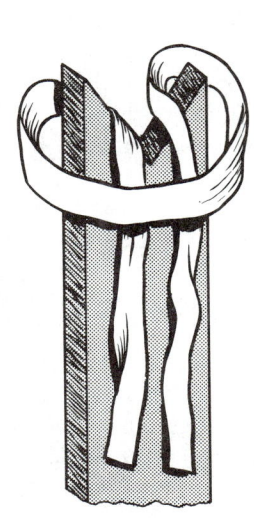

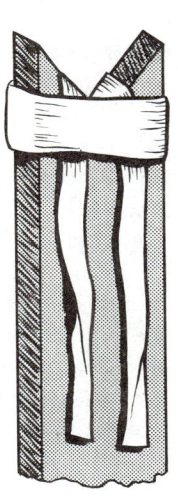

FIGURE 22.30 Securing cravat on improvised splint.

Essential Techniques to Master: Bandaging and Splinting

Leg—Improvised Wooden Splint One would expect to find the Thomas splint at school, in industry, or on a rescue truck. If it is available, it should be used. However, broken legs occur in many places, and if the Thomas splint is not at hand, it becomes necessary to improvise. Putting the leg in traction by means of an improvised splint is not difficult and it is effective. These are the steps to follow:

1. A splint should be prepared from four-ply plywood, a one-by-four-inch piece of wood, or if need be a tree limb. It should be long enough to extend about one foot beyond the victim's feet and one foot beyond the victim's crotch. There should be a notch or "V" cut down into each end of the splint, two to three inches deep.
2. The victim should be placed in a supine position and protected against shock.
3. The first-aider's helper must grasp the victim's foot, one hand on the toes and the other on the heel, and maintain a constant pull or traction until splinting is finished.
4. The first-aider, with a triangular bandage folded as a cravat, should apply an ankle wrap snugly on the victim's foot. It must be tight or it will pull off and not serve the purpose intended.
5. With another triangular bandage folded as a cravat, the first-aider should form a loop from the crotch; the loop should extend around the leg and above the hip. The upper end of the splint will be placed in this loop.
6. With another triangular bandage folded as a cravat, the first-aider should form a loop and secure the bandage to the foot end of the wooden splint with a lock-type hitch. (See Figure 22.30.)
7. The first-aider should put the splint in place, tuck the two ends of the cravat that have been attached to the foot end of the splint beneath the portion of the ankle wrap which goes under the foot. He should pull toward the end of the splint to tighten, then pass around the splint and tie with a square knot.
8. The first-aider should place a twisting device, a broom handle or other strong material, between the two ends of the cravat between the end of the splint and foot and apply traction.
9. The splint should be secured to the leg with neckties, cravats, or elastic wraps.
10. The foot should be elevated a reasonable distance from the floor and protected from sagging.
11. The victim should be transported to the hospital in a reclining position when suitable transportation is available.

ACTIVITIES

1. Prepare several triangular bandages of different sizes and demonstrate the six uses you consider to be the most important. Be prepared to defend your choices.
2. Demonstrate to fellow classmates the use(s) of the roller gauze bandage.
3. Demonstrate the figure-of-eight bandage for the wrist, ankle, and knee.
4. Demonstrate recurrent bandaging of a finger and the spiral reverse bandaging of the forearm or lower leg.
5. Prepare fixation splints of different sizes from wood or other materials. Demonstrate the use of these splints on different body parts.
6. Prepare improvised traction splints for splinting the upper leg. Demonstrate to the class traction splinting on the leg.

QUESTIONS TO ANSWER

1. What is the difference between a bandage and a dressing? Give examples of each.
2. How is a fractured pelvis protected by splinting?
3. How is a fractured kneecap protected by splinting?
4. Describe the Thomas splint. What is it used for?
5. What precautions should be followed in protecting an elbow that is fractured or dislocated?
6. What protection is given the upper arm or collarbone that has been fractured?
7. Why are fractures of the upper arm or leg more dangerous than fractures of the lower arm or leg?
8. Why is it important to keep the victim of a pelvic fracture from standing? What are the indications of such a fracture.
9. What are some of the provisions that a first-aider can make to splint a fracture of the lower arm or wrist?
10. How should a first-aider protect suspected broken ribs if he has nothing to work with but triangular bandages?

SELECTED REFERENCES

AMERICAN NATIONAL RED CROSS, *Advanced First Aid and Emergency Care*. New York: Doubleday, 1973.

AMERICAN NATIONAL RED CROSS, *Standard First Aid and Personal Safety*. New York: Doubleday, 1973.

Cole, Warren H., and Puestow, Charles B., *First Aid: Diagnosis and Management.* New York: Appleton-Century-Crofts, 1965.

Henderson, John, *Emergency Medical Guide*, 4th ed. New York: McGraw-Hill, 1978.

Potthoff, Carl J., "First Aid—Fractures of the Ankle." *Today's Health*, January, 1963.

Potthoff, Carl J., "First Aid—Fracture of Pelvic Bone." *Today's Health*, November, 1963.

Potthoff, Carl J., "First Aid—Finger and Thumb Injuries." *Today's Health*, April, 1963.

23. TRANSPORTATION FOR PROTECTION

In a recent year there were 15 million disabling accidents in the United States, and in almost every case the victim had to be transported either to his home or to medical help. In some cases an assist from another person was sufficient; in others, a litter with several helpers and an ambulance with trained attendants were needed.

The mode of transportation used to assist an accident victim may endanger his life if proper care is not taken. Usually the victim should not be moved unless there is immediate danger, such as fire, a falling wall, or other such condition. In some situations speed is an essential part of the protection for injuries, but speed should not aggravate the victim's injuries.

The American National Red Cross has suggested two objectives that should be applied in transportation of a victim.

1 Avoid subjecting the patient to unnecessary disturbance during planning, preparation, and transfer.
2 Prevent injured body parts from twisting, bending, and shaking.[1]

To these two objectives, a third objective should be added:

3 Fit transportation to the injury.

A basic rule is to carefully check the victim to determine the problem, protect the problem, and then make certain the transportation meets the victim's needs. "When an individual has been injured, he should not be

---

[1] American National Red Cross, *First Aid*, 4th ed. New York: Doubleday, 1957, p. 97.

[355]

[356] Transportation for Protection

hastily put in the back seat of a car and taken to the hospital until it is determined what may be the extent of his injury." [2]

The American Red Cross has gone on to say

> It should be recognized that more harm can be done through improper rescue and transportation than through any other measures associated with emergency assistance. In the majority of situations, rescue from confinement or pinning should be carried out by ambulance or rescue personnel. Pending their arrival, the first-aider should gain access to the victim, give him emergency care, reassure him, and avoid ill-advised or foolhardy attempts at rescue that might jeopardize the safety of the victim as well as that of the first aider.[3]

GENERAL PRECAUTIONS AND DIRECTIONS

The necessary directions and recognized precautions in transporting a victim are summarized as follows:

1. All first-aid measures should be carried out: control bleeding, bandage wounds, and immobilize fractures, sprains, and dislocations before transporting the victim. A first-aider should protect against shock, try to minimize pain, and make the person comfortable.
2. A first-aider should make all movements gently, deliberately, and calmly. Tension by the first-aider in the situation can cause emotional strain in the victim. Also, hasty or careless handling of the victim may result in a more severe injury. The first-aider should not allow the victim's body to jacknife. Support should be provided for the legs, arms, head, and back.
3. It is best to use an approved stretcher, if one is available. If an improvised stretcher is to be made, it should be strong enough to hold the victim. Two persons are usually essential to give adequate transportation, but with minor injuries one person can transport a victim.
4. The means of transportation, i.e., stretcher, should be brought to the victim instead of carrying the victim to the transportation device.
5. One person should take charge and give the proper orders and directions.
6. The victim should be fastened to the mode of transportation (stretcher) so he cannot slip off.
7. The victim should be transported in the position suited to his situation or injury. Normally the victim is moved while lying on his back. A person who has a breathing problem should be transported in a semireclining position. A sitting-up or upright position can be utilized for a victim who has no serious injuries.

---

[2] W. J. Gillesby, "Transportation of the Injured." *First Aid: Diagnosis and Management*. Warren H. Cole and Charles B. Puestow (eds.). New York: Appleton-Century-Crofts, 1965, p. 135.

[3] American National Red Cross, *Standard First Aid and Personal Safety*. New York: Doubleday, 1973, p. 225.

8   If the victim is being carried in a reclining or horizontal position, he should be moved feet first.
9   If a motor vehicle can be used for transportation, an ambulance is best. Passenger cars and even station wagons or panel trucks are impractical and can result in further injury through improper handling. If a vehicle of this type must be used it should be driven with utmost care and at a reasonable speed.
10 The attending physician should be informed as to what actually happened to the victim, i.e., a fall from a tree or a traffic accident.

METHODS OF TRANSPORTATION

The purpose of this section is to present and explain the better manual methods of transporting the accident victim. Methods requiring one man, two men, and three or more men will be presented. Also, transportation by air and vehicle will be discussed. These methods need to be practiced until the first-aider is proficient in their use.

One-Man Methods

There are several one-man methods that are all satisfactory, especially when the victim has no body injuries. If the victim is overcome by gas, is unconscious from water, has fainted, has a sprained ankle, or is intoxicated, the type of transportation does not present a problem. The following are considered as being satisfactory one-man methods of transportation.

Blanket Drag This is an easy way to move a person from a burning building. It is also commonly used in hospitals to move patients during emergency situations.

1   Place the victim on a blanket or sheet. If the victim is on the floor, the blanket can be placed beneath the victim by rolling the victim to one side and putting the blanket beneath, then rolling him to the other side and moving the blanket across. If the victim is in bed he can be taken from the bed and placed on the blanket.
2   Gather the blanket about the victim's head; then gently pull or drag him on the floor.

Fireman's Drag This is another one-on-one method, especially for the burning building, the hospital, or in the home. The method works best if the floor is smooth.

1   The victim is placed on his back (supine) on the floor.
2   The victim's arms are folded across his waist and the wrists tied securely with a cravat or necktie.

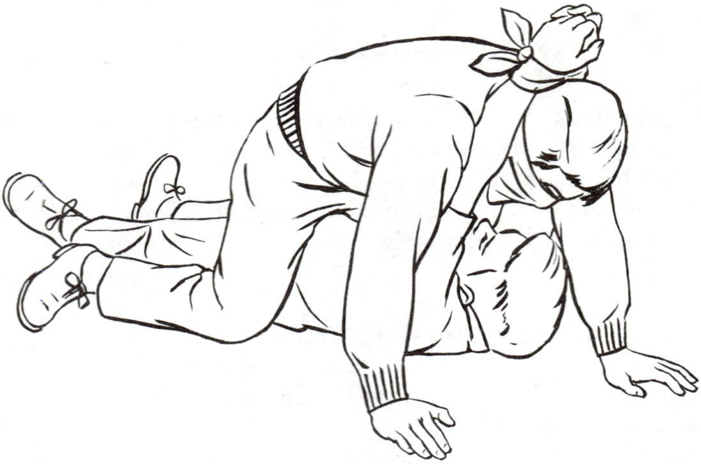

[358] Transportation for Protection

FIGURE 23.1 Fireman's drag.

3. The rescuer gets down, straddles the victim's body at the waist, raises the victim's arms, and places his head into the arch made by the arms, the yoke.
4. The rescuer crawls on the floor on his knees and drags the victim to safety.

Fireman's Carry This is an excellent method for carrying a victim, especially from a burning building where a ladder is involved. The rescuer has one hand free for climbing. The rescuer should

1. Get the victim in an erect position with the victim facing the rescuer.
2. Grasp the victim's left wrist with your right hand.
3. Pull the victim's left arm over your shoulder.
4. Bend your knees, stoop, and allow the victim's abdomen to rest on your left shoulder and back.
5. Put your left arm between the victim's legs.
6. Bring the victim's body across your back.
7. Take hold of the victim's left wrist with your left hand.
8. Stand, using powerful leg muscles to lift, then adjust and balance the victim's weight across your shoulders.
9. Climb or descend and walk carefully.

Arm Carry This is a satisfactory method for a person with minor injuries, who is sick or faint. It would serve for a sprained ankle or bad cut on the foot.

1. Kneel on one knee.
2. Have the victim sit on your bended knee.
3. Place your arm under the victim's knees.
4. Grasp the victim around the waist with your other arm.

Methods of Transportation [359]

5 Stand slowly, holding the victim securely against your body. Have the victim place his arm about your neck.
6 Walk slowly and carefully.

One-Man Support and Carry This method is good for helping a victim with minor injuries who can partially help himself.

1 Assume a position on the victim's side away from the injury.
2 Draw the victim's good arm across and over your shoulder.
3 Hold the victim's arm at the wrist with one hand.
4 With the other hand, support the victim by encircling his waist.
5 Walk slowly and carefully and if possible get your shoulder beneath the victim's armpit for better support. The rescuer and the victim should keep in step.

One-Man Piggyback This method can be used on the victim whose injuries are not severe. It should not be used if there is a possibility of skeletal or internal injuries.

1 Place yourself in front of the victim with your back to the victim.
2 Stoop or get down on one knee.
3 Have the victim put his arms around your neck and grasp one wrist with the other hand.
4 Put your arms beneath the victim's legs at the thighs and grasp your hands.
5 Stand up carefully, using your leg muscles to lift.
6 Adjust the victim's body and weight on your back.
7 Walk carefully and slowly.

Two-Man Methods

If two rescuers are available there are several methods for transporting the injured which are satisfactory when the injuries are minor. These methods involve moving the victim in a standing, sitting, or reclining position. It is also possible for two rescuers to improvise several devices for transporting a victim, such as a chair, belt, blanket, jacket, or sack.

Two-Man Support In this method the two rescuers serve as supports and help the victim walk. The victim must be able to use his arms. The steps to follow are

1 Rescuers assist the victim to his feet.
2 Victim extends an arm around each rescuer's neck.
3 Rescuers place their inside arm next to the victim and around his body.
4 Rescuers grasp the victim's wrists with their hands away from the victim.
5 Rescuers assist the victim as he walks slowly and carefully.

[360] Transportation for Protection

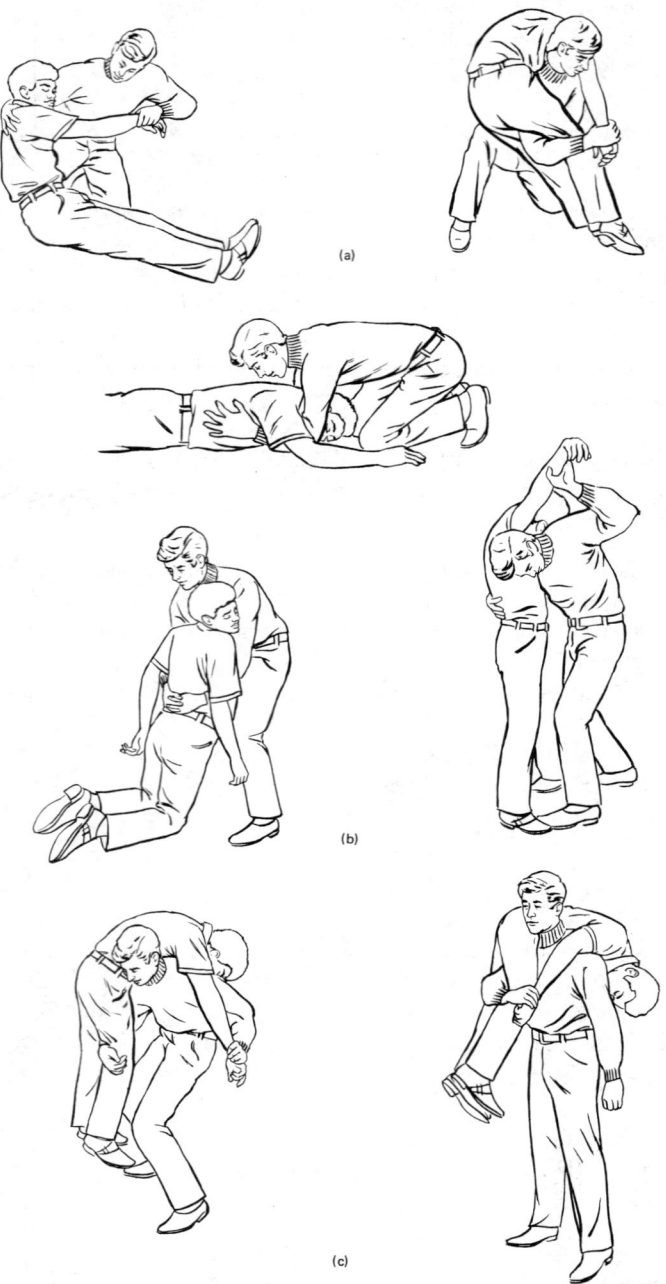

FIGURE 23.2 Fireman's carry: (a) steps in loading the victim from reclining position; (b) steps in loading with rescuer in kneeling position; (c) final carrying position with hand free.

Methods of Transportation [361]

Fore-and-Aft Carry This is a good way to carry a sick person who does not have an injury. It should not be used if there are broken bones, dislocations, or internal injuries of the abdomen or chest. The steps to follow are

1. Rescuers elevate the victim to a semireclining position.
2. One bearer stoops and places his hands beneath the victim's arms and across his chest, then locks his hands or wrists.
3. The second bearer places himself between the victim's legs, facing the victim's feet, and grasps the victim's knees from the outside.
4. The two bearers on a predetermined signal stand, using their leg muscles to lift the victim.
5. The bearers step off on different feet to transport, thus keeping the victim's body moving in a straight line.

Pack Saddle—Four Hands In the event that the victim has a leg injury and cannot walk, it is possible for two bearers to form a pack saddle with their hands and carry the victim. Two bearers can transport a victim of their own size a reasonably long distance. The steps to follow are

1. Rescuers raise the victim to a sitting position.
2. Rescuers kneel on one knee facing each other, one on each side of the victim.
3. Victim places his arms over the shoulders of the two rescuers.
4. Rescuers grasp their own right wrist with their left hand; then with their right hand they grasp the other rescuer's left wrist.
5. Victim puts his weight onto the saddle that has been formed by the four hands.
6. Rescuers lift the victim on command, adjust the victim, and step off with opposite feet, out of step.

Chair Carry Straight chairs with or without legs provide a good support for transporting a victim through a narrow passageway or up and down steps. Chairs with legs are most desirable as they provide a safe holding place for the rescuer. When using the chair carry method, the bearers should

1. Elevate the victim to the standing position.
2. Move the chair into place and assist the victim as he seats himself in the chair.
3. Tilt the chair backward, the bearer in front facing away from the chair, and each grasp the chair legs.
4. Lift on command, adjust their load, step off, and keep in step as they transport the victim.

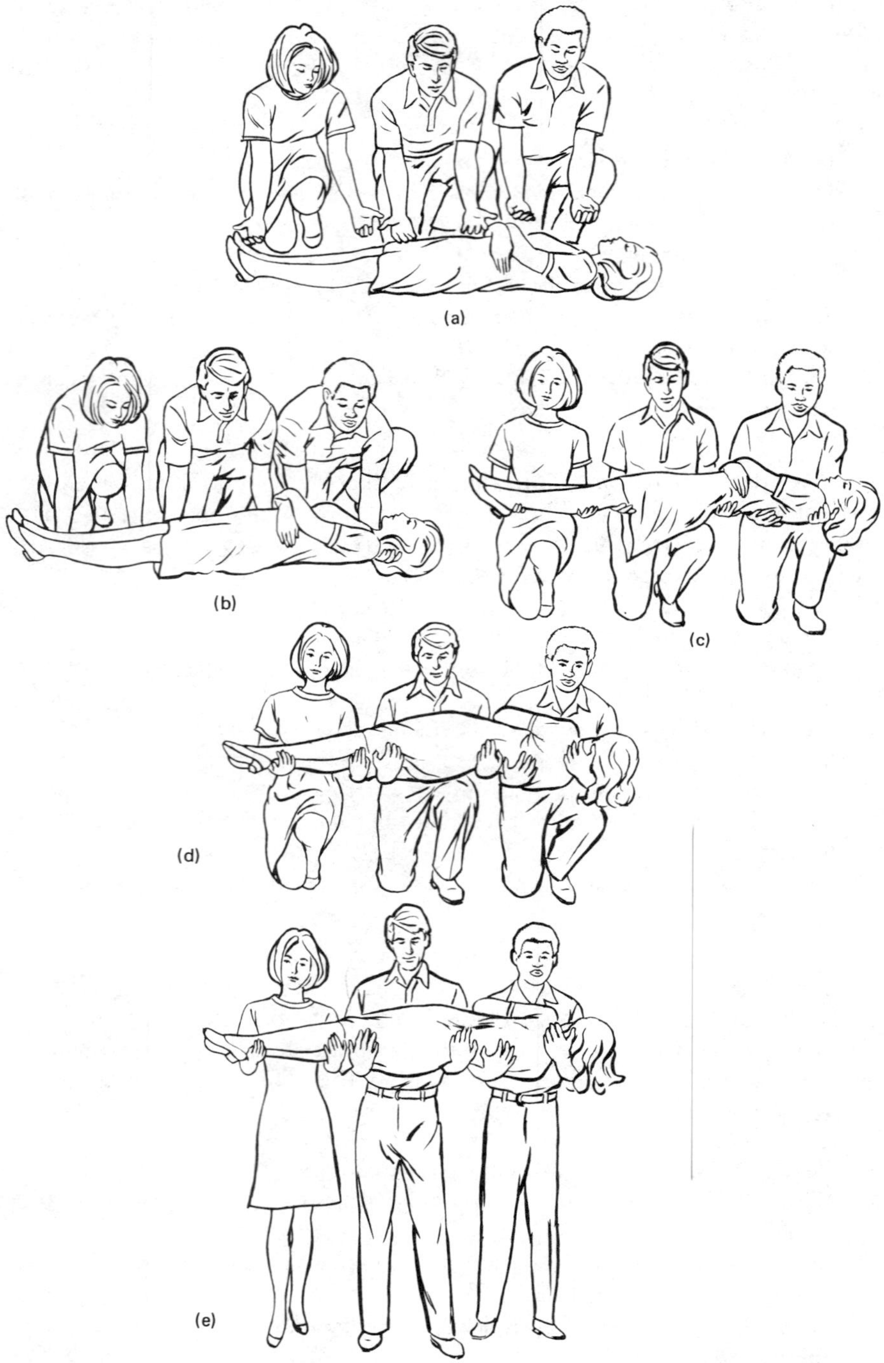

[362] Transportation for Protection

FIGURE 23.3 Steps for three-man lift —one side: (a) practicing correct position; (b) placing hands beneath victim; (c) victim raised to bended knee; (d) victim rotated and held firmly; (e) final walking position.

Three-Man or More Carries

There are two excellent three-man carries, the three-man lift from one side and the hammock carry. Each of these methods has several advantages. These carries are easy to execute. If one person knows the method and the others will assist him, the helpers can be quickly informed as to their specific roles. These methods should be taught to all emergency care groups.

Three-Man Carry from One Side This carry is desirable for picking a person up and carrying abreast in a straight line or for passing through a narrow place. It is an excellent way to place the victim on a litter, put the victim in bed, or take the victim out of bed. It is possible to keep the victim's body in a horizontal position and to protect his head, neck, and entire body. The steps to follow are

1. The victim is placed on his back, and if he is unconscious, his wrists and hands are secured.
2. Rescuers take a kneeling position all down on the knee that is nearer to the victim's feet.
3. Rescuers place their hands in position, first above the victim to make sure of the position. The bearer at the shoulders places one hand above the victim's head and shoulder and one above the victim's upper back; the bearer at the hips places one hand above the hips and the other above the thighs; the third bearer places one hand above the knees and the other at the ankles.
4. The bearers check the position of the hands, then place their hands directly beneath the victim.
5. The bearers on command lift the victim onto their bended knees.
6. From this position the bearers can place the victim on a litter for transportation.

Or

7. The bearers can turn the victim toward their bodies and hold securely.
8. The bearers lift on command and rise to a standing position and transport the victim in a straight line or step to the side, step-close, step-close, and pass through narrow places.
9. To unload the victim the bearers return the victim to their bended knees and rotate the victim to the face-up position.
10. The bearers on command lower the victim to a litter for transportation.

Three-Man Hammock Carry This method provides a good means of transporting the victim, and it can be used for moving the victim a reasonably long distance. An advantage of this technique is the position of the bearers. The bearers are free to walk in any direction, and the feet of each bearer are out of the way of the other bearers. Two bearers are

[364] Transportation for Protection

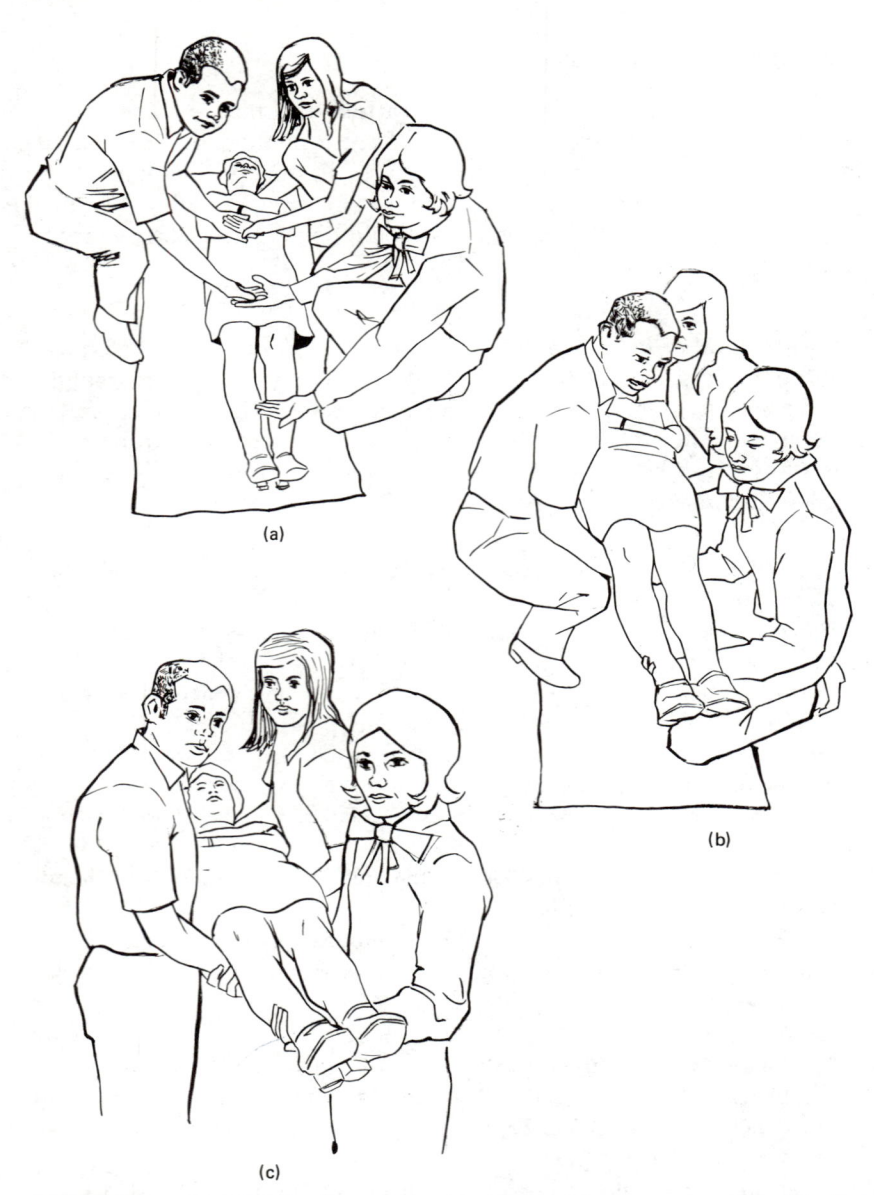

FIGURE 23.4 Steps for three-man hammock: (a) practicing correct position; (b) placing hands beneath victim; (c) final walking position.

placed on one side of the victim, one at the head and shoulders, the other at the knees and feet. The third bearer is positioned at the hips of the victim on the other side. The two strongest bearers should be placed opposite the head and shoulders and the hips. They will bear most of the weight. The steps to follow are

Methods of Transportation [365]

1. The rescuers place the victim on his back and secure his hands and feet if unconscious.
2. The rescuers assume a kneeling position, two on one side at the shoulders and knees and one on the opposite side at the hips. The rescuers should be down on one knee, the knee nearer to the victim's feet.
3. Rescuers place their hands above the victim to indicate the position.
   a. Rescuer at shoulders places his first arm and hand beneath the neck and head, grasping the victim's shoulder and cradles the head. The other arm passes beneath the back at an angle.
   b. The rescuer at the hip passes one arm beneath the victim and upward toward the back, the other beneath the victim's hips and downward toward the thighs.
   c. Rescuer at the knees passes one arm beneath the victim and upward toward the thighs, the other beneath the legs, grasping the legs at the ankles.
4. The rescuers on command lift the victim to a position resting across their bended knees.
5. The rescuers lock their wrists; the rescuer at the hips locks his wrists with the other two bearers, one in the region of the thighs, the other in the region of the back.
6. The rescuers on command rise, lifting with their legs.
7. The rescuers step off and move in any direction.
8. The rescuers or bearers unload the victim in the same manner, first by lowering the victim to the bent knees, then down to the litter, bed, or floor.

Four-Man Carry If the victim is heavy, it is advisable to have sufficient help before attempting to move him. This method is suitable for moving a victim a short distance or for placing a casualty on a litter. The steps to follow are

1. The rescuers place the victim on his back and secure his hands and feet if he is unconscious.
2. Two rescuers assume kneeling positions on each side of the victim. All bearers should be down on the knee nearer to the victim's feet.
3. The rescuers place their hands over the victim's body, starting at the head or feet, alternating their hands. The hands should be evenly spaced and the palms should be upward.
4. The rescuers move their hands directly beneath the victim from the preceding positions, making a platform of their hands from the victim's head to his feet.
5. The rescuers on command lift the victim, keeping his body level, to a position across their bended knees.
6. After adjusting their hands, the rescuers rise on command with the victim resting on the platform of hands in a horizontal position.
7. The rescuers move the victim to safety or a litter; as they move they keep in step.

[366] Transportation for Protection

(a)

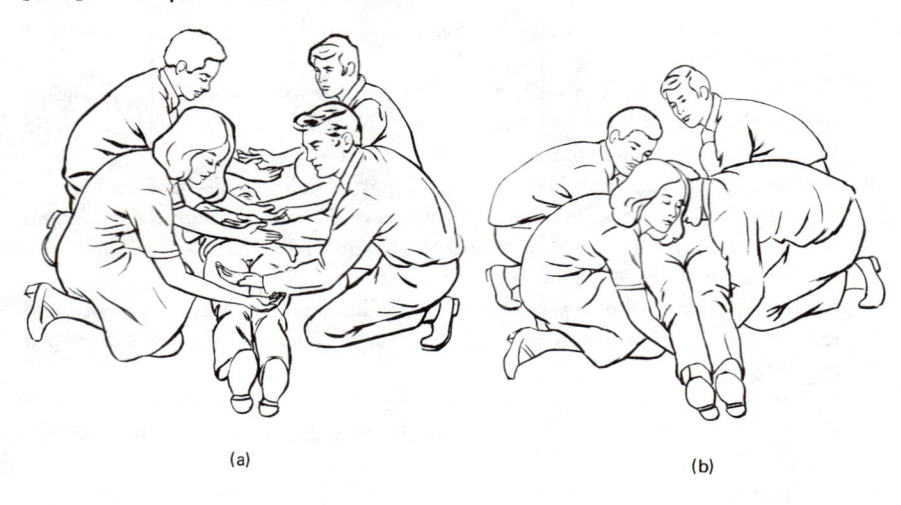

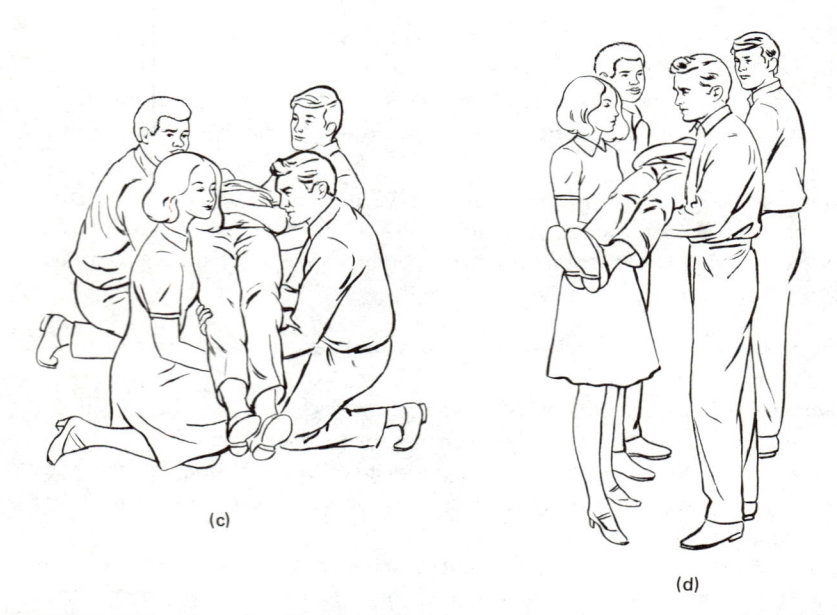

(b)

(c)

(d)

FIGURE 23.5 Steps for four-man lift: (a) practicing correct position; (b) placing the hands in correct position; (c) lifting victim to position of bended knee; (d) final walking position.

8 The rescuers unload the victim in the same manner, lowering the victim to the bended knee, then to the floor or litter.

Methods of Transportation [367]

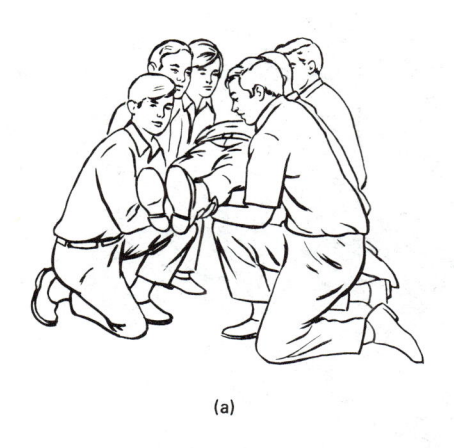

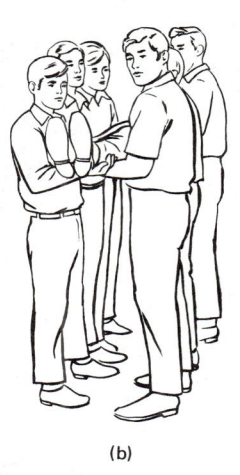

FIGURE 23.6 Steps for six-man lift: (a) lifting victim to position of bended knee; (b) final walking position.

Six-Man Carry This method is exactly like the four-man carry except there are three bearers on each side of the victim and the hands are placed closer together. If the victim is a very large person, it is well to use the six-man carry if enough bearers are available.

Types of Litters

There are several ways to improvise a litter that will be adequate for transporting the victim. Two heavy coats or jackets, two heavy sacks, a blanket, two chairs, an army cot, a platform, or a small bed can be used as a litter.

From the standpoint of first aid and emergency care the ideal litter is the army-type stretcher. Such a litter should be readily available at a school, a play area, an industry, and on rescue vehicles. Large schools and industries should have several litters conveniently placed, and rescue vehicles should have two or more litters. Litters that can be easily improvised are as follows:

Blanket Litter The blanket litter can be easily and quickly made from two wooden poles and one blanket. Figure 23.7 demonstrates how this litter is made.

Also, blanket litters can be prepared with just one substantial blanket. The victim is placed in the center of the blanket. The blanket is rolled up from the edges, as close to the victim and as tight as possible. Two or three bearers on each side can life and transport the victim.

[368] Transportation for Protection

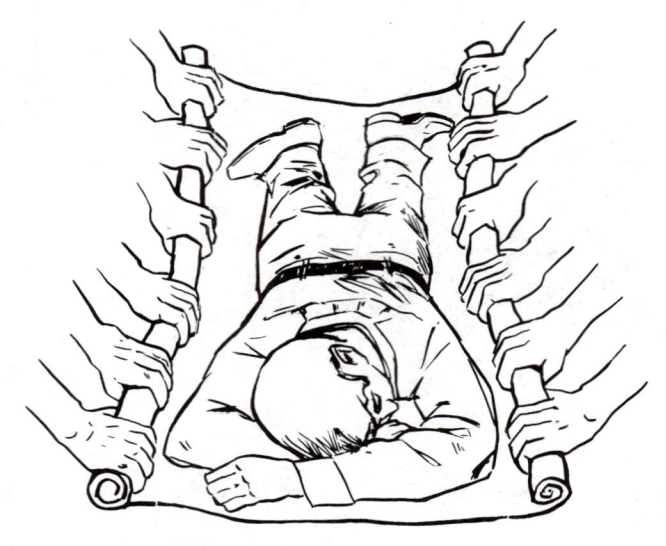

FIGURE 23.7 Improvised blanket litter.

Jackets or Hunting Coat Litter This litter requires two or three jackets or hunting coats, depending upon the size and height of the victim, and two poles strong enough to support the victim's weight. The sleeves of the jackets are reversed (pulled inward) and the poles are passed through the sleeves, then the jackets are buttoned or zippered. The jackets are moved as close together as possible to prevent sagging.

Two-Sack Litter Two heavy burlap sacks or grain sacks and two poles can provide a suitable litter. It is best that the sacks be of the same size and that the poles be six to seven feet long and strong enough to support the victim.

Holes are made in the bottom corners of the sacks; the poles are passed through the sacks and out of the holes. The sacks should overlap, and three sacks are preferred to two, especially for a tall person.

Two-Chair Litter Two chairs and sufficient rope or cravats to secure them together will provide an emergency-type litter. This litter would need some padding with blankets or pillows. The chairs are placed in a downward position with the chair backs overlapping. The backs are secured with rope or cravats.

Army Cot Many homes, schools, and recreational areas have army cots available at all times. The cot can be opened and used as a litter. The victim can be placed on the cot. There are locations at the corners and on the sides for the bearers to take hold and carry. The cot will support several hundred pounds of weight.

Methods of Transportation [369]

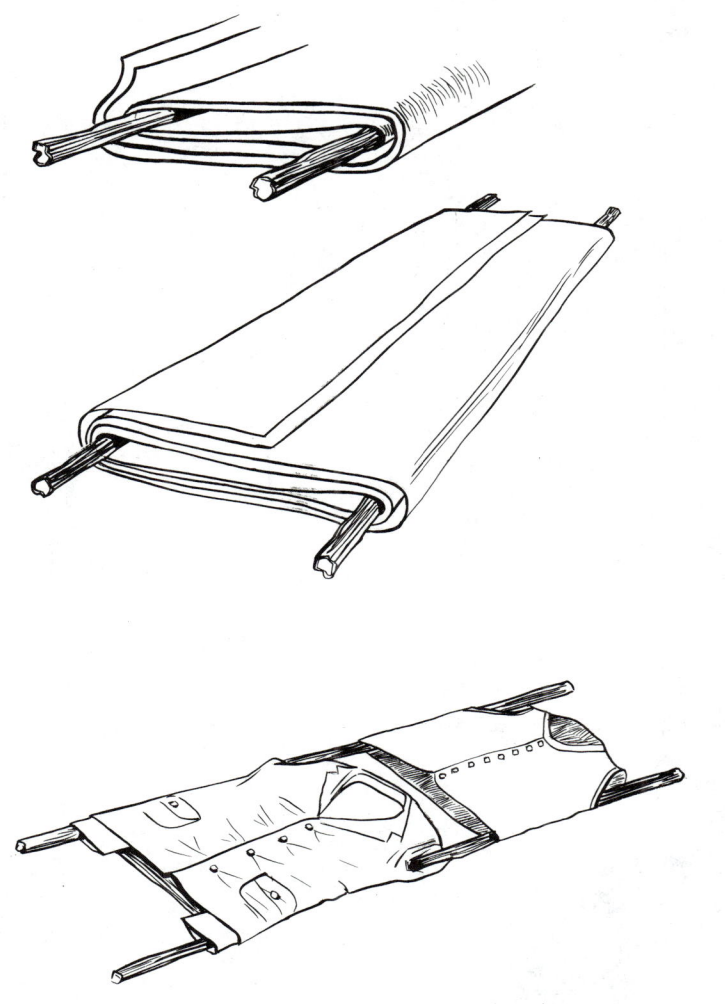

FIGURE 23.8 Improvised litters made from blanket and from jackets and coats.

   Platform Litter A rigid platform is needed for transporting victims with suspected neck and back injuries. A door can provide such a litter, or the litter can be quickly assembled from two boards some seven feet long, six to eight inches wide, and at least one inch thick. The boards are placed in the long position, side by side and about two inches apart. Four cross boards at the locations of the ankles, knees, hips, and shoulders are placed beneath the long boards at right angles and parallel with each other. The four short cross boards are nailed to the long boards to provide the rigid platform. Industries and schools should have such a litter available at all times, and they should have trained personnel who know how and when to use it.

[370] Transportation for Protection

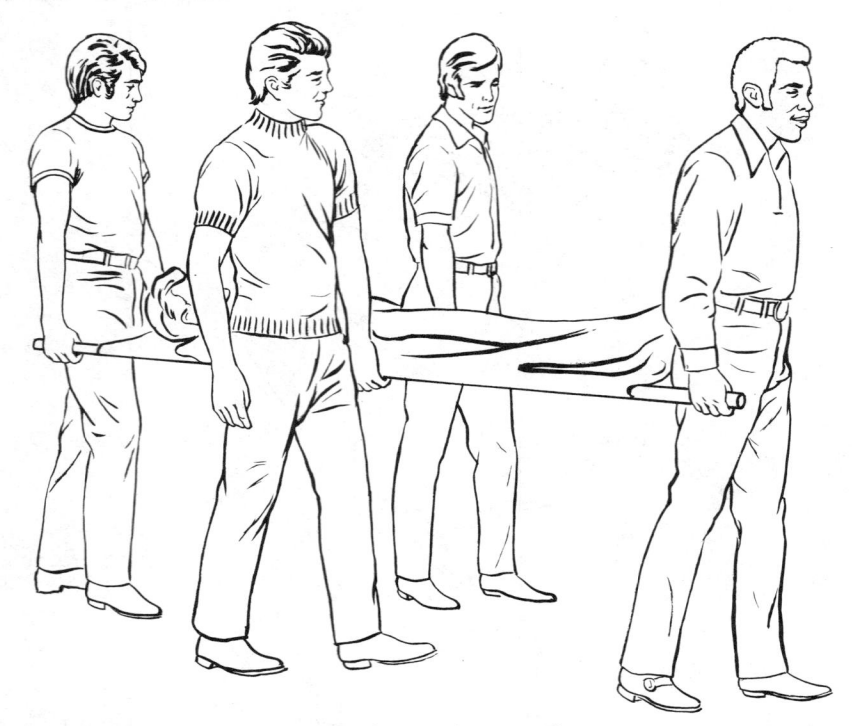

FIGURE 23.9 Position of carriers, showing feet out of step.

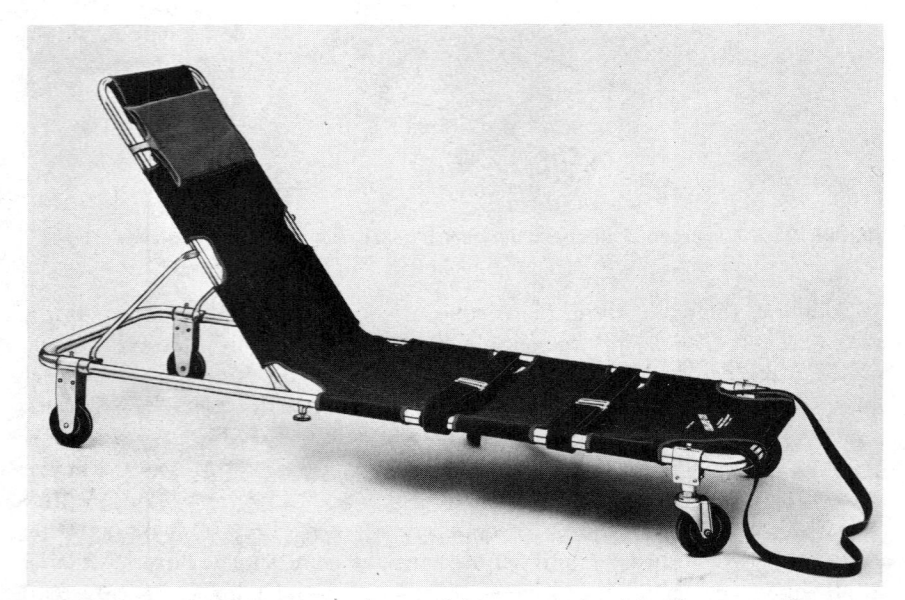

FIGURE 23.10 Collapsi-cot stretcher used for transporting injured persons. (Emergency Aids Company)

TRANSPORTATION BY VEHICLE

As was discussed previously in this chapter, the best means of vehicle transportation is by ambulance which has trained first-aid and rescue personnel. If an ambulance is not available, a passenger car or truck would have to be used. Cars in which the front right seat can be folded down make an ideal vehicle for transporting a victim on a stretcher. A station wagon can become an excellent substitute ambulance. Persons with fractures of the upper extremities can sit up in the car, but they should be watched for signs of shock. In all cases, someone must sit near the victim in order to prevent further injuries. If at all possible, a person with a back or neck injury should not be moved in a passenger car, station wagon, or truck. An ambulance is the best type of vehicle for these injuries. (The ambulance and its equipment are discussed in more detail in Chapter 25.) The vehicle should be driven carefully to avoid jolting and jarring the victim. The vehicle should not be driven recklessly or too hurriedly. Too many accidents are caused by people who are in a hurry to get an injured person to the hospital.

TRANSPORTATION BY AIR

In view of the fact that airplanes and helicopters are now being used in transportation of the injured, first-aiders and rescue crews should be aware of their uses and advantages. The major advantages of air transportation are primarily speed and the ability to reach remote areas. Many times accident victims need medical aid that only a special hospital may provide. This is when a helicopter or airplane is of great benefit. A medical hospital two hundred miles away is too great a distance in many situations for ambulance transportation. Under these circumstances a helicopter or airplane could travel the distance in a hour or two.

> . . . a 25-year-old pilot, James Long, was practicing aerial stunts when his single-engine plane suddenly went into a dive, hit the ground, and flipped end-over-end across a plowed field, inaccessible to a conventional ambulance. Within minutes, the Ohio State University Hospital medicopter (helicopter) answered the call, a doctor-nurse team aboard.
>
> Following the doctor's instructions, the rescue party carefully removed the pilot from the wreck and placed him aboard the helicopter. Long had suffered multiple fractures. Swift transportation, medical attention at the scene and en route, and the care of the alerted medical team at the hospital culminated in completely recovery.[4]

A helicopter can fly from 120 to 150 miles an hour and reach a desolate place where typical modes of transportation are unusable. Also, helicopters

[4] Morton J. Schultz. "Help Is a Helicopter." *Today's Health*, April, 1969, p. 21.

that are used for rescue can accommodate two or four victims. First-aid and medical equipment are essential on these helicopters.

Schultz has identified three conditions that must be present before a rescue helicopter can be successful in a community:

1. Crews of the helicopter rescue program must include medical personnel who can help at the accident scene and en route to the hospital.
2. Landing sites must be provided by hospitals in order that no delay in proper medical treatment results.
3. The helicopter program must be a part of the emergency network of the community. Communication is needed between the police and fire departments, ambulance services, and helicopter program.[5]

ACTIVITIES

1. Prepare a rigid-type litter and demonstrate how to secure and transport a victim with a broken neck or back on this type of litter.
2. Visit a local fire or police department rescue unit. Report to the class the transportation facilities they utilize for accident victims.
3. Demonstrate to the class two different types of one-man carries.
4. Demonstrate the two-man support, fore-and-aft carry, and chair carry to the class.
5. Select five persons from class and teach them the three-man lift from one side, the hammock lift, the four-man lift, and the blanket lift. Then demonstrate these lifts to the class.

QUESTIONS TO ANSWER

1. What are the three objectives of transportation? Can they be applied to all accident situations? Why?
2. In what situations would it be necessary to move a victim before preparing him for transportation?
3. What parts of the body need to be supported during transportation? Why?
4. What is the difference between the fireman's drag and the blanket drag?
5. Discuss the steps needed to perform the one-man support and carry.
6. When would first-aiders use the three-man carry from one side? Four-man carry?
7. Discuss the various types of litters. Discuss when and how each can be utilized.

[5] Ibid., p. 73.

8 What is the best type of vehicle transportation for a person with a broken back?
9 What are the advantages of air rescue?
10 If you had to transport an accident victim over a great distance by yourself, what considerations are necessary? Why?

SELECTED REFERENCES

AMERICAN NATIONAL RED CROSS, *Standard First Aid and Personal Safety*. New York: Doubleday, 1973.

GILLESBY, W. J., "Transportation of the Injured," *First Aid: Diagnosis and Management*. Warren H. Cole and Charles B. Puestow (eds.). New York: Appleton-Century-Crofts, 1965.

HAFEN, BRENT Q., and KARREN, KEITH J., *First Aid and Emergency Care Workbook*. Denver: Morton Publishing Co., 1977.

HAFEN, BRENT Q., and PETERSON, BRENDA, *First Aid For Health Emergencies*. St. Paul, Minn.: West Publishing Co., 1977.

HENDERSON, JOHN, *Emergency Medical Guide*, 4th ed. New York: McGraw-Hill, 1978.

KENNEDY, ROBERT H. (ed.). *Emergency Care*. Philadelphia: Saunders, 1966.

MAHONEY, ROBERT F., *Emergency and Disaster Nursing*, 2nd ed. New York: Macmillan, 1969.

OLSON, LYLA M., *Prevention, First Aid and Emergencies*. Philadelphia: Saunders, 1946.

SCHULTZ, MORTON J., "Help Is a Helicopter," *Today's Health*, April, 1969, pp. 21–23, 72–73.

U.S. NAVY, *Standard First Aid Training Course*. Washington, D.C.: Bureau of Naval Personnel, U.S. Government Printing Office, 1955.

24. FIRST-AID SUPPLIES

There is no known solution for keeping people free from accidents or various health disorders and their sudden onset. Therefore, it is essential that people be prepared to give emergency care and that facilities and first-aid supplies be available. These first-aid supplies should be in as many locations as possible, for they are needed everywhere people are present. Appropriate quantities of the necessary items should be stocked in accordance with the needs in various areas, such as home, school, motor vehicle, industry, and recreation.

LOCATION AND CARE OF SUPPLIES

First-aid supplies should be convenient. They should be located in an area with good lighting and a safe water supply. In the home the kitchen or the bathroom is a typical location. Schools and industries should have a specially designed room for this purpose. First-aid kits should be carried in all motor vehicles, and recreation leaders and participants should have such supplies readily available. It is helpful if a first-aider can take a victim to a nearby first-aid facility, but in various situations it is necessary to take the supplies to the victim. If possible there should be means for carrying all the needed supplies in one trip.

The container for the first-aid kit is extremely important. If the unit is to be kept in a motor vehicle, at the recreation area, carried on the person, or kept on some unit of farm equipment, it is necessary to keep the contents free from dust and contamination. The container should close tightly. It should have rubber seals. A heavy plastic bag will guarantee the safety of the first-aid container and contents.

First-aid kits and supplies should be checked regularly for quality and quantity. If supplies become old, contaminated, or unsafe, they should be destroyed and replaced by a new supply. Usually it is a mistake to buy large quantities of antiseptics. It is better to obtain a smaller fresh supply at regular and shorter intervals. Also, it is better to purchase supplies such as petrolatum in tubes rather than jars. All adhesive tape products should be kept in a reasonably cool place; otherwise, the tape may deteriorate faster and this is an unnecessary waste. Many supplies are available in prepared packages and are desirable from the standpoint of convenience and safety. It is advantageous to purchase sterile pads, Band-Aids, and compresses already closed in sterile unbroken packages so the contents will remain safe and sterile. First-aid supplies should be labeled well and kept in their proper containers. It is important that all supplies be returned to their designated location and used items be replenished after each use.

Improvised Supplies

One of the important tests for the first-aider is whether or not he can improvise satisfactorily when there is little at hand with which to work. He must use his imagination and ingenuity to make use of whatever is available to give protection to the injured. This may mean that a clean handkerchief will serve as the compress, a shoestring will be a constricting band, a shirt the arm sling, and an undershirt or belt the tourniquet. Too frequently there are no first-aid supplies at the accident scene.

HOME AND FARM

Every home should make adequate provision for first-aid supplies. It must be remembered that more accidents happen in the home than anywhere else. Falls, burns, and small wounds are quite common in the home. The first-aider will need to give protection for these and other problems.

A well-supplied first-aid kit can be most helpful in protecting injuries sustained at home. It should be large enough to contain all the necessary items. It should be kept in a convenient location, preferably mounted on a wall and kept locked so children cannot get into it. The first-aid kit and supplies should always be kept in the same location so adults in the family can find and use them instantly. Moreover, the key should be kept in the same place at all times.

It is important that items such as flashlight, sharp knife, razor blade, tweezers, and constricting band be kept in the first-aid kit. Though they are available in most homes these items cannot always be found at a moment's notice. Time can be very important when it is a matter of protecting a badly injured person. The following items are suggested for the home first-aid kit and supplies:

[376] First-Aid Supplies

Adhesive compresses—(Band-Aids) different sizes
Adhesive tape—1-, 1½-, and 2-inch rolls of each size
Air way—1 S-type
Alcohol—70%, 1 pint bottle
Ammonia—aromatic spirits, 1 ounce
Ammonia—inhalant ampules, 6
Antiseptic—1 ounce Merthiolate or Metaphen
Antiseptic—6 ounce hydrogen peroxide
Aspirin—1 box
Baking soda—small container
Boric acid—small container for preparing eye wash
Burn ointment—1 tube
Calamine lotion—4- to 6-ounce bottle
Constricting band—rubber tubing
Cotton sterile applicators—1 package
Cotton—sterile, ½-ounce box
Drinking cups—1 package
Elastic wraps—(Ace) 2- or 3-inch width, 1 can
Eye cup
Emergency telephone numbers, doctor, hospital, fire and police departments, Poison Control Center
Flashlight—and extra batteries
Ice bag
Manual—first aid
Measuring cup
Mineral oil—4 ounces
Paper and pencil
Petrolatum—small tube
Poison universal antidote—packaged from druggist if available
Safety pins
Salt—small container
Scissors—1 pair
Sharp knife or razor blade
Splints—2 or 3 of different lengths
Sterile compresses—(gauze) in paper packages, sizes up to 6-inch square
Sterile eyepads—3 or 4
Sterile gauze—rolls in widths up to 3 inches, 1 each
Sterile soap—(liquid) 4 to 6 ounces
Sugar—small container
Syrup of ipecac
Thermometer—1 oral, 1 rectal
Tongue depressors—1 dozen
Triangular bandages—2 or more with material for making additional units
Tweezers—2 or 3 different sizes
Vinegar—2 ounces

These items and possibly more should be included in the farm first-aid kit. A stretcher and large compresses are additional items that might be helpful on a farm. Perhaps special emphasis should be given to the matter of a sharp knife or other fast-cutting instrument being kept within reach of any power take-off equipment. Clothes are sometimes caught in such equipment and a fast-cutting instrument could be used to free a person of the entangled clothing.

Farm safety measures are of special significance because, on the farm, the opportunities are many for accidents and injuries. A basic problem with farm accidents is that it takes longer to get medical services in the event of an injury or serious illness, regardless of whether the victim is taken to help or help is called to the accident scene. This tends to compound the farm accident situation and makes it more serious than if the accident had occurred in an urban area. A well-supplied first-aid kit and a trained first-aider are a necessity for each farm family if reasonable and adequate protection is to be given to the farm accident victim.

SCHOOL

There is a need for a special room or facility for emergencies in every school. If there is a school nurse, usually a nurse's office or first-aid emergency room is assigned to her. A school without a nurse should have a designated emergency room with cots or beds and emergency supplies available at all times. It is usually a good policy for each teacher to have some first-aid supplies in his room. This is particularly true for the shop, home economics, and physical education teacher. If a teacher has an epileptic child in his room, he might want to have a folding screen and bed in the room; of course, this would depend on whether or not the school had an emergency room, the distance of the classroom from the emergency room, and whether or not the classroom had the space for such items.

Teachers and particularly coaches who accompany schoolchildren on trips would find it advantageous to take a first-aid kit and supplies with them.

Certainly a school first-aid kit and supplies should be all-inclusive. If the school is in a rural area or in a community without a physician, the problem of adequate supplies becomes all the more acute.

The following first-aid supplies are suggested for the school:

Adhesive compresses—(Band-Aids) all sizes and in boxes of 100
Adhesive tape—several tubes assorted cuts
Airway—3, S-type
Alcohol—70%, several pint bottles
Ammonia inhalant ampules—several dozen
Antiseptic—have M.D. recommend

[378] First-Aid Supplies

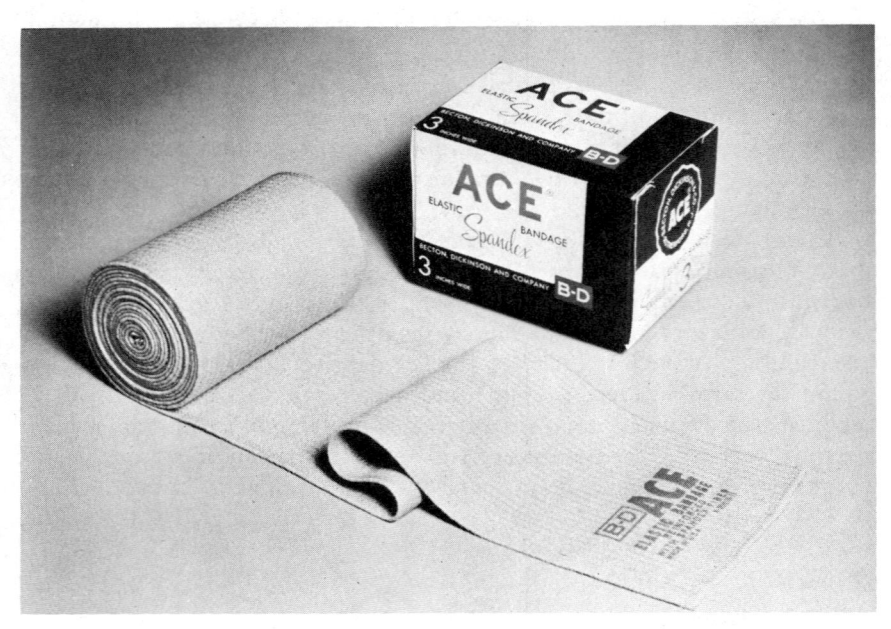

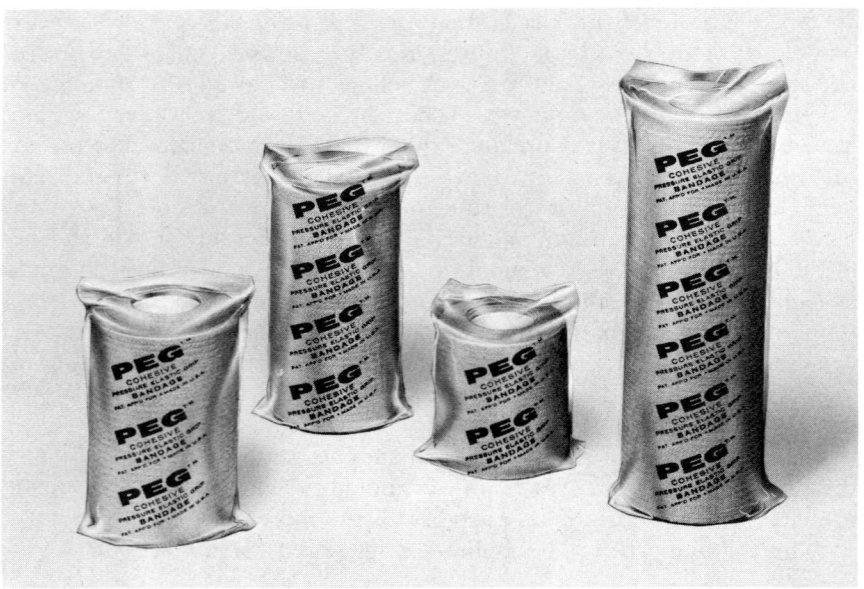

FIGURE 24.1 ACE elastic bandage and cohesive bandages. (Becton, Dickinson and Company)

Antiseptic—hydrogen peroxide
Aspirin—reasonable quantity, doctor's orders
Baking soda—1 box

Blankets—heavy woolen, at least 6
Boric acid—1 box
Burn ointment—several small tubes
Calamine lotion—1 pint
Compresses—packaged, different sizes
Constricting band—rubber tubing, 2
Cots or beds—at least 2
Cotton sterile applicators—1 gross
Cotton (sterile)—½-oz boxes, 3 or 4
Drinking cups—100 or more
Elastic bandage—(Ace), 2-, 2½-, and 3-inch widths, 2 each
Emergency telephone numbers
Eye cup—2 or 3 for eye wash
Eye pads—1 dozen
Ice bags—several, plastic
Insect sting kit
Litter—(army type), at least 2
Knife or razor blade
Manual—first aid
Measuring cup
Mineral oil—1 pint bottle
Petrolatum—6 small tubes
Poison universal antidote—prepared from druggist
Safety pins—reasonable supply, all sizes
Salt—1-pound box or several small units
Scissors—2 or 3 pairs
Splints—plastic, orally inflated, assorted sizes
Splints—several wooden padded for arms and legs
Splints—1 Thomas or several improvised for traction
Spinal board
Soap—liquid, 1 pint
Syrup of ipecac
Thermometer—6 oral
Tongue depressors—1 gross
Towels—1 dozen cotton
Tweezers—2
Twisting device—strong broom handle
Vinegar—1 pint bottle

MOTOR VEHICLE

The emergency care situation on the nation's highways needs much improvement. Surely it would be helped if more motor-vehicle operators were first-aid-trained, especially all commercial drivers, and if all motor vehicles carried first-aid kits or equipment. At many motor-vehicle acci-

[380] First-Aid Supplies

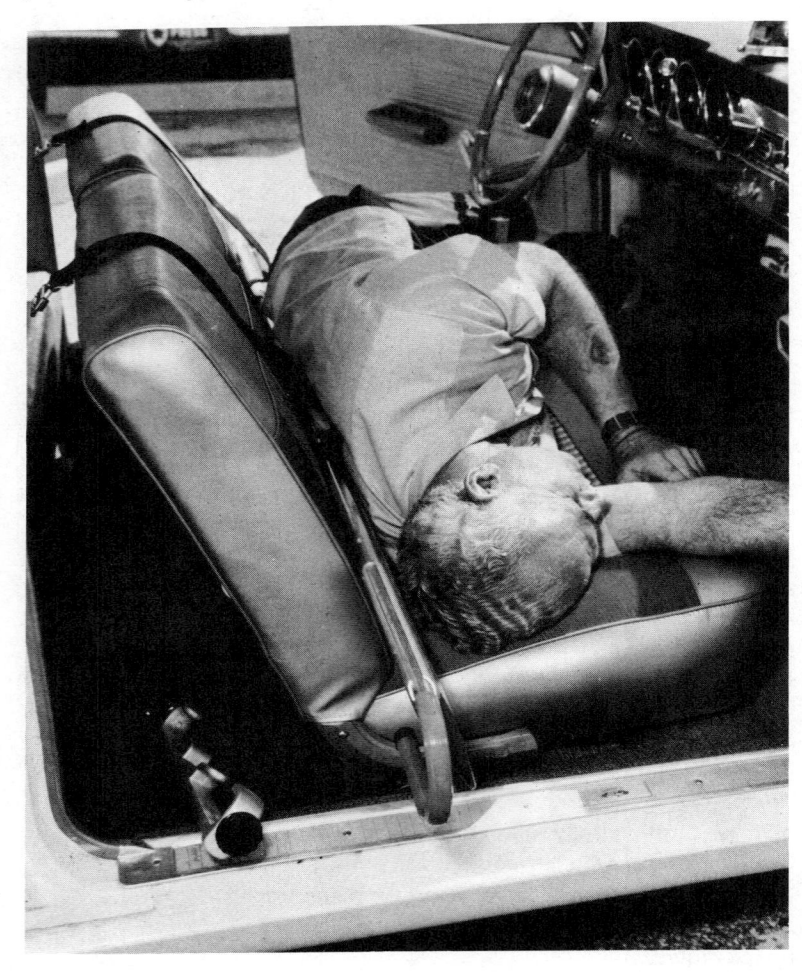

FIGURE 24.2A Use of a Scoop Stretcher in a motor vehicle: inserting the stretcher. (Sarole, Inc. and Fort Lauderdale News. Scoop Stretcher®)

dent scenes there are badly injured persons with few emergency supplies to use. It would be helpful if the motor-vehicle manufacturer would include a special compartment with a first-aid kit and a first-aid manual in each new car. This would add a few dollars to the original cost; however, it might help to save many lives. The following items are suggested for the automobile first-aid kit:

Adhesive compresses—(Band-Aids) assortment of sizes
Adhesive tape—1½-inch roll
Ammonia inhalant ampules—several
Antiseptic—Merthiolate or Metaphen

Motor Vehicle [381]

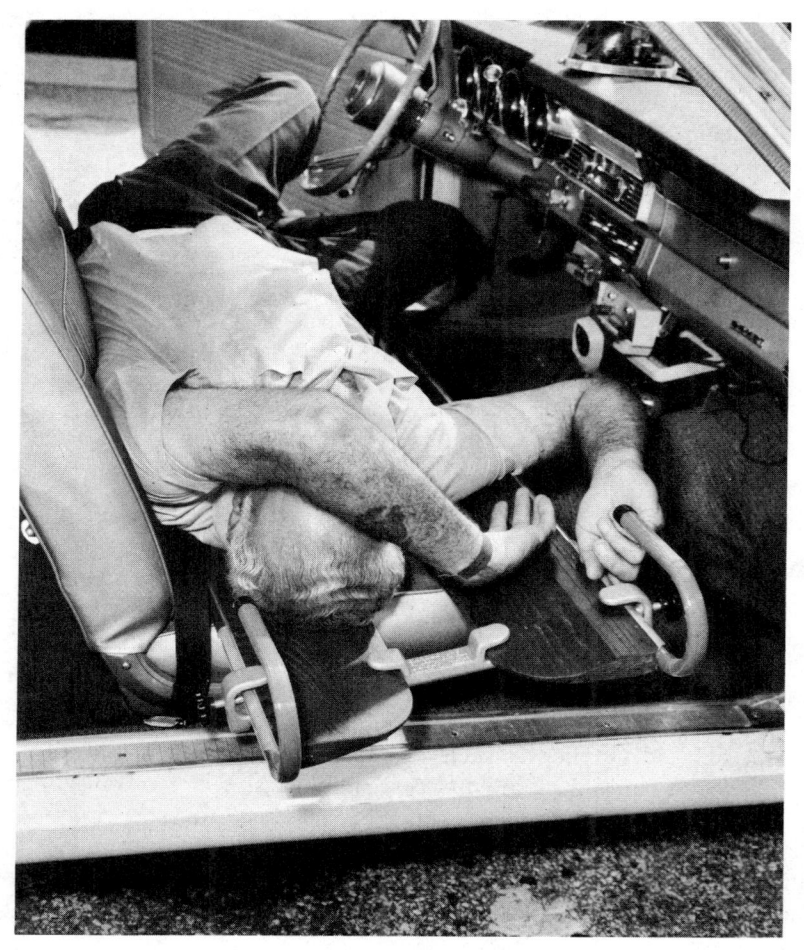

FIGURE 24.2B Use of Scoop Stretcher in a motor vehicle: the patient on the stretcher. (Sarole, Inc. and Fort Lauderdale News. Scoop Stretcher®)

Baking soda—small container
Blanket—1 or better, several
Burn ointment—small tube
Compresses—sterile packaged, assorted sizes
Constriction band—rubber tubing, 1
Cotton applicators—several
Cotton (sterile)—½ ounce
Cutting device—knife or razor blade
Drinking cups—6 plastic
Emergency telephone numbers—include name of town
Flashlight—with extra batteries

[382]   First-Aid Supplies

    Flares—for warning, several
    Manual—first aid
    Matches—several pads
    Paper and pencil
    Petrolatum—small tube or 2
    Safety pins—small and large, supply of each
    Salt—small container
    Scissors—1 pair
    Splints—2 or 3 padded wooden for fixation
    Sterile compresses—(small), 2-, 3-, 4-, and 6-inch, in sterile packages
    Sterile gauze—(rolls), 1-, 2-, and 3-inch widths
    Sterile soap—(liquid), small container
    Sugar—small container
    Towels—1 or more
    Triangular bandages—4 to 6
    Twisting device—for tourniquet or for applying a traction leg splint

RECREATION

More first-aid supplies would be on hand to use in recreational activities if the idea of having such supplies in every car was accepted and practiced.

Families or groups going on vacation in their cars or campers should include first-aid supplies. In such an undertaking it is a good idea to delegate the emergency planning and care supply task to a particular member of the family or party. If any member has had first-aid training, this responsibility should be given to him. Playgrounds, swimming pools, gymnasiums, and other recreational areas need to have trained leaders or supervisors and adequate first-aid supplies at all times. The following first-aid supplies are suggested:

    Adhesive compresses—(Band-Aids) assortment of sizes
    Adhesive tape—1 tube, assorted cuts
    Alcohol—70%, 2 or 3 bottles
    Ammonia inhalant ampules—1 dozen
    Antiseptic—Merthiolate or Metaphen
    Baking soda—1 box
    Blankets—(army type), at least 2
    Burn ointment—several tubes
    Compresses—sterile, packages of assorted sizes
    Cotton applicators—1 box of 100
    Cutting device—sharp knife or razor blade
    Elastic wraps—(Ace) 2, 3, and 4 inches wide
    Emergency telephone numbers

Recreation [383]

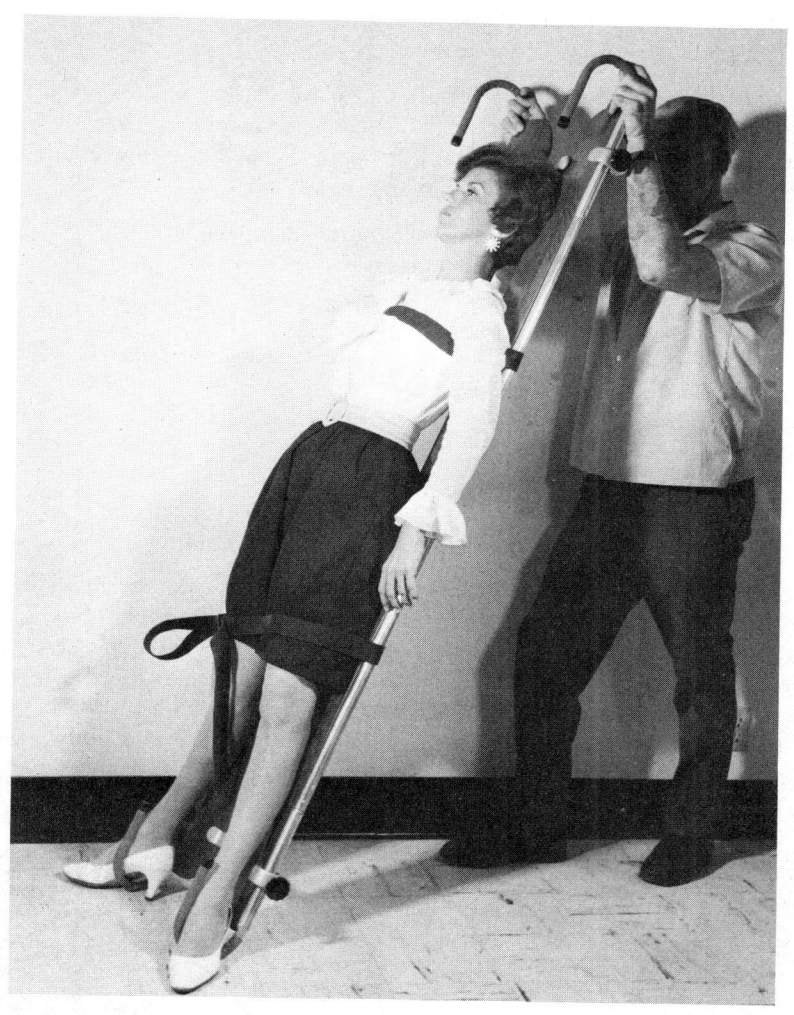

FIGURE 24.3 A patient being lifted on the Scoop Stretcher. (Sarole, Inc. and Fort Lauderdale News. Scoop Stretcher®)

Eye pads—packaged, 1 dozen
Flashlight—with extra batteries
Gauze—sterile rolls, 1, 2, and 3 inches wide
Insect sting kit
Litter—(army type), at least 2
Manual—first aid
Petrolatum—several small tubes
Salt tablets—bottle of 100
Soap—(liquid), 4 to 6 oz.

[384] First-Aid Supplies

Splints—padded wooden, several lengths
Triangular bandages—6 or more

The person who hunts, fishes, hikes, or camps will want a small first-aid kit, often called "lost kits." It must be remembered that the hunter could need supplies for his hunting dog, himself, or his companion. Suggestions for the kit to carry on the person are

Antiseptic—small amount of Merthiolate or Metaphen
Band-Aids (sterile adhesive compresses)—3 or 4
Compresses—sterile packaged, 2, 3, and 4 inches
Constriction device (could use shoestring)
Matches—paraffin-treated, so they will burn longer and can be used for starting a fire, if necessary
Petrolatum—very small tube
Roller gauze—2-inch roll
Sharp knife or razor blade
Small tube or piece of soap
Triangular bandage—1 (handkerchief could be used)

The number of items could be reduced somewhat, but in each case they can be placed in a small container and carried in a tackle box, saddle bag, knapsack, hunting cot, or game bag. The total weight of these items is less than one pound and could save a life. For the person who fishes it is extremely important to have pliers or snips to remove the barbs from fishhooks, which then can be removed without tearing the body tissues. The pliers belong in the tackle box or first-aid kit.

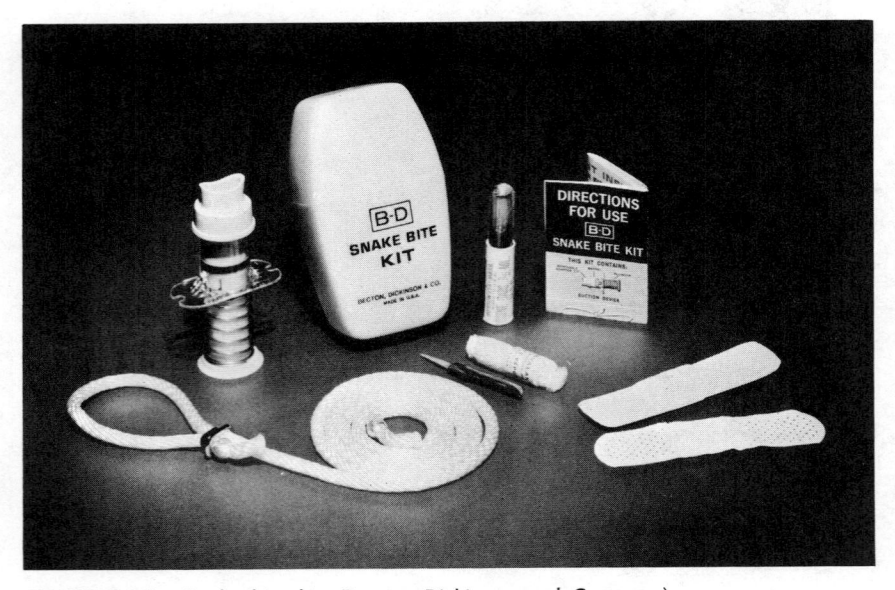

FIGURE 24.4 Snake bite kit. (Becton, Dickinson and Company)

WORK OR INDUSTRY

In no segment of the American population is the idea of first aid so widely accepted and practiced as in industry. Industry has been the leader in the entire field of accident prevention through the years, and it is in industry that some of the best accident records are found.

Large industries have superior facilities and a well-trained staff for taking care of the injuries and other health problems that occur on the job. Smaller industries also should have provisions for taking care of all emergencies. It is suggested that the smaller industries have the following first-aid supplies:

Adhesive compresses—(Band-Aids) all sizes and in boxes of 100
Adhesive tape—several tubes, assorted cuts
Alcohol—70%, several bottles
Ammonia inhalant ampules—several dozen
Antiseptic—have M.D. recommend
Antiseptic—hydrogen peroxide
Aspirin—reasonable quantity, doctor's orders
Baking soda—1 box
Blankets—army type, at least 6
Boric acid—1 box
Burn ointment—several small tubes
Calamine lotion—1 pint
Compresses—sterile packaged, assorted sizes
Constricting band—rubber tubing, 2
Cotton (sterile)—½-oz. boxes, 3 or 4
Cotton applicators—1 gross
Cots or beds—at least 2
Drinking cups—plastic
Elastic bandage—(Ace), 2-, 2½-, and 3-inch widths, 2 each
Emergency telephone numbers
Eye cup
Eye pads—1 dozen
Knife or razor blade
Litter—(army type), at least 2
Measuring cup
Mineral oil—1 bottle
Oxygen supply—for heart and breathing problems
Petrolatum—6 small tubes
Poison antidote—available from druggist
Safety pins—reasonable supply, all sizes
Salt—1 box or several small units
Scissors
Soap—liquid, 1 pint
Splints—plastic, orally inflated

[386]   First-Aid Supplies

Splints—wooden, padded for arms and legs
Splints—Thomas, or several improvised for traction
Thermometer—several
Tongue depressors—1 gross
Towels—1 dozen
Tweezers—2 or more
Twisting device, such as strong broom handle, several
Vinegar—1 bottle

DISASTER SHELTER

Since the concept of Civil Defense has shifted somewhat in the past few years, preparedness for disaster has changed also. Preparedness for disaster at the present time has emphasis upon the natural problems rather than man-made catastrophes. There is increased concern for the problems of tornado, hurricane, flood, earthquake, and fire. These concerns are more meaningful and realistic to our citizenry.

Still there remains the need for areas of safety in our homes, schools, factories, businesses, and industries. Such areas need to be marked well, and drills need to be practiced. It is sensible that these areas be stocked with a minimum of necessary items in the event of a problem. The emergency items which were included in the Civil Defense shelter are still desirable supplies for such areas:

Medication

Ammonia inhalant
Aspirin
Bismuth subcarbonate tablets
Calamine solution
Cascara sagrada extract tablets
Eugenol
Phenobarbital sodium tablets
Soap, surgical
Sulfadiazine tablets

Dressings

Adhesive plaster, surgical
Bandage, absorbent, adhesive
Bandage, gauze rolls
Bandage, muslin
Compresses—packaged, assorted sizes
Cotton, purified

Ear drops
Eye, nose drops
Isopropyl alcohol
Lubricant, surgical
Pad, gauze, surgical
Pad, sanitary, heavy
Penicillin G tablets
Tetracaine, ointment

Other

Applicator, wood, cotton-tipped end
Belts, sanitary
Depressor, tongue, wood
Forceps, splinter, tweezer
Thermometers, human, clinical, oral and rectal
Pin, safety, medium
Syringe, fountain, plastic and attachments
Scissors, pocket
Splints—plastic and orally inflated
Splints—for arms, legs, and back

ACTIVITIES

1 Prepare a first-aid kit for the home or ranch. Carefully select the container and the items to be placed in it. Keep a complete record of the cost.
2 Prepare a first-aid kit to carry on the person when hunting, hiking, fishing, or bicycling. Limit the kit to one pound in weight.
3 Visit the rescue and emergency care units of the community or area and observe the emergency care supplies carefully. Report the findings to the class.
4 Visit a disaster shelter in the community and determine the first aid and medical supplies included. Find out how old the supplies are and how they are kept up to date.
5 Visit the industries in the community or area and study their first-aid programs with special consideration given to facilities and equipment for emergency care.

QUESTIONS TO ANSWER

1 Where should the first-aid kit be kept in the home? School? In sports?
2 What items should be included in the first-aid kit for the automobile?

First-Aid Supplies

3 Why should every teacher have a first-aid kit? What items should be in the kit?
4 What are the basic first-aid supplies a school should stock?
5 What first-aid equipment should the hunter carry for his protection? For his dog's protection?
6 If a person is working or playing in an area where there are poisonous reptiles, what first-aid equipment should he have available? Why?
7 What first-aid supplies does the U.S. Government place in the Civil Defense fallout shelter?
8 What first-aid materials could a person reasonably improvise from his clothing?
9 What bandages should be included in the first-aid kit for the home and school? Why?
10 What first-aid supplies should be included in the first-aid kit for preventing infection? Why?

SELECTED REFERENCES

AMERICAN MEDICAL ASSOCIATION, *Today's Health Guide*. Chicago: AMA, 1965.

AMERICAN NATIONAL RED CROSS, *Advanced First Aid and Emergency Care*. Garden City, N.Y.: Doubleday, 1973.

AMERICAN NATIONAL RED CROSS, *Standard First Aid and Personal Safety*. Garden City, N.Y.: Doubleday, 1973.

COLE, WARREN H., and PUESTOW, CHARLES B., *First Aid: Diagnosis and Management*. New York: Appleton-Century-Crofts, 1965.

HENDERSON, JOHN, *Emergency Medical Guide*, 4th ed. New York: McGraw-Hill Book Co., 1978.

OFFICE OF CIVIL DEFENSE, *Family Guide Emergency Health Care*. Washington, D.C.: U.S. Dept. of Defense and U.S. Dept. of HEW, 1963.

POTTHOFF, CARL J., "First Aid—Automobile First Aid Supplies." *Today's Health*, May, 1963.

U.S. DEPT. OF AGRICULTURE, *First Aid Guide for USDA Employees*. Washington, D.C.: U.S. Government Printing Office, 1963.

25. ORGANIZING EMERGENCY CARE SERVICES

Throughout this text the scope of the nation's accident problems has been emphasized. With our industrial and highly mobile society it can be expected that accidents and other types of emergency care problems will continue to occur at an alarming rate.

> As the era of mechanization advances, the number of injuries will increase. More vehicles on the streets and highways will further add to the number of those injured and killed annually. Acute medical emergencies, which occur as a result of oral poisoning, heart attack, stroke and so forth, are also mounting.[1]

In order for school personnel, industrial personnel, homeowners, police units, or emergency crews to handle such emergencies in an appropriate manner, first-aid and emergency care services must be organized.

NEED FOR ORGANIZATION

Because of the complexity and the nature of first-aid and emergency care problems, all facets of a state must be organized to handle these emergency conditions. Such organization will require a good deal of planning and training to prepare the school personnel, police, etc., to fulfill their responsibilities to members of the community.

[1] Carl B. Young, *First Aid for Emergencies Crews.* Springfield, Ill.: Charles C Thomas, 1965, p. 3.

[390] Organizing Emergency Care Services

FIGURE 25.1 SCORE SHEET FOR COMMUNITY EMERGENCY MEDICAL CARE

IF YOU'RE STRUCK by a car this evening on the way to the drugstore, how quickly and well will you be cared for? Here's a checklist to score your community on availability of ambulances, training of attendants, coordination with hospitals, and the equipping and staffing of emergency wards. Every "no" answer indicates a point of weakness in your community program.

☐ Can you call an ambulance at any hour, any day of the year?

☐ Are all ambulances dispatched through a central agency by a dispatcher trained in first aid?

☐ Do ambulances carry crews of two or more, trained in advanced first aid, in handling their equipment and in dealing with common emergency situations?

☐ Can you call a service that is trained and equipped for rescue and extrication operations?

☐ Do ambulances carry equipment that meets the list of Minimal Equipment for Ambulances approved by the American College of Surgeons?

☐ Do ambulances have two-way radios that can reach hospitals and police?

☐ Does your community, county, or state have a law equivalent to the model ambulance ordinance?

☐ Are hospital emergency departments open 24 hours a day throughout the year?

☐ Is a physician assigned to the department at all times and supported by a second physician when necessary?

☐ Are medical specialists available for consultation?

☐ Are there enough nurses regularly assigned to give immediate care to urgent cases without delaying attention to other cases?

☐ Are additional nurses available for peak hours and unusual situations?

☐ Are emergency department doctors and nurses trained in first aid and procedures for common emergencies?

☐ Are there x-ray and laboratory facilities in or near the emergency department?

☐ Is the department equipped and organized to meet the Standards for the Emergency Department in Hospitals, as approved by the American College of Surgeons?

☐ Do ambulance services and emergency departments keep permanent records of their work?

☐ Does your community have agreements with neighboring areas for mutual support in emergency medical care?

☐ Does the community train its citizens in first aid?

☐ Has your community surveyed its emergency care needs and determined if present facilities meet these needs?

☐ Do you have a community council or emergency medical care?

Information about ambulance and emergency department services should be available directly from ambulance operators and hospital administrators, from police, fire, and health departments, and from medical societies and other interested private organizations.

Source: Reprinted from *Journal of American Insurance*, American Mutual Insurance Alliance, 20 North Wacker Drive, Chicago, Illinois 60606.

HIGHWAY SAFETY PROGRAM STANDARDS

A great many persons die or become permanently disabled because they do not receive immediate and proper emergency medical care following an accident, especially automobile accidents. Few areas in the United States now have sufficient emergency care services to cope with the countless numbers of persons injured on our highways, at home, at work, in school, or while engaging in a recreational activity.

As some funeral directors, fire departments, and commercial ambulance services are discontinuing emergency care services at an alarming rate, today individual communities must evaluate needs and plan ways to compensate for the services lost. A fundamental question in providing emergency medical service is "Who shall pay for it?" States are exploring this problem and in some instances are suggesting financing through taxation, local subsidies, or individual health care plans. In order to have a network of facilities for emergency care purposes, local hospitals are assuming this responsibility in some areas while trauma centers are being established in some states.

Any plan for emergency medical service should provide enough equipment and personnel to ensure that any victim can be reached within a matter of minutes. Some studies recommend that service should be within 20 minutes of any person, no matter where he is injured or becomes incapacitated. States that are presently developing statewide emergency medical service plans are attempting to meet this requirement as nearly as possible.

In most states there has been inadequate planning for emergency services, including transportation and communications facilities. Usually, owners of ambulance services, drivers, and attendants are not required to be trained in first aid, and in most areas their vehicles do not have the essential equipment. For example, hospitals and ambulances seldom have radio communications with each other or with police.

Recognizing that emergency medical services are important in saving lives, especially of those injured in highway accidents, the U.S. Congress approved the Highway Safety Act of 1966 including a standard related to this area, the "Highway Safety Program Standard No. 11—Emergency Medical Services." [2] The intent of this standard is to assure that when a highway accident occurs every resource will be mobilized to save lives, lessen the severity of injuries, protect property, and restore normal traffic flow.

Specifically, the standard requires that each state, in cooperation with its local political subdivisions, is to have a program to ensure that persons involved in highway accidents receive prompt emergency medical care.

[2] "Highway Safety Program Standards." U.S. Dept. of Transportation, National Highway Safety Bureau, Washington, D.C.: Dec., 1968, pp. 18–19.

Each state is to have a program that shall provide the following as a minimum:

1. Training, licensing, and related requirements for ambulance and rescue vehicle drivers, attendants, operators, and dispatchers.
2. Requirements for types of and number of emergency vehicles, including equipment and supplies to be carried.
3. Requirements for the operation and coordination of ambulances and other emergency care systems.
4. First-aid training programs and refresher course for emergency service personnel, with the general public being encouraged to take first-aid courses.
5. Criteria for the use of two-way communication systems.
6. Procedures for summoning and dispatching aid.
7. Up-to-date, comprehensive plans for emergency medical services, including facilities and equipment, definition of areas of responsibility, agreements for mutual support and communication systems.
8. Program to be evaluated periodically by the state, with the National Highway Traffic Safety Administration being given a copy of the evaluation.

THE SCHOOL

The role of the school in the prevention of accidents and in caring for accident victims should be a major concern to each community. School personnel must be organized to handle emergency situations. All schools should have trained nurses or nurses' aides on hand to care for the victims of school accidents. If they are not available, it is of extreme importance that the school have several teachers or employees who have had first-aid training and will assume this responsibility. Quite likely at the elementary level the trained first-aid persons will be regular classroom teachers; however, at the junior and senior high levels they could well be the home economics teachers, the shop teachers, the physical education teachers, the athletic coaches, or others. It would be reasonable for this responsibility to be delegated to a teacher or several teachers by the school administrator.

In addition to trained personnel, each school needs a well-stocked, centrally located first-aid facility. Adequate supplies are necessary to take care of the many cuts, bruises, sprains, and other injuries sustained by schoolchildren. Each school should have a communications system that will permit instant contact with hospital and transportation personnel. Transportation should be planned for and available for immediate use in times of emergency. The school can be used to communicate emergency care plans, procedures, projects, etc., to the community. Schools should be an integral part of any community action plan. Furthermore, because schools have facilities and equipment, they can serve as the training center for first-aiders. Principles upon which an emergency care program should be based are discussed in Chapter 3.

THE POLICE

Police departments across the nation are called upon to perform many different tasks. Taking care of gunshot wounds, burn victims, traffic victims, and drowned persons are among the many types of problems that police personnel are asked to handle as a normal part of a routine assignment. Organization and training to meet these emergency situations are vital to the success or failure of such assignments. To function during emergencies police need to be tied into a communications system that permits contact with hospital and ambulance services. Training that prepares policemen to use first-aid techniques and procedures and emergency equipment should be an integral part of their preparation.

EMERGENCY CREWS

In many communities there are special units that have the responsibility for handling all community emergency situations where a life is at stake. Such crews are specially trained and have the finest equipment, supplies, and transportation vehicles available for local emergencies. The type of situations handled range from drowning incidences to traffic accidents, from fires to cave-ins, from heart attack to emergency childbirth.

Emergency crew members may be selected from the police or fire department, or be appointed as a part of the city's Civil Defense program. Still the emergency crew unit may be independent of these governmental agencies.

DISASTER PREPAREDNESS

The value of a community disaster preparedness program is discussed at length in Chapter 16. However, the emergency care aspect of such a program needs to be reemphasized. First-aid and rescue services can be provided by disaster preparedness units when no other group is available to serve a community. Usually disaster preparedness units have available much of the equipment necessary to serve the total emergency care needs of a community. Therefore, their services can be utilized with a minimum of difficulty.

FUNERAL DIRECTORS

A great many communities depend upon the local funeral directors for all emergency care services. The operators of such businesses have usually been cooperative in providing such services, although many times it has taken money and effort for which they were not compensated, and the personnel asked to handle various situations for which they often are not trained to give the necessary aid to the injured person. As a result the aid provided has been nothing more than a "pick-up" service and a quick ride to the local hospital. If funeral directors are to continue with such service, they should have well-trained personnel (paraprofessionals who can render first aid and emergency care while en route to the hospital) and well-equipped ambulances.

INDUSTRY

Industry, with its large and small machinery, its hard surfaces, such as metal and concrete, its heating processes and its chemicals, is a constant source of accidents. Always, industries must have an emergency plan in force. A doctor and nurse, employed full time or on call at all times, and an adequately supplied first-aid facility should be a part of this plan. Large industries in particular could provide emergency transportation for their employees. They might elect to do this for off-the-job emergencies as well as those on the job. A communications system with hospitals or emergency transportation is highly recommended. Many small industries without their own tranportation or doctor might find such a system essential.

Many industries require their employees to take first-aid courses, because first-aid-trained workers have fewer accidents. Industry accepts and promotes the concept that "individuals can develop a safety consciousness," and one of the ways to help develop this greater awareness is to give safety instruction, including first-aid training, to their employees. A first-aid and emergency care program for industry is a must for the well-being of all employees.

EVALUATING EMERGENCY CARE NEEDS

To determine the emergency care needs of a community some evaluative criteria are needed. Various groups have attempted to identify and define the needs of the community regarding training, equipment, and facilities. The "20-point checklist" depicted in Figure 25.1 can be used to help a community identify its needs and shortcomings relative to an adequate community emergency care program. A few of the criteria mentioned are (1) Hospital emergency departments open 24 hours a day throughout the year. (2) Ambulances available at any hour of any day of the year. (3) Citizens of the community trained in first aid. And (4) enough nurses regularly assigned to give immediate care to urgent cases without delaying attention to other cases.

Evaluating Emergency Care Needs [395]

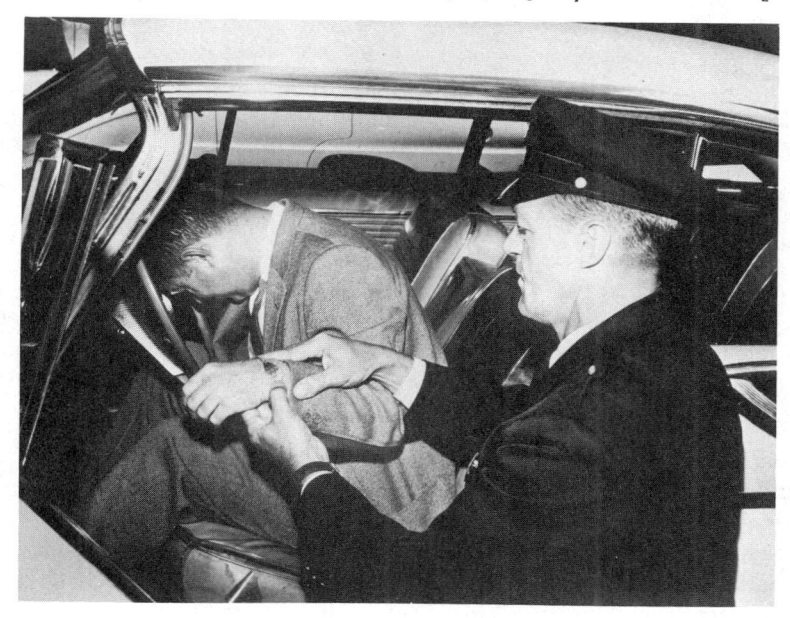

FIGURE 25.2 A Medic Alert bracelet helps to identify individual medical problems and suggested procedure to assist the person in times of emergency. (Medic Alert Foundation International)

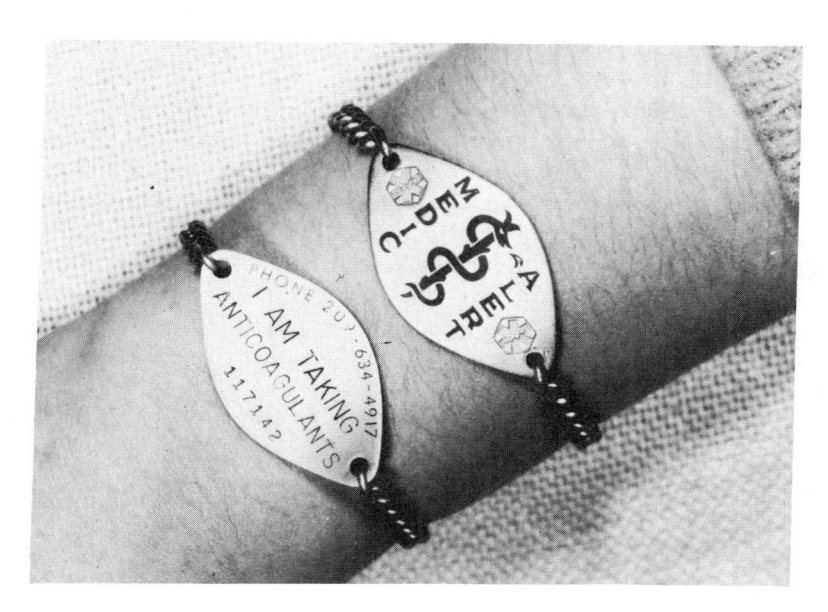

FIGURE 25.3 The two sides of the Medic Alert bracelet. (Medic Alert Foundation International)

MEDIC ALERT

Persons with health disorders who experience sudden attacks often lose their lives because rescuers do not know the victim's problem. One possible solution to this problem is suggested by the Medic Alert Foundation International, Turlock, California:

> This foundation is a charitable, nonprofit, tax-exempt organization whose main purpose is to educate and encourage all members of the population to wear on their person an indestructible and ordinarily inseparable means of identification of any medical problems that should be known in an emergency, and to encourage doctors and nurses to advise persons of the importance of wearing such identification.[3]

Numerous people are prone to conceal any medical problem that might label them as "abnormal" or "unusual." However, means of identifying their problem during times of emergency is necessary.

There are many conditions that could benefit from emergency first-aid protection or medical assistance. Among these are people suffering from diabetes, epilepsy, unusual blood type, allergy, arthritis, cardiovascular disorders, and hemophilia.[4] More than 200,000 persons wear Medic Alert emblems so that their problem can be easily identified.

AMBULANCE DESIGN AND EQUIPMENT

One of the primary concerns of various organizations is the standards for ambulances. There are many types of vehicles being used as ambulances, but most of them do not meet acceptable standards for ambulance design and have incomplete fixed equipment, carry inadequate supplies, and are manned by untrained personnel. The National Academy of Sciences–National Research Council Committee on Emergency Medical Services has enlisted the assistance of a great number of professional and lay persons to develop nationally acceptable standards for ambulance design and equipment. The following is a discussion of their recommendations.

The Ambulance

By definition, an ambulance is a

> vehicle that provides space for a driver, two attendants, and two litter patients, so positioned that at least one patient can be given intensive

---

[3] *Why Medic Alert?* Turlock, California: Medic Alert Foundation International, pp. 1–7.

[4] Ibid., pp. 1–7.

Ambulance Design and Equipment [397]

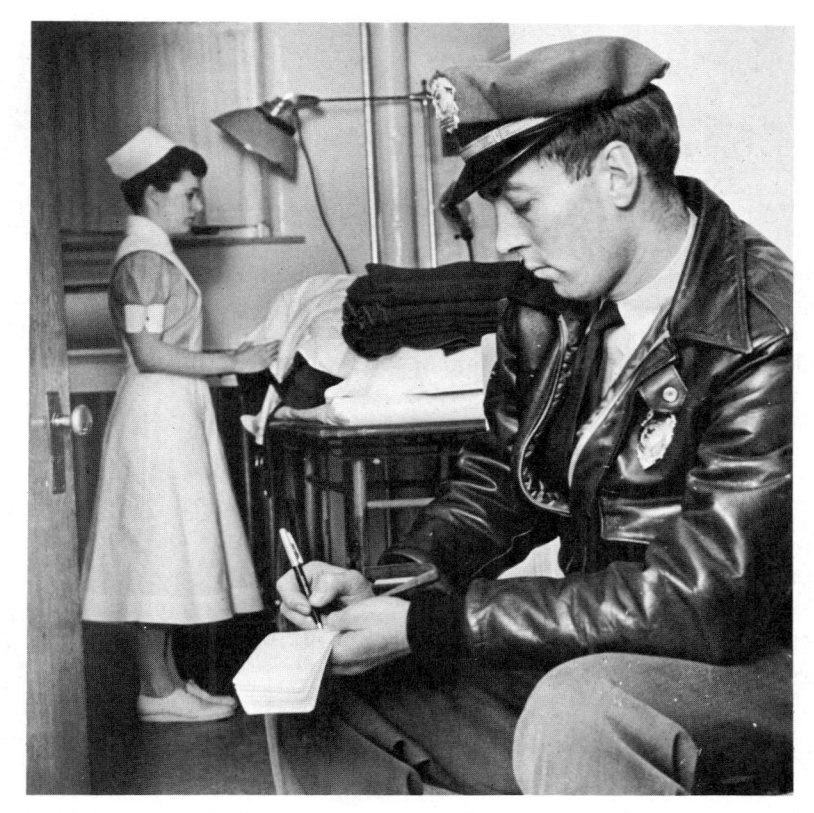

FIGURE 25.4 Well-trained personnel are essential to a community's emergency medical services program. (National Safety Council)

life-support during transit; carries equipment and supplies for two-way radio communication, for safeguarding personnel and patients under hazardous conditions, for light rescue procedures and for optimal emergency care outside the vehicle and during transport; and is designed and constructed to afford maximum safety and comfort and to avoid aggravation of the patient's condition, exposure to complications and threat to survival.[5]

General Safety Standards The ambulance must comply with motor-vehicle safety standards as may be issued by the U.S. Department of Transportation. Each vehicle should be identified by a nationally uniform color, signal, emblem, and flashing roof light. The vehicle should ride smoothly, gently, and comfortably while in transit. To protect occupants in the event of an accident collision, reinforcing bars should be in the sides and rear, and roll bars incorporated in the roof.

[5] National Academy of Sciences, *Medical Requirements for Ambulance Design and Equipment*. Washington, D.C.: The Academy, 1968, p. 7.

[398] Organizing Emergency Care Services

The Driver Area The driver area should be separated from the patient area to afford privacy for radio communication and to protect the driver from unruly patients. The area should include restraining devices, dash padding, collapsible steering wheel, and other safety devices as prescribed by the Department of Transportation.

The Patient Area This area must be large enough to accommodate two litters, two attendants, space for administering life-supporting care, and all equipment and supplies not carried in the driver area or on the outside of the vehicle. Litters should be secured with crash-stable fasteners. Supplies should be stored close to the attendant area for ready access. Both visual and voice communication between the patient area and the driver area should be provided.

Security and Rescue Equipment

Providing for the safety of patients and ambulance personnel at the scene of an accident requires equipment to direct and control traffic and bystanders, to isolate areas, and to remove victims from hazardous situations. Such equipment includes flares, reflectors, flashlights, floodlights with extension cords, a fire extinguisher, voice-amplification devices, gas masks, and disposable gauntlets.

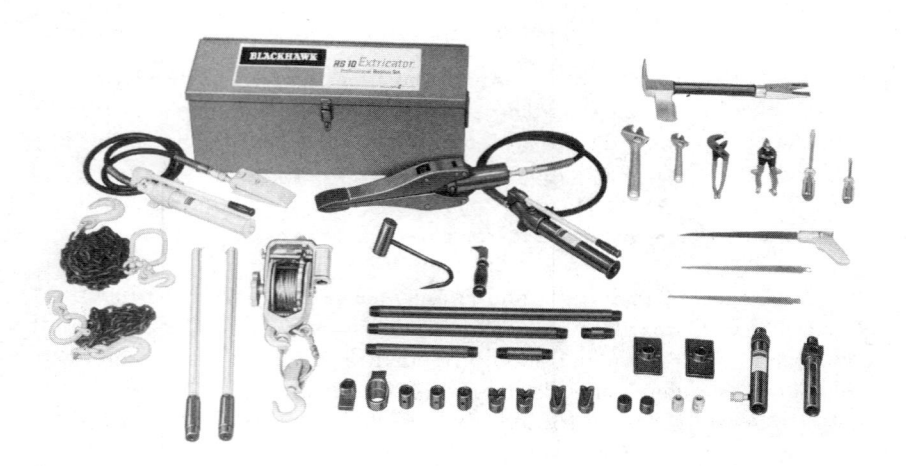

FIGURE 25.5 A display of extrication equipment, vital to saving traffic victim's lives. (Dyna-Med, Inc., Carlsbad, California)

Emergency Care Equipment and Supplies

In order to take care of the first-aid and emergency care problems, each ambulance needs to be designed with adequate space to accommodate necessary equipment and supplies. Each ambulance should be equipped with a wheeled litter, folding litter, and a collapsible device that enables attendants to carry a patient over stairways and in narrow spaces where a rigid litter cannot be used. In addition there needs to be artificial-ventilation devices such as airways, oxygen inhalation equipment, and appropriate suction equipment. A backboard for effective external cardiac compression and a supply of splints, bandages, and other accessories for immobilizing fractures or suspected injuries of the spine are also useful. Supplies for wounds include sterile gauze pads, roller and elastic bandages, all purpose dressings, tape, safety pins, and shears. Special supplies for handling shock patients include sterile intravenous agents, such as isotonic saline solution or dextran, and sterile disposable intravenous administration sets and injection kits (needles, catheters, syringes, antiseptic sponges, venous tourniquet, and tape). Dressings and towels for emergency childbirth should also be carried.

Snakebite kits are needed in areas where the hazard of snakebite exists. Also supplies for poison victims need to be among the basic supplies aboard the ambulance.

Additional equipment and supplies needed include blankets, pillows, sheets, tissues, emesis basin, urinal, bedpan, thermometer, aneroid blood-pressure manometer and cuff, stethoscope, drinking water, disposable cups, and sandbags. If it is anticipated that a physician or others with special training will ride in and use the equipment aboard the ambulance, wherever possible the following special-purpose equipment should be available: tracheal intubation kit, pleural decompression set, drug injection kit, tracheostomy kit, portable cardioscope/external defibrillator, and cardiac compression machine.[6]

ACTIVITIES

1. Make a study of the emergency care facilities of the community. Develop a report of the findings.
2. Organize an emergency care plan for a school, including all necessary equipment, supplies, facilities, and personnel.
3. Write to the U.S. Department of Transportation and request a copy of their standards for emergency medical services. Make an oral presentation of these standards in class.
4. Review daily the emergency accident problems reported in local

[6] National Academy of Sciences, ibid., pp. 16–21.

[400] Organizing Emergency Care Services

newspapers. Attempt to determine the strengths and weaknesses of the emergency care provided to each accident victim.
5 Write a paper on the subject "Emergency Medical Services Are a Valuable Asset to Every Community."

QUESTIONS TO ANSWER

1 Briefly discuss the role of the school in providing first aid and emergency care to all students.
2 Why is it necessary to have organized community care services? Discuss briefly.
3 Identify five major components of the National Highway Safety Standard Emergency Medical Services.
4 Identify four types of accident victims for which a police officer might need to provide first-aid protection.
5 A cave-in victim would most likely receive first-aid attention from (1) a policeman or (2) an emergency crew?
6 Develop a brief statement on the value of the Medic Alert concept of emergency care.
7 What are some of the important design features of an ambulance?
8 List ten evaluative criteria of a good community emergency medical care program.
9 Identify 15 pieces of equipment or supplies necessary for an ambulance to be considered well-equipped.
10 How may a Civil Defense unit fit into a community emergency medical care program? Briefly discuss.

SELECTED REFERENCES

AMERICAN ACADEMY OF ORTHOPAEDIC SURGEONS, COMMITTEE ON INJURIES, *Emergency Care and Transportation of the Sick and Injured*. Chicago: The Academy, 1971.

AMERICAN MUTUAL INSURANCE ALLIANCE, "Score Sheet for Community Emergency Medical Care." *Journal of American Insurance*, 1969.

BRENNAN, WILLIAM T., and LUDWIG, DONALD J., *Guide to Problems and Practices in First Aid and Emergency Care*, 3rd ed. Dubuque, Ia.: Wm. C. Brown Co., 1976.

ERVIN, LAURENCE W., *First Aid and Emergency Rescue*. Beverly Hills, Calif.: Glenco Press, 1970.

HENDERSON, JOHN, *Emergency Medical Guide*, 4th ed. New York: McGraw-Hill, 1978.

MAHONEY, ROBERT F., *Emergency and Disaster Nursing*, 2nd ed. New York: Macmillan, 1969.

MEDIC ALERT FOUNDATION INTERNATIONAL, *Why Medic Alert?* Turlock, Calif.: The Foundation.

NATIONAL ACADEMY OF SCIENCES, *Medical Requirements for Ambulance Design and Equipment.* Washington, D.C.: The Academy, 1968.

U.S. DEPARTMENT OF TRANSPORTATION, *Highway Safety Program Standards.* Washington, D.C.: National Highway Safety Bureau, 1968.

YOUNG, C. B., *First Aid for Emergencies Crews.* Springfield, Ill.: Charles C Thomas, 1965.

APPENDIX—
STATE-BY-STATE EMS SURVEY

Appendix

State	What are the minimum state requirements?	What is most recent law regulating ambulance services?	Are there minimum state requirements governing ambulances and equipment?	What are minimum state requirements for EMT/paramedical training?	Where are EMT/paramedic training sites?	What is EMT/paramedic course curriculum?
ALABAMA	Must be 18, high school graduate and complete ARC first aid course or equivalent.	EMS rules, regulations and standards amended 8/15/76. Regulates ambulance and personnel.	Yes	DOT courses. EMT, 81 hrs. EMT-II, 120 hrs.; Paramedic, 280 hrs.	Universities, hospitals, jr. colleges.	DOT outline.
ALASKA	None	None	No	None, regulations presently being drafted.	Community Colleges, Public Safety Academy, Southern Region EMS Council.	No current standard. DOT EMT-A is accepted standard course. Brady's Emergency Care.
ARIZONA	Valid driver's license, certified by state corporation commission.	General Order R-14-5-316 established personnel and equipment standards.	Yes	DOT standards for EMTs, 500 hrs. of training for paramedics.	Jr. colleges, universities, hospitals, and community colleges.	DOT curriculum.
ARKANSAS	EMT certified, no minimum age.	1977 legislation established vehicles standards, equipment and licensing.	Yes	DOT, slightly revised.	EMT trained at 45 vo-tech schools statewide; paramedics at four area hospitals.	DOT curriculum slightly revised.
CALIFORNIA	Must be EMT.	Title 17, Subchapter 12 effective 12/28/74 states general requirements and program approval.	Yes	EMTs must complete a 96-hr. course, including 10 hrs. of emergency room service. 80 hrs. of classroom. No state requirements for paramedics, governed by counties, but minimum 500 hrs.	EMTs are trained at community colleges, universities and high schools. Hospitals for paramedics.	EMTs follow DOT curriculum plus added state requirements. Paramedics adhere to DOT plus added county requirements.
COLORADO	No state requirements. Several state programs for training. Locals may choose from these for their jurisdiction (SB 454).	SB 454, HB 1119. SB 454 set minimum state standards for ambulance personnel training. HB 1119 — County commissioners may provide for ambulance in budget. Sets standards for ambulance.	SB 454 — ambulance must meet state vehicle code requirements. Have a minimum number of ALS — recommended equipment. County commissioner may make more stringent requirements.	No state requirements.	Hospitals, medical society.	DOT Draft curriculum. No information on texts.
CONNECTICUT	Two licensed EMTs for community services. One certified EMT and driver with CIM for private service.	1977 legislature adopted numerous laws that formalized bi-monthly meetings between coordinators and EMS office, extended the Good Samaritan Act to include those trained in CPR but unaffiliated with provider, and allow paramedics to administer IVs and defibrillate under doctors' orders.	Yes	Based on DOT requirements.	Hospitals, community colleges and providers.	DOT course curriculum.
DELAWARE	Ambulance attendant must be certified by the state fire prevention commission. Must recertify every 3 yrs. Complete the state fire school emergency care course.	Operation permit required by Title 16, Chapter 67, effective since 1972.	Minimum 1 valid certified ambulance attendant from state fire prevention commission.	Paramedic program consists of 400 hrs. of didactic and 320 hrs. of internship, totaling 720 hrs.	Wilmington Medical Center, School of EMTs/Paramedic Program.	Total 320 hrs. Texts include *Emergency Cardiac Care*, *Practical Electrocardiography* and *Rapid Interpretation of EKGs*.
DISTRICT OF COLUMBIA	Completion of DOT 81-hr. basic EMT course, 18 yrs. old, and good health and moral character.	Amendment of Good Samaritan Act to include EMT/paramedic and physician directing activities when providing ALS. Amendment of ambulance regulation to allow for training certification and functioning of EMT-Ps. Effective 7/8/77.	Yes	Certified EMT-A, successfully passed the National Registry Examination and sponsored and recommended by a local based ambulance company that provides MIC services.	Teaching hospitals approved by the DC Department of Human Resources.	15 module curriculum recommended by the DOT and DHEW. Text determined by course medical director and coordinator.
FLORIDA	EMT, State Certified CPR.	Paramedic certification in ALS.	Yes	81-hr. EMT DOT course; DOT course will most likely be established for paramedic program.	Vo-tech schools, jr colleges.	DOT regulations.
GEORGIA	18 yrs. old, 125-hr. DOT course, successfully complete didactic certification examination.	Senate Bill 99 defines training and duties of EMTs cardiac technicians, and advanced EMTs. Provides for recertification, and the standard performance of licensed ambulance services and emergency medical personnel. Effective 3/11/77.	Yes	Advanced EMT training requires DOT advanced course level training and certification via Georgia State Composite Board of Medical Examiners.	28 area vo-tech schools. Georgia State University, DeKalb Community College.	For EMTs — DOT 125-hr. basic EMT course. For cardiac technicians — similar to DOT cardiac module but somewhat more extensive. For advanced EMTs — generally DOT level courses or better.

[404]

State-by-State EMS Survey [405]

How can an EMT get paramedical training?	What qualifications must be met by an EMT instructor?	How often must EMTs/ pamedics be recertified or refreshed?	With which states do you have a reciprocity agreement?	Are functions that an EMT/paramedic performs outlined by law? Do they need physician guidance?	Are EMTs/paramedics protected against malpractice litigations?	Do state laws protect volunteers as well as paid personnel?	Are there any other laws pending in regard to EMS?
Apply to one of training institutions.	Must be either a doctor, nurse with 2 yrs. ER experience, or paramedic with 2 yrs. experience.	Beginning January, 1978; EMT-I must take refresher every 3 yrs. No recertification requirements for others.	None	May defibrillate, administer drugs, start IVs, etc., but only under guidance of physician.	Only the Good Samaritan Law.	Yes	None
Anchorage Community College, Fairbanks Memorial Hospital.	No specific state requirements.	Paramedic refresher will be required when regulations are completed.	None, there are no regulations.	CPR, administer drugs under oral supervision of physician, administer IV solutions by direction of doctor.	Yes, by statute from litigation. Good Samaritan Law covers those who provide care w/o compensation.	Good Samaritan Act covers volunteers.	Legislation will be sought in 1978 to define and certify levels of emergency care personnel with less training than the paramedics.
Apply to training institutions.	EMT/A practicing for 2 yrs., teach one course annually, pass instructors exam.	20-hour refresher course required every 2 yrs.	None	Yes, but must perform ALS by doctor guidance.	Good Samaritan Law.	Good Samaritan Law.	None
Must be affiliated with provider of ALS and apply to one of four hospitals with training program.	Trained in CPR, certified EMT, and complete EMS department's instructor course.	In 1979, will have to recertify every 2 yrs.	Any state with DOT course or equivalent providing applicant passes written and practical exam.	Yes, but ALS must have physician guidance.	No	Good Samaritan Act.	No
Apply to state directors.	Must be an RN or MD.	Recertification every 2 yrs.	Nevada and Oregon.	Yes. ALS requires physician guidance.	Paramedics are protected, EMTs are not.	Good Samaritan Act.	Woodward-Townsend Act extended the paramedic pilot program 2 yrs.
Private contract with agencies offering program.	Approval of EMT training center administration, course medical advisor and state health department.	No legislation as of yet, no legislation to even certify paramedics.	None	No state legislation.	No legislation for paramedics. EMTs are covered under state law.	No such laws.	None
Apply to trainers.	Certified EMT and completed instructor training program.	Paramedics must be recertified annually; EMTs, every 2 yrs.	New England states are formulating reciprocity program.	May defibrillate and start IVs by doctors' orders.	No	Good Samaritan Act.	New England states reciprocity program.
Send resume and application to Wilmington Medical Center, Paramedic Program Advisory Board, P.O. Box 1668, Wilmington, DE 19899 (tuition program).	Must be 21, have 5 yrs ambulance attendant fire I, II, III and basic rescue or vehicle rescue, 200 hrs. certified training, and successfully complete emergency care examination.	Not required by law, but recertify every 6 mos.	None	Not written into law, but require physician approval.	Yes, by Good Samaritan Law.	Yes	None
Members of the DC fire department who meet requirements of certification.	Certified EMT/As or medical professionals with teaching abilities. Courses and instructors are monitored by the EMS branch of the Department of Human Resources.	Annually	None	Yes. They may defibrillate, administer drugs, pass airways, apply MAST. Physician guidance provided by telemetry, radio communications and written protocol.	Good Samaritan Act.	Yes, however, no volunteer system.	None
Must be EMT with 1 yr. field experience.	DOT standards.	Yes, every 3 yrs.	None	ALS must be performed with physician guidance.	State Statute.	Good Samaritan Act.	None
DeKalb Community College, Georgia State University, Valdosta area vo-tech school; Dalton area vo-tech school; DeKalb County fire department, Clayton County fire department.	Generally advanced EMT, physician's assistant, RN, MD. All must have emergency ambulance or ER experience.	Yes, every 2 yrs.	Certified EMT with valid credentials may challenge Georgia test. A passing grade earns certification. Those failing may challenge after completing 60-hour refresher course.	Administer drugs, cardioversion, gastric suction by intubation for advanced EMT. Order of physician is universal, though protocols differ.	EMTs protected during training by state statute. No protection once on duty except by Good Samaritan Act if volunteering.	Yes	New rules and regulations being drafted covering more stringent requirements for EMT certification, vehicle specifications, equipment, communications system, decertification of EMTs, delicensing of ambulance services, and ambulance service record keeping.

State	What are the minimum state requirements?	What is most recent law regulating ambulance services?	Are there minimum state requirements governing ambulances and equipment?	What are minimum state requirements for EMT/paramedical training?	Where are EMT/paramedic training sites?	What is EMT/paramedic course curriculum?
HAWAII	2 EMTs aboard each ambulance.	Chapter 48 became effective on 7/1/76. It regulates both ambulance personnel and equipment.	Yes	State has no minimum. Presently must have completed 1,215 hrs. MIC training or 640 hrs. based on DOT curriculum.	By the State Department of Health.	Paramedic course curriculum is the DOT course plus an internship in Los Angeles. MIC course is structured with 4 mos. clinical training and 4 mos. internship.
IDAHO	All ambulance attendants must have 81-hr. DOT.	The Idaho EMS Act, which includes minimum standards for ambulance services, effective 7/1/77. Includes provisions to define the levels of EMS personnel, certification standard, minimum standards for ambulance services, and liability protection for life-support personnel.	Yes. The Idaho EMS Act includes uniform requirements for ambulance vehicles, ambulance equipment and personnel.	The State Board of Medicine adopted the DOT EMT/paramedic curriculum as the minimum standard of training.	The EMS Bureau of the State Department of Health & Welfare works with regional hospitals that provide clinical facilities for paramedic training.	The National DOT EMT/paramedic curriculum.
ILLINOIS	None, program is voluntary.	No	No	Completion of state approved training program, required field experience, prior EMT/A certification.	Area hospitals.	82-hr. Dunlap course. Texts include *Rapid Interpretation of EKGs*, *Practical Electrocardiography*, *Understanding Electrocardiography*, and *Respiratory Care*.
INDIANA	One EMT in patient compartment when transporting, one EMT at scene if ambulance responds.	P.L. 142 of 1975 authorized EMS commission to develop standards for certification of paramedics; P.L. 183 of 1977 authorizes development of certification standards for an intermediate level of care.	Same as DOT/NHTSA, except 48-inch minimum interior head room.	Successful completion of DOT EMT/P curriculum, as a minimum, approval by course director and passage of state exam.	Statewide network of hospital and vocational schools involving 32 agencies.	Utilize DOT EMT/P curriculum. Textbooks left to discretion of training institution.
IOWA	None	None	None	116-hr. course and 5 ambulance runs.	Area community colleges with physician involvement.	Expanded version of DOT curriculum.
KANSAS	Must have 81-hr. EMT training approved by the University of Kansas Medical Center.	1977 Senate Bill 56 amended ambulance attendant regulations to include RNs, MDs and MDs' assistants.	Yes, for those serving populations of more than 20,000. By 1980 all ambulances will be regulated.	EMT — 81-hr. DOT course. EMICT — 1,200 hrs. at the University of Kansas Medical Center.	Colleges, universities, jr. colleges for EMT; University of Kansas Medical Center for EMICT.	EMT — DOT curriculum. EMICT differs from DOT in that 80 percent of didactic program must be taught by MDs.
KENTUCKY	DOT course extended to 87 hrs.	Amendment to 902 KAR 20:115 effective 4/14/76. Amendment defines personnel, ambulance and equipment.	Yes	DOT course extended to 87 hrs. for EMT; DOT course for paramedic.	Hospitals, universities, medical schools, jr. colleges, state universities and vo-tech schools.	DOT curriculum.
LOUISIANA	Must hold first aid certificate or EMT certificate.	Act 626 of the 1977 Regular session, will redefine and revamp the EMS system effective 11/8/77.	Yes	18, high school diploma or equivalent, 81-hr. DOT course, member of an ambulance squad for a minimum 1 yr.	Tentatively at area hospitals.	Module DOT course guidelines.
MAINE	Minimum 15 yrs. old apprentice with Adv. ARC.	As of 1977 physicians' assistants may be considered ambulance attendants by virtue of their licenses.	Yes	EMT-DOT 81-hr. course; EMT advanced is based on DOT but coupled with additional state requirements.	EMT training at vo-tech schools. EMT advanced at hospitals.	DOT curriculum coupled with additional state formulated curriculum.
MARYLAND	Adv. ARC	Prehospital cardiac care law effective since 1976, provides for certification of paramedics from the board of medical examiners.	No	Minimum 81-hr. course for EMT, 140-hr. course for paramedic.	State Institute for Emergency Services thru hospitals, jr. colleges, and fire academies.	DOT curriculum
MASSACHUSETTS	Must be EMT with 81-hr. DOT course.	The 1973 Ambulance Laws and Regulations Act, adopted in 1975 established standards for EMT training and ambulances.	Yes	Presently no state program for paramedics. EMTs follow DOT guidelines.	Department of Health sponsored courses at universities, jr. colleges and hospitals	DOT curriculum.
MICHIGAN	ARC or equivalent.	Acts 288, 290, 330, P.A. 1976, as amended. Revamps the EMS system.	Yes	Successful completion of the EMT program. Other requirements as determined by the respective training center for admission.	Delta College, University Center; Madonna College, Livonia; Oakland Community College, Auburn Heights; Lansing Community College, Lansing; Grand Valley State Colleges, Allendale; St. Mary Hospital, Saginaw.	EMT must complete an expanded version of DOT curriculum totaling 120 hrs. EMT/A must meet 120 hrs. of field work plus 2 semesters at one of the approved colleges.
MINNESOTA	Adv. ARC	A 1977 amendment to Section 144.801 regulates ambulance services and licensing.	Yes	DOT regulations.	Community Colleges, hospitals, local EMS systems.	DOT curriculum.
MISSISSIPPI	18 yrs. old, completion of EMT training program, pass national registry exam, valid driver's license.	Section 41, Chapter 59 of the state code which redefines and revamps EMS system, effective 1976.	Yes, establishes minimum equipment standards.	Paramedic requirement not established. EMTs must be 18 and possess a valid driver's license.	Through the jr. college system.	Paramedic training being considered. DOT program.

How can an EMT get paramedical training?	What qualifications must be met by an EMT instructor?	How often must EMTs/pamedics be recertified or refreshed?	With which states do you have a reciprocity agreement?	Are functions that an EMT/paramedic performs outlined by law? Do they need physician guidance?	Are EMTs/paramedics protected against malpractice litigations?	Do state laws protect volunteers as well as paid personnel?	Are there any other laws pending in regard to EMS?
Available to personnel from the government and private sectors, but must be sponsored by service promising job at end of course.	No specific standards, usually MDs or RNs.	Recertify yearly after 40-hr. retraining.	None	Start IVs, administer basic emergency drugs, perform intubation. Rural islands do not have telemetry, paramedics have received adequate training to perform without physician approval.	Yes, by state statute.	Yes	Considering establishing paramedic minimums.
No regular course. City or county makes decision to initiate a community level ALS project, and then train the necessary personnel.	EMT instructor must be a physician. Overall course instructor must be at least an EMT-A with 2 yrs. field experience and completed the necessary Idaho EMS instructor course.	Yes, EMT/paramedic recertification is on annual basis.	No reciprocity with any other state. Must take Idaho tests for EMT/paramedic. Basic EMT will accept Washington and Oregon certification.	Fluid therapy, drug therapy, defibrillation, endotracheal intubation are sanctioned by law. State Board of Medicine requires all intensive care paramedic programs have biomedical telemetry. Local physicians establish protocols for specific procedures requiring telemetry.	Yes, by the Idaho EMS Act and the Idaho Paramedic Law.	Yes, there is no differentiation made in the law.	None
By applying to training institutions.	State employed EMS coordinator or approved on individual basis.	Every 2 yrs.	No formal agreement, discretion of project medical director.	Yes, but require telemetry for ALS.	No	Good Samaritan Act applies only to those volunteering.	None
Apply to one of the 32 hospitals or colleges.	State certified EMT, 1 yr. experience, attend commission approved workshop, teach at least one class a year.	EMT recertification every 3 yrs., 20 hrs. in service each of the first 2 yrs.; DOT refresher third year.	Equivalent training but must pass state exam.	Paramedic may perform defibrillation, endotracheal intubation, pareteral injections, EKGs, but require telemetry sanction, although occasionally may proceed without upon petition of provider medical director.	Yes, under Good Samaritan Law.	Yes	None
State has no established paramedic program.	EMT-A with instructional background in coordination with physician.	Annually EMTs must complete 9-hr. refresher course and basic life support.	Presently none.	No	No	Good Samaritan Act.	A total emergency service bill is being formulated to regulate personnel and equipment, establish paramedic program and outline responsibilities.
Apply to training institutions.	Must be certified by UK Medical Center and recertified annually.	Yes, annually.	None. Must take written and oral test if previous training approved.	Yes, must have system to provide guidance for ALS procedures but operate on standing orders.	Good Samaritan Act.	Yes	None
Apply to training institutions.	Must be an EMT recommended by an instructor, must assist an instructor for 6 mos. and must be approved by Department of Human Resources.	Yes, every 2 yrs.	None, if training approved may take exam on one shot basis; if fail, then must go through state training.	No, regulated by the state EMS training committee.	Yes, by state statute.	Good Samaritan Act.	Legislation to strengthen the entire EMS system.
Through the Bureau of EMS.	Currently re-evaluating these criteria.	Not at present time.	Not at present time.	Yes, under DOT guidelines.	By state statute.	Yes	None
Must be affiliated with some service providing ALS.	Must be an EMT and approved by the vo-tech school and the state EMS department.	EMT every 3 yrs.; EMT advanced every 2 yrs.	New England states.	No. Under advanced rules and regulations of the Department of Human Services. Physician guidance preferred for ALS but operate on standing orders.	No	Good Samaritan Act.	Establishing rules and regulations for ambulance equipment.
Selected thru ambulance companies.	Cardiac rescue technician, hold current certification as instructor.	EMT every 3 yrs., paramedics yearly.	Accept NREMTs. Paramedics are reviewed on individual basis	Administer drugs, defibrillate, start IVs. All procedures are physician directed, with allowance for standing orders.	Good Samaritan Law.	Yes	None
An EMT cannot get paramedical training until such a program is established.	NREMT, 1 yr. field experience, registered CPR instructor, and serve as an instructor intern for 50 hrs.	EMTs must be recertified every 2 yrs.	New England states.	No. ALS prohibited by lack of paramedic program.	Good Samaritan Act.	Yes	The First Responder Law of 1974 regulates the training of emergency personnel beginning July 1978. Amendment to Good Samaritan Law would specifically include EMTs and private individuals trained in CPR.
By applying to the colleges.	Must be licensed MD, RN, paramedic, approved by the department of public health.	Recertification every 2 yrs. by completing continuing education program and by passing a written and practical examination.	One who meets training requirements would be eligible to take state exam. If training not equivalent, must successfully complete an EMT/A refresher program and then pass examination.	Yes, may perform CPR, airway and gastric intubation, defibrillation, start IVs, and administer drugs. Telemetry required to administer cardiac related drugs.	Yes, by state legislation.	Yes	Yes; an act regulating ambulance services, Act 330, P.A. 1976.
The 916 Vo-tech institute and Mankato State University offer courses open to the public. St. Paul-Ramsey Hospital and Hennepin County Medical Center have private courses. Inver Hills offers paramedic courses for credit.	81-hr. emergency care course.	EMTs must be recertified every 2 yrs., no established rule for paramedics.	All NREMTs, not yet established for paramedics.	Yes, as outlined in the state credential process. No statewide paramedic bill.	Good Samaritan Law.	Yes	None
No paramedic training program.	Teachers of adult education.	No	None	EMTs, No; Paramedics, when instituted will be allowed to administer parenteral medications under supervision of MD or RN.	EMTs are covered by state statute.	Yes	None

State	What are the minimum state requirements?	What is most recent law regulating ambulance services?	Are there minimum state requirements governing ambulances and equipment?	What are minimum state requirements for EMT/paramedical training?	Where are EMT/paramedic training sites?	What is EMT/paramedic course curriculum?
MISSOURI	State funded ambulance attendants must be EMT/As, private must be Red Cross first aid certified.	1974 law established standards for ambulance equipment and personnel.	Yes	291-hr. course.	Universities, jr. colleges and hospitals.	EMT/A is the DOT course curriculum.
MONTANA	Currently certified at the level of advanced ARC first aid or equivalent.	Definition of patient was redefined. "Patient" refers to the sick, injured, wounded or helpless.	Yes	List too extensive, contact EPN for information.	Approach to training has not been developed.	DOT standards.
NEBRASKA	EMT; or advanced first aid and CPR; or 5 yrs. experience and recommendation of a doctor.	L.B. 418 establishes ambulance requirements, licensing and certificate of competency for ambulance attendants effective 7/1/77.	Yes	EMT — DOT program; paramedic program currently being revamped.	EMTs trained at local fire stations, community colleges. Undetermined for paramedics, most likely Creighton University Medical School or thru hospitals.	DOT curriculum for EMTs; undetermined for paramedics, most likely based upon DOT.
NEVADA	Age 18, advanced first aid, good health and driving record, no felonies in previous 10 years, no drug/alcohol abuse, understand English.	Amendment changes advanced EMT/A regulations in operating ALS units. Also affects training certification and reciprocity. Effective since 1976.	Yes	EMT 81-hr. DOT course Paramedic 300-hr. didactic, 200-hr. clinical, 4 to 6 mos. observed field practice.	Courses state funded in local community for EMS responders. Advanced EMT restricted to employees of EMS providers. Open course at Clark County Community College.	EMT, AAOS curriculum. Paramedics, DOT curriculum.
NEW HAMPSHIRE	Advanced first aid and emergency care and CPR.	New Hampshire revised Statutes Annotated 151-B as established in 1971 and as amended in 1975 and 1977. This law declares policy for the state of New Hampshire and regulates the New Hampshire EMS Coordinating Board, EMS Districts, and ambulance service, ambulance vehicle and ambulance attendant licensure.	Accomplished through regulations issued under the authority of New Hampshire RSA 151-B.	High school diploma or equivalent with course work in chemistry and biology, age 18, current certification as a basic EMT, 1 year experience in field of emergency medicine, member of a provider service, completion of a pre-screening examination	New Hampshire Technical Institute, Concord, New Hampshire.	Text: Schmidt's Paramedical Dictionary; Emergency Medical Care; Handbook of Emergency Care and Rescue; Emergency Psychiatric Care; Emergency Cardiac Care; Introduction to Clinical Pharmacology.
NEW JERSEY	EMT/A or equivalent.	Highway Safety Act of 1971 set requirements for personnel and established equipment minimums.	No	EMT/A, certification with minimum grade of 80, 18, three references satisfactory psychological profile, high school graduate or equivalent.	All training under the state health department. Training at selected medical schools, community colleges and hospitals.	Original DOT curriculum, new DOT curriculum to be implemented.
NEW MEXICO	Adv. ARC or the 40-hr. DOT course. Refresher training course each year.	The Ambulance Standards Act of 1974 provided requirements for ambulance design, equipment and operation.	Yes	No minimum requirements for paramedic training. 81-hr. DOT course for EMTs.	University of New Mexico School of Medicine, Albuquerque, New Mexico, volunteer instructor program operating statewide.	The DOT 81-hr. EMT/A curriculum and the DOT paramedic curriculum.
NEW YORK	Commercial ambulances, and those of municipalities with populations larger than 1 million must have one EMT on board. No regulations for volunteer services or smaller municipalities.	Act 30 of the Public Health Laws established ambulance regulations and licensing.	Yes	DOT requirements.	Hospitals, universities colleges, jr. colleges.	DOT course curriculum.
NORTH CAROLINA	Must be a DOT certified EMT.	General Statute 130-233 establishing minimum standards for ambulance services. Effective since July, 1977.	Yes	DOT approved courses.	Local services, Guilford Technical Institute, Western Carolina University.	DOT course curriculum.
NORTH DAKOTA	Standard Red Cross, First Aid, and Personal Safety.	None since 1973, mandates vehicle equipment.	Only on equipment, none on vehicle design.	No legislative requirements.	Local communities, wherever possible.	Text — Emergency Care and Transportation, Wonderful Human Machine.
OHIO	Must be 18, have a high school diploma or equivalent, valid driver's license, good health and character, and EMT certification.	Amended substitute House Bills 832 and Number 1 Second Special Session require that all new EMT/As and paramedics complete minimum requirements for training before they can function as such. Those who function in either capacity prior to 8/31/76, have until 8/31/78, to complete training requirements.	No, unless vehicle and equipment purchased with DOT funds.	An EMT/A must complete 196 additional hrs. of didactic and clinical training above the 90-hr. EMT course to receive paramedic certification.	EMT/As trained in technical and vocational schools and some EMS headquarters. Paramedics are trained through institutions accredited by the Ohio Board of Regents.	EMT/A course curriculum follows DOT guidelines. There is no standardized curriculum or text for paramedic training.
OKLAHOMA	None	May, 1977, legislation permits the health department to survey and categorize skills and equipment of all providers.	No	No formal state program. Requirements currently being defined, most likely will follow DOT regulations.	None	Not officially determined as yet, likely DOT.
OREGON	DOT standards.	ORS 485.500 amended requires district EMS committees to develop ambulance service districts and a plan for the need and coordination of ambulance service. Effective 7/1/77.	Yes	Paramedic instructor must have successfully completed paramedic course and been certified by Board of Medical Examiners.	University of Oregon Health Sciences Center.	Based on DOT standards.

How can an EMT get paramedical training?	What qualifications must be met by an EMT instructor?	How often must EMTs/paramedics be recertified or refreshed?	With which states do you have a reciprocity agreement?	Are functions that an EMT/paramedic performs outlined by law? Do they need physician guidance?	Are EMTs/paramedics protected against malpractice litigations?	Do state laws protect volunteers as well as paid personnel?	Are there any other laws pending in regard to EMS?
Write to training institutions.	EMT, teach a minimum of one course a yr.	Yes, every 3 yrs.	Any state that has equivalent standards.	Yes, physician guidance required for some life support procedures.	Yes	Yes	None
N/A	Approval of local course committee.	Every 2 yrs. for EMT/Advanced National Registrar Criteria. Applies to basic EMTs.	No states have been identified.	Yes, administer drugs and medication for which trained and certified. Requires voice contact or written standing orders.	No	Yes	None
EMTs apply to local rescue squads, paramedics to training institutions.	Must be an EMT and meet department of EMS approval.	Not mandated. Recommended every 2 yrs.	None. If training approved must pass state exam.	Yes, by state law paramedics will be allowed to start IVs, defibrillate, administer drugs under physician guidance.	Good Samaritan Act.	Yes	The Board of Advanced Emergency Care is currently formulating policy to govern paramedics.
Available only to employees of municipalities or private provider upgrading to ALS status.	EMT, or qualified professional with instructor training, CPR certified, monitored teaching, recommendation of regional EMS council.	Yes, every 2 yrs.	States with equivalent certification standards but must take Nevada exam.	EMT by regulations. Advanced EMT by law. Can administer drugs, start IVs, draw blood, perform needle aspiration of chest, administer airway intubation. Voice contact or telemetry allowed, but not mandated.	EMT and volunteer covered by Good Samaritan Act. Advanced EMTs thru insurance of provider.	Yes	Definition of emergency vehicle. Audible and visual warning systems.
New Hampshire Technical Institute, Concord, New Hampshire.	Currently NREMT, high school graduate or equivalent, 6 mos. ambulance or rescue experience.	Has not been determined.	New England states.	Currently in the process of being defined in regulations. Yes.	Yes, by the New Hampshire Good Samaritan Law.	Yes	The Medical Practice Act regulates physicians (N.H. RSA 329). The Nursing Practice Act regulates registered nurses. (N.H. RSA 326-B). Chapter 106 — Law of 1977 regulates paramedics.
By participating in an approved pilot program conducted by the hospitals.	EMT certification, complete instructor training thru state department of health, and instruct 2 EMT courses as a teacher's aide.	Not by law.	None for paramedics. For EMTs, must have completed the 81-hr. DOT course with verification from the appropriate state agency.	Yes, can administer drugs but in ALS areas, need telemetry approval.	Yes, during the pilot program.	Yes	None
By applying to the University of New Mexico School of Medicine. The Academy of EMS, 2701 Frontier Place, NE Building 3-A, Albuquerque, NM 87131.	Attend an EMT instructor course conducted by the University of New Mexico School of Medicine.	EMT refresher training is required by law yearly. There is no requirement for paramedical recertification.	From all states.	No, not addressed by statute.	No	Yes	Yes, an EMS Act to establish a comprehensive EMS program in the department of health and environment.
Must be part of a system offering ALS.	DOT standards.	Yes, every 3 yrs.	Reciprocity with Pennsylvania; will accept any DOT trained.	Any functions above EMTs' must be performed under MD guidance.	State Statute.	Good Samaritan Act.	None
Local hospital and education institution.	Determined locally.	Every 2 yrs.	Must meet DOT curriculum and pass state exam.	Yes, outlined in rules and regulations. ALS requires telemetry.	No	Yes	None
United Hospital in Grand Forks.	Physician	No	All states if proof of certification is established equivalent to National Registry.	No	No	N/A to EMTs but pertains to all attendants, volunteered or paid.	39-0804.1 — shall not be held liable if acting in good faith.
Apply at training institutions.	5 yrs. experience as EMT/A, attended one instructor conference each yr., instruct two classes per yr., pass interview committee, complete minimum 99-hr. instructor course.	Recertification for both EMT/A and paramedics every 3 yrs. Paramedics must obtain 153 hrs. of continuing education every 3 yrs.	Only those who have set up residence in Ohio and completed a DOT approved EMT/A course and meet National Registry of EMTs requirements.	Governed by DOT guidelines.	Yes, by state statute.	Yes	None
No official training sites established.	No official standards determined.	No recertification since no state recognized program.	None	No	No	Good Samaritan Act	The Technical Medical Direction Committee, recently authorized by state legislature to do so, is in the process of defining and establishing an EMS system.
Apply to: VOHSC; 3181 SW Sam Jackson Park Rd., Portland, OR 97201. Attention Paramedic Coordinator.	Recommendation by local EMS committee based on EMS experience, teaching experience and skills, and completion of EMS instructor workshop.	Yes — 40 hrs. refresher training every 2 yrs. with recertification.	Reciprocity arrangements are not yet worked out on paramedic level. EMT — Reciprocity with any state using 81-hr. DOT EMT-I course of basic level.	Defibrillation, intubation, various drugs on written or oral authorization. No.	Protected under common law of any negligence suit.	Yes	N/A

State	What are the minimum state requirements?	What is most recent law regulating ambulance services?	Are there minimum state requirements governing ambulances and equipment?	What are minimum state requirements for EMT/paramedical training?	Where are EMT/paramedic training sites?	What is EMT/paramedic course curriculum?
PENNSYLVANIA	No minimum state requirements.	None	None	No minimum state requirements. 81-hr. EMT DOT program, EMT/Paramedic program under U.S. DOT.	Hospitals, community colleges, vo-tech schools.	Curriculum of the U.S. DOT.
PUERTO RICO	First aid by department of health.	Ambulance Services Act 225, regulates the ambulance services.	Yes	Completion of department of health course, 18, high school diploma, and valid driver's license.	Department of health and the San Juan Community Technological Institute.	360-hr. course. Texts include *Emergency Care and Transportation of the Sick and Injured*.
RHODE ISLAND	18 yrs. of age. Completion of 81- hr. DOT approved EMT course.	Basic Ambulance Law, Paramedic Law.	Meet KKK-A-1822 standards and carry minimum equipment as recommended by American College of Surgeons.	Program approved by director of health. 75 hrs. classroom, 75 hrs. clinical and 100 hrs. OJT.	Rhode Island Jr. College for classroom instruction at one of five hospitals throughout the state.	Standard 81-hr. DOT training course.
SOUTH CAROLINA	Must be EMTs	Act 1118 of 1974 allows the SC Department of Health and Environmental Control, with the advice of the State EMS Advisory Council, to develop EMS standards and prescribe regulations governing ambulance services, vehicles and personnel.	State law authorizes the promulgation of regulations that mandate minimum standards for vehicles and equipment.	EMT — completion of first aid course, read, write and speak English, 18 yrs. old. Paramedic — Six mos. EMT experience, sponsorship by 2 physicians, recommendation by ambulance service provider, and screening exam.	EMTs are trained in technical education centers throughout the state. Paramedics are trained in regional hospitals.	EMT course curriculum is the DOT curriculum extended to 97 hrs. Paramedic course curriculum is the DOT curriculum at 425 hrs.
SOUTH DAKOTA	Must complete emergency care course approved by department of health.	Legislature currently revamping entire EMS system.	Only applicable to mechanical (brakes, lights, etc.) Sec. 34-11-7.	Presently being developed.	Being developed.	DOT Standards.
TENNESSEE	Basic EMT course, no felony convictions, 6 mos. emergency field experience, 18, and a valid driver's license.	Telecommunication act provides quality control over communications and frequency utilization.	Yes	EMT must pass 93-hr. course. EMT/A must be an EMT for 1 yr., member of NREMT, personal interview and letter of recommendation from employer which uses or plans to use telemetry, and completion of 480-hr. course.	Health services and schools approved by the Division of EMS, department of health.	Advanced course requires use of *Tabors Medical Dictionary*, *Rapid Interpretation of EKGs*, *Emergency Cardiac Care*, *Life Science for Health Technologies*, and *Drugs and Solutions*.
TEXAS	Yes	Vernon's Civil Statutes 4590B, SB 230 1943.	Yes	None	Colleges, jr. colleges.	—
UTAH	2 EMTs on all ambulance runs (industrial services excluded).	Utah Ambulance Control Act, 1973, as amended 1976. Rules and Regulations of the Utah Ambulance Control Act, 4/15/77. Provide minimum standards for control inspection and regulation of services, personnel and equipment.	Yes. Vehicle design and minimum equipment standards are clearly specified.	At least 480 hrs. of training and a satisfactory score on the state certification examination. Actual training standards include 6 wks. didactic, 6 wks. clinical, and 6 wks. internship.	Weber State College, Ogden, Utah.	Information not available.
VERMONT	Advanced first aid required but almost 100% have 1 EMT.	24-1969 Legislative Session, statute provides for political subdivision with responsibility of coordinating prehospital care.	No	EMTs must meet DOT standards. No paramedic program, only rural ALS which is based on DOT module.	At the ambulance district level.	DOT course curriculum.
VIRGINIA	ARC	Current rules and regulations governing ambulance services last amended in 1975.	Yes	18 yrs. old, certified EMT/A. Member of agency providing ALS.	Health department holds courses at local hospital.	Intermediate program called "Cardiac EMT" Paramedic program being established.
VIRGIN ISLANDS	18 yrs. old high school graduate, valid driver's license, National Registry as EMT-A.	Amendment to Good Samaritan Act (Pending). Ambulance Ordinance (Pending). GSA — to include REMTs and PAs. AO — to regulate ambulance services including personnel.	Pending	EMT — National Registry. Paramedic — under development.	EMT — department of health. Paramedic — under development.	EMT — DOT standard 81-hr., Emergency Care, Brady and/or EC & TSI, AAOS. Paramedic — under development.
WASHINGTON	EMT 81-hr. DOT Program.	ALS Training (paramedic) under the state medical practices act. Definitions & guidelines for certifying 3 levels of ALS personnel.	Chapter 18.73, Revised Codes of Washington.	EMT 81-hr. DOT curriculum; paramedic — 3 levels, based on DOT paramedic training curriculum.	EMT — 23 community colleges. Paramedics — University of Washington, Central Washington State College, jr. colleges and hospitals.	Course outline DOT program.
WEST VIRGINIA	Advanced first aid as certified by the department of health.	HB 705. Attendant in patient compartment during transport Effective since 1974.	No	82-hr. EMT course. 100-hrs. MICP course.	Emergency hospitals, vocational schools, colleges, all supervised by the health department.	EMT text, AAOS and Brady.
WISCONSIN	18 yrs. old, good moral character, physically and emotionally capable of performing the required task and be a certified EMT.	Assembly Substitute Amendment 2 to the 1977 Assembly Bill 447 sets requirements for ambulance attendants and equipment.	Yes	Complete a course of instruction prescribed by the department of health.	Universities, colleges, hospitals, jr. colleges.	Based on DOT but own program.
WYOMING	Effective 1/1/78, ambulance attendants must be certified by the state of EMTs or similarly qualified.	EMS Act of 1977 revamps system.	Yes, effective 1/1/78 through the "EMS Act of 1977."	To be established 1/1/78, will mandate minimum qualifications for the student, medical director, sponsoring facility, and ambulance operator.	EMTs — through the health department, jr. colleges, universities, high schools. EMT-Adv. will most likely be through the health department at hospitals.	Effective 1/1/78, EMT-Advanced program will contain approximately nine of the full national paramedic modules.

How can an EMT get paramedical training?	What qualifications must be met by an EMT instructor?	How often must EMTs/paramedics be recertified or refreshed?	With which states do you have a reciprocity agreement?	Are functions that an EMT/paramedic performs outlined by law? Do they need physician guidance?	Are EMTs/paramedics protected against malpractice litigations?	Do state laws protect volunteers as well as paid personnel?	Are there any other laws pending in regard to EMS?
Contact a local EMS Council.	Physician coordinator chooses qualified EMTs to assist.	Not required by law. EMT certificate valid for 3 yrs., paramedic for 2 yrs.	No paramedics. EMTs from New York, Maryland, Virginia and West Virginia.	Yes. Can render pulmonary resuscitation, CPR, establish and maintain airways, perform defibrillation, administer pharyngeal intubation.	Good Samaritan Law.	Yes	Ambulance Licensure Bill pending. Amendment to Good Samaritan Law to provide protection when performing in the line of duty.
At the Puerto Rican Technological Institute of Emergency Medicine and thru the department of health.	None by law, but use only MDs and RNs.	None	None	May perform all life support systems without MD approval or telemetry.	By statute.	Yes	None
Apply to Rhode Island Dept. of Health, Division of EMS.	EMT instructors must have at least 10 years experience as an EMT and pass a special instructors examination.	EMTs are recertified every 3 yrs. by accumulating 100 points in a continuous education program. Paramedics recertified every 2 yrs. by completing 25-hr. refresher.	New England states.	EMT functions are not "spelled out." Paramedics may administer medications, defibrillation, cardioversions and gastric suction by intubation. Administer intravenous saline or glucose solutions. Yes	Yes, by state law.	Pertains to both volunteer and paid EMTs.	None
Paramedical training is provided on selective basis at various locations in the state. EMTs meeting minimum qualifications should contact state office of EMS for location and dates.	EMT for 1 yr., 21 yrs. old, completion of 16-hr. state evaluation course.	Recertification required every 2 yrs.	EMT — if completed 81-hr. course, will be permitted to take SC certification exam. Paramedic — Must submit curriculum outline and after review, is tested orally and in writing.	No. Certain functions require physician supervision.	No. Good Samaritan Act valid only when volunteering services.	Yes	None
Being developed.	Approval of EMS office.	20 hrs. during certification program.	Anyone completing DOT course.	Being adopted. Yes.	Yes, if present legislation passes.	Yes	Many being considered.
Contact the Division of EMS, Tennessee Department of Health.	Information not provided.	Yes, every 2 yrs.	None at present.	Administer drugs, start IVs, perform defibrillation, CPR, intubation. Doctor approval necessary for some functions.	Yes, by state statute.	Yes	None
Apply to institution or department of health resources.	—	Recertification every 2 yrs.	None	No	No	No	None
By direct application to Weber State College.	Must be an EMT with 1 yr. service, knowledge of working EMT subjects, 20-hr. instructor training program and recertification once a year.	Both EMT and paramedic recertification is required every 2 yrs.	None, we reserve the right to review credentials and give applicant a state examination.	Yes, parenteral medications, defibrillation drugs, IVs, intubation needle aspiration of the chest, surgical exposure of vein, phlebotomy, intracardiac puncture. EMTs may perform IVs under the direction of a physician. Definitive therapy requires voice contact or telemetered electrocardiogram monitored by a licensed physician or registered nurse.	Paramedics protected by statute. EMTs have no legal protection.	Yes, volunteers by Good Samaritan Law.	None
Can't. No paramedic program.	No requirements, usually MD or RN.	Recertify every 2 yrs.	Reciprocity with the New England States Council effective January 1.	ALS requires physician guidance.	No	Good Samaritan Act.	None
By being member of rescue squad that is preparing to offer ALS service.	Certified EMT — 5 yrs. ambulance experience, 40 hrs. instructor institute.	Every 2 yrs.	Individual must pass Virginia final examination if equivalent training.	Start IVs, defibrillate, administer drugs. Need physician approval for all ALS.	Good Samaritan Law.	Yes, if performing in good faith w/o compensation.	Proposed legislation being drafted for one EMT aboard each ambulance.
Through department of health. Must have 3 yrs. experience as IV EMT.	REMT-A, three classes as instructor aide, certification by instructor trainer.	EMT — yes, REMT standards plus 8 hrs. a month ER service. Paramedic — under development.	None at present. Plan to use National Standards.	EMT — basic life support. Paramedic — under development. Not applicable at this time.	Good Samaritan Act.	Yes	No other specific laws.
Direct contact with training agency.	Acknowledged skill and expertise in EMS. Previous teaching experience of EMS, certified EMT recognition by physician coordinator.	EMT — Every 3 yrs. paramedic — 2 yrs. with additional skill maintenance requirements.	EMT — Any state following DOT guidelines. Paramedic — determined on individual basis.	Included in DOT program. Physician option — not required by law.	Written into the law.	Yes	None
Be a West Virginia certified EMT, active on ambulance service or emergency squad with paramedic capability.	MD or RN with emergency care background.	EMT every 3 yrs. after 20-hr. refresher. MICP every 2 yrs. after 75 hrs. of continuing education.	Maryland, Pennsylvania, Virginia reciprocity for EMTs. Only Maryland for MICP.	Yes. Drugs can be administered, IV started, defibrillation. Some procedures require voice contact with MD.	Yes, by state legislation.	Yes	None
Submit an application to training institutes or contact health department.	Minimum certified EMT; each institution sets additional qualifications.	No	None	Advanced support therapy, by state law, requires physician guidance.	Yes, by state statute.	Yes	None
None at present. After 1/1/78 only through state sanctioned programs.	Must have served as local course coordinator for 3 complete programs, an active responder with an ambulance service for 3 yrs., nationally registered EMT	2 yrs. certification program.	None	EMT-Adv. should allow for intubation, some cardiac drugs and defibrillation. The full EMT/paramedic shall be consistent with course outlines.	Good Samaritan Act	Yes	None

INDEX

Abdominal thrust, 123, 124, 125
Abrasions, 71–72
Accident, defined, 31
Accident prevention. *See* Safety movement
Accident records and reporting, 44–45, 314
  school accidents, 314
  system, 44–45
Accidents, 3–19, 295, 300–310, 303, 304
  causes, 16–19
    energy cause theory, 18–19
    unsafe behavior, 17
    unsafe environment, 18
  costs, 3, 6, 300–301
  number of deaths and disabling injuries, 3
  off-the-job, 13, 15, 295, 301, 303, 304
  types, 6–7, 11, 13, 15–16
  motor-vehicle, 6–7
  public, 11
  school, 15–16
  work, 13, 15
    See also Farm accidents; Home accidents; Industrial accidents; Motor vehicle accidents; Office accidents; Public-recreational accidents; School accidents
Acclimatization, 138
Acid poisoning, 136, 137, 138, 153–56
  common acids, 153, 155
    list of, 154, 155
    protection, 155
    symptoms, 155
  eyes, emergency care, 137, 138, 156
  skin, emergency care, 137, 138, 156
Activated charcoal, use of, 152

Airway obstruction, foreign body, 121–26
  chest thrust, 126
  complete, 122–25
    conscious victim, 123
    victim losing consciousness, 123–24
    unconscious victim, 124–25
  partial, 122
  prevention, 122
  protection of
    infants and small children, 125
    obese victim, 126
    pregnant victim, 126
  symptoms, 122
Alcohol, and traffic accidents, 248–49, 274
Alcohol poisoning, 157, 159
Alkali poisoning, 136, 137, 138, 155–56
  common alkalis, 155
  eyes, emergency care, 137, 138, 156
  protection, 156
  skin, emergency care, 137, 138, 156
  symptoms, 156
Allergic reaction, 44, 64, 197, 208, 211, 214
  snake antivenin, 208
  stinging insects (Hymenoptera), 44, 64, 197, 211
    See also Hives; Poisonous plants, skin irritation
Ambulance program, 257–58
  See also Emergency care services, ambulance design and equipment *and* ambulance service
American Association for Health, Physical Education and Recreation (AAHPER), 30
American Driver and Traffic Safety Education Association (ADTSEA), 31

[413]

Index

American National Red Cross (ANRC), 29–30, 257, 355, 356
  Advanced course, 257
  Standard course, 257
American Society of Safety Engineers (ASSE), 30
Ammonia poisoning, 163
Anaphylactic shock, 95–96
Angina pectoris, 108
Anoxemia, 105
Apoplexy, 239–41
  little strokes, 239
  protection, 240–41
  symptoms, 240
Appendicitis, 245–47
Arachnids. See Poisonous bites and stings
Arsenic poisoning, 160
Arterial bleeding, 81–83
  control of, 81–83
  by tourniquet, 84–85
Artificial respiration, 105, 106
  recovery chances according to time lapse, 106
    See also Cardiopulmonary resuscitation
Artificial resuscitation, 106
  See also Cardiopulmonary resuscitation
Artificial ventilation, 109, 114, 127–28
  method, chest-pressure arm-lift, 127–28
    See also Cardiopulmonary resuscitation
Asphyxia, causes of, 63–64
  See also Respiratory arrest
Assumption of risk, 51
Atropine poisoning, 158
Aura, 244–45
Avulsions, 75

Bandaging material, 319
Bandaging techniques, 319–36
  anchoring the bandage, 320–21
  closed spiral turn, 321
  complete turn, 321
  figure-of-eight, 322–23
  four-tailed, 324
  open turn, 321
  recurrent turn of finger, 323–24
  spiral reverse, 324–26
  spiral turn, 321
  triangular bandage, 321–36
    ankle wrap, 335
    arm sling, 333–34
    ear and chin, 332
    elbow and knee, 331–32
    eye injury, 336
    forearm, 332
    fractured or dislocated jaw, 335
    hand and foot, 327–28
    head, 328–29
    hip and shoulder, 330–31
    material for, 326–27
    pressure bandage—hand, 334–35
    torso—chest and back, 329–30
    versatility of, 326
Barbiturates, poisoning by, 157
Belladonna poisoning, 158
Biological death, 113
Bites, poisonous. See Poisonous bites and stings
Bleeding, 43, 79–86
  arterial
    control of, 81–83
    and tourniquet, 84–85
  capillary, control of, 79
  internal, 79, 83–85
    symptoms, 83–84
  venous, control of, 80
  See also Hemorrhage
Body parts, injuries to. See Industrial accidents, parts of the body injured
Body temperature, methods of taking, 145
Boils, 86–87
Bone injuries. See Dislocations; Fractures
Boric acid and borates, poisoning by, 159
Botulism, 164
Brachial artery, 83
Breathing stoppage. See Asphyxia
Breathing system, 103–104, 105
  breathing or respiration, defined, 103
  inspiration, 104
  internal respiration, 103
  expiration, 104
  external respiration, 103–104
  oxygen need, 105
Bruises, 75–76
Burns, 44, 64, 130–37
  chemical, 136, 137
  first-degree, 131
  second-degree, 132
  third-degree, 133–34
  fourth-degree, 134
  number of deaths from, 130
  position of victim, 134
  principle for protection, 44, 64

Camphor poisoning, 159
Capillary bleeding, 79
Carbon monoxide poisoning, 106, 107, 110–11, 149, 161
  cause of asphyxia, 106, 107, 110–11, 149, 161
  precautions, 110–11
  protection, 161–62
  symptoms, 111, 161
Carbon tetrachloride poisoning, 162
  mentioned, 149

Index [415]

Carbuncles, 86-87
Cardiac arrest, 107-12
  angina pectoris, 108
  causes, 108
  definition, 107
  heart attack, 108-109
    protection, 109
    symptoms of, 108-109
  problems, 110-12
    carbon monoxide, 110-11
    compression, 112
    drugs, 111-12
    electricity, 112
    hanging, 111
    gases, 111
  results of, 107
  symptoms of, 109-10
Cardiopulmonary resuscitation (CPR), 103-128
  certification and training, 103
  need to up-date, 103
  procedure, 113-21
    ABC steps of, 113
    one first-aider, 113-18
    two first-aiders, 118-19
    infant, 119-21
    options, 114-18
Cardiovascular drugs, poisoning by, 158
Cardiovascular system, 105-106
  definition, 105
  functions of, 105
Carotid artery, 82
Castor bean poisoning, 225, 227
Certification, CPR, 103
Chemical burns, 136, 137, 138
  See also Poisons, corrosive
Chemical poisoning. See Poisoning, drugs and chemicals
Chemical warfare gases, 163
Chest-pressure arm-lift, 127-28
Chest thrust, 126
Chiggers, 197, 210-11
Circulatory system. See Cardiovascular system
Civil defense. See Disaster Preparedness and Civil Defense
Civil Defense, 254, 255, 256, 257, 386
  name change, 254
  See also Defense Civil Preparedness Agency
Clinical death, 113
Cole, W. H., and C. B. Puestow, 175, 177
Colorado tick fever, 210
Community emergency medical care, score sheet, 390
Concussion, 241-42
Contusions (bruises), 75-76
Convulsions, 242-43
Cursory check of injured at scene of accident, 65-67
  rules to follow during and after check, 68
Cyanide poisoning, 161

Dalrymple, Byron W., 209
Defense Civil Preparedness Agency (DCPA), 254-60
  administered by, 254
  disaster shelter, 255-56
  disaster supplies, 258-59
  disaster volunteer, 256-57
  disaster warning signals, 260
    attack warning signal, 260
    attention or alert signal, 260
  purpose, 254, 255
  radiological monitors, 258
Depressant drugs, poisoning by, 157
Diabetes, 98-100
  coma, 100
    protection, 100
    symptoms, 100
  insulin shock, 98, 99-100
    protection, 99-100
    symptoms, 98, 99
Digitalis poisoning, 158
Disabling injury, defined, 31
Disaster preparedness, 254-60, 393
  community services, 393
  emergency care training, 257-58
    American National Red Cross courses, 257
    Ambulance Program, 257-58
    Emergency Medical Technician (EMT) course, 257
    Heliocopter Program, 258
    Trauma Program, 257-58
  problems relating to area, 254, 255
    man-made, 254
    acts of nature, 254
Disaster shelter, 386-87
  need for, 386
  supplies, 386-87
Disaster supplies, 258-59
  emergency care items, 258-59
  shelter equipment, 259
Disaster volunteer, 256-57
Disaster warning signals, 260
  attack, 260
  attention or alert, 260
Dislocations, 180-82
  protection, 181-82
  signs and symptoms, 181
Dislocations, specific, 181-82
  elbow, 182
  finger, 182
  knee, 182
  kneecap (patella), 182
  lower jaw, 181
  shoulder, 182

[416] Index

Dislocations, specific (cont.)
　thumb, 182
　　See also Dislocations
Drivers, age of, 271, 273
Drug overdose, 111
Drug poisoning. See Poisoning, drugs and chemicals
Duck Embryo Vaccine, 198

Electric shock, 96–98, 112
　causes and prevention, 96–97
　protection, 97–98, 112
　symptoms, 97
Emergency Cardiac Care (ECC), 103
Emergency care, 32, 61–68
　defined, 32
　hurry cases, 63–64
　at scene of accident, 61–68
　　cursory physical check, 65–66, 67
　　procedure after check, 67–68
　　See also Emergency care services; Emergency childbirth; First aid; First-aid principles; Psychological first aid
Emergency care services, 46, 389–99
　ambulance design and equipment, 396–99
　　ambulance, defined, 396–97
　　driver and patient areas, 398
　　equipment and supplies, 399
　　safety standards, 397
　　security and rescue equipment, 398
　ambulance service, 46
　community score sheet, 390
　disaster preparedness, 393
　emergency crews, 393
　evaluating needs of, 394
　funeral directors, 393–94
　highway safety program, 391–92
　industry, 394
　Medic Alert, 392
　need for, 46, 389
　police, 393
　school, 392
　　See also Defense Civil Preparedness Agency; Emergency Care Training
Emergency care training, 103, 257–58
　Ambulance Program, 257–58
　certification and training in CPR, 103
　Emergency Medical Technician (EMT), 257
　Heliocopter Program, 258
　Red Cross First Aid program, 257
　Trauma Program, 257
Emergency Medical Technician (EMT) course, 257
Emergency childbirth, 251, 252
Energy cause theory, 18–19
Epilepsy, 243–45, 289–90

Epsom salts, use of, 152
Eye, 44, 76–77, 137, 138, 156, 303, 336
　bandaging, 336
　corrosive acids and alkalis, emergency care, 137, 138, 156
　foreign body, 44, 76–77
　injury, frequency in work accidents and on the farm, 303

Facial artery, 82
Fainting, 95, 247–48
　causes, 95
　protection, 248
　symptoms, 248
Farm accidents, 7, 281–82, 304
　farm home, 7
　farm-home-related deaths and injuries, 281–82
　farm-related occupations, deaths and injuries, 304
　Occupational Safety and Health Administration, 7
Femoral artery, 83
Fever, 145, 146
　medication for reducing, 146
　methods of taking temperature, 145
Finger, 78, 182, 302, 303, 321–24, 342–43
　bandaging techniques, 321–24
　　figure-of-eight, 322–23
　　recurrent turn, 323–24
　　special turns, 321–23
　injuries, 78, 182
　　dislocation, 182
　　kinds of, 78
　　percent of injuries, 302
　splinting, 342–43
First aid, 32, 35–37
　defined, 32
　prevention of emergency care errors, 37
　reasons for, 35–37
　　See also Emergency care; Emergency care services; First-aid principles; Psychological first aid
First-aid principles, 37, 39–44
　general, 37, 39
　home, 42
　industrial, 42–43
　public accidents, 43–44
　school accidents, 40–41
　　administrative role, 41
　　teacher's role, 41
　traffic collisions, 39
First-aid supplies, 374–87
　disaster shelter, 386–87
　home and farm, 375–77
　improvised, 375
　location and care of, 374–75
　motor-vehicle first-aid kit, 379–82

Index [417]

recreational activities, 382–84
school, 377–79
work or industry, 385–86
Fishhook wounds, 78
Fixation splinting. *See* Splinting
Food poisoning caused by bacteria, 163–65
   botulism, 164
   prevention, 163–64
   protection, 164, 165
   salmonella, 164–65
   staphylococci, 165
   symptoms, 164, 165
   See also Poisonous plants, oral
Foreseeability, 51, 52
Fractures, closed (simple), 169–73
   defined, 169–70
   examples of cases, 171–73
      clavicle or collarbone, 172
      elbow, 172
      forearm and wrist, 171
      hand and foot, 172
      hip or pelvis, 173
      kneecap (patella), 172
      neck and back, 172–73
      ribs, 172
      skull and face, 173
      upper arm (humerus), upper leg (femur), 172
   kinds, of, 169–70
   protection, 171–73
   signs and symptoms, 171
   See also Fractures, open
Fractures, open (compound), 174–76
   defined, 174
   protection, 175–76
   signs and symptoms, 174–75
   types of, 174–75
   See also Fractures, closed
Frazier, Claude, 211
Frostbite, 140–41

Gas poisoning, 111, 156, 161–63, 280
   ammonia, 163
   carbon monoxide. *See* Carbon monoxide poisoning
   carbon tetrachloride, 149, 162
   chemical warfare, 163
   hydrogen sulfide, 162
   methane (marsh gas), 163
   number of deaths annually, 280
   petroleum distillates, 156, 162
      See also Petroleum products and distillate poisoning
   protection same for all kinds, 161–62
   symptoms vary for different gases, 111
Gastric distention, 126–27
   effects of, 126–27
   protection, 127

Gila monster, 197
Glass, Thomas G., 208
Good Samaritan laws, 55–56
Grand mal (epilepsy), 243–45, 289–90
Gunshot wounds, 77–78

Heart Association, 103
Heart attack, 108, 109
   symptoms of, 108–109
   See also Cardiac arrest
Heart resuscitation. *See* Cardiopulmonary resuscitation
Heat cramp, 142
Heat exhaustion (heat prostration), 142, 143
Heat fatigue, 142
Heat stroke, 141–42
Heat problems, 138, 139–45
   acclimatization, 138
   causes, 142–43
   frostbite, 140–41
   heat cramp, 142
   heat exhaustion (heat prostration), 142, 143
   heat fatigue, 142
   heat stroke, 141–42, 143
   hypothermia, 139
   muscle cramp, 142
   suggestions for protection against, 142–45
   sunstroke, 141–42
Heliocopter Program, 258
Hemorrhage, 64, 65, 79
   control by tourniquet, 84–85
   triangular bandage as tourniquet, 326
   See also Bleeding
Henderson, John, 83–84, 173, 179
Hernia (rupture), 249–50
Highway Safety Program Standards, 28, 61, 271, 391–92
Hives (urticaria), 250
Home accidents, 7, 42, 278–82
   adults, 281
   causes, 280
   children, 281
   cost, 7, 278
   farm, 7, 281–82
   first aid, 278–79
   general principles, 42
   types, 279–80
Hurry cases, 63–64
Hydrogen sulfide poisoning, 162
Hydrophobia. *See* Rabies
Hymenoptera (stinging insects), 44, 64, 197, 211
Hypothermia, 139

Idiopathic epilepsy, 244
Incised wounds, 72–74

[418] Index

Industrial accidents, 13, 15, 42–43, 294–304
  causes, 302
  cost, 13, 300–301
    lost time, 13, 301
  deaths and disabling injuries, number of, 13, 294, 295
    by types of industry, 295
  falls, 295
  farm-related occupations, deaths, and disabling injuries, 304
  first-aid principles, 42–43
  lifting, 297, 298–300
  Occupational Safety and Health Act, 13
  office accidents, 296, 297
  off-the-job accidents, 13, 15, 295, 301, 303, 304
  parts of the body injured, 302–303
    deaths and permanently disabling work injuries, number of, 302
    frequency of injury, 302–303
    severity of injury, 303
  See also Accidents
Infant CPR, 119–21
Infections, 72, 74–75, 78–79, 86–87
  boils, carbuncles, pimples, 86–87
  tetanus. *See* Tetanus infection
Insects, stinging (Hymenoptera), 44, 64, 197, 211
Insulin shock, 98, 99–100
Internal bleeding, 79, 83–84
Intoxication, 248–49
Iodine poisoning, 159
Iron poisoning, 158
Israel, Kenneth, 290

Joints, injuries to. *See* Sprains

Lacerations, 74
L-C technique (protection for scorpion sting), 209
Lead poisoning, 160
Legal responsibility, 52–55
  agencies, 53–54
    state agencies, 53
  homeowners, 55
  industries, 54
  physicians, 54–55
  police, 53
  school system and administrator, 52–53
  teacher, 53
  See also Liability, legal
Liability, legal, 49–52, 55–56
  basis for, 51–52
  definitions, basic, 50–51
  Good Samaritan laws, 55–56
  immunity laws, 52
  personal liability, 49–50
    application of protection concept, 50
    trends in, 49
  See also Muscle strain
Ligature-Cold Technique (protection for snakebite), 206–207
Litters. *See* Transporting the injured
Lizard (Gila monster), 197

Marsh gas (methane) poisoning, 163
Means, Bruce, 207, 208
Medic Alert Foundation International, 396
Methane (marsh gas) poisoning, 163
Methyl alcohol (wood alcohol) poisoning, 159
Migraine headache, 241
Mistletoe poisoning, 229–30
Mites. *See* Chiggers
Motorcycle accidents, 268, 270–71
Motor-vehicle accidents, 6–7, 248–49, 265–76
  age of drivers, 271, 273
  causes, 248–49
    alcohol, 248–49, 274
    violation of traffic laws, 274
  collisions, 6, 266, 268, 270
    involving animals, animal-drawn vehicles, streetcars, 270
    motor vehicle-bicycle, 268, 270
    motor vehicle-fixed object, 270
    between motor vehicles, 266, 268
    pedestrians, 266
    total number of collision accidents, 6, 266
  cost, 6
  death rate, 6–7
    by age range, 268
  growing problem, 265–66
  motorcycle accidents, 268, 270–71
  noncollision (overturning, running off roadway), 268
    causes, 268
    death rates, by age group, 268
  parts of the body most frequently injured, 269, 270
Muscle cramp, 142
Muscle strain, 179–80
  causes, 179
  protection, 180
  signs and symptoms, 180
  See also Lifting
Mushroom poisoning, 225, 227–29

Narcotics poisoning, 157
National Safety Council (NSC), 30
Negligence, 50, 51–52
  comparative, 52

Index [419]

contributory, 52
defined, 50
Negligent acts, 49
Nosebleed, 76

Occupational Safety and Health Act, 13
Occupational Safety and Health Administration, 7
Office accidents, 296, 297
Off-the-job accidents, 13, 15, 295, 301, 303, 304
Oleander poisoning, 230
Organizations behind the safety movement, 29–31

Parrish, Henry, 196, 197
Petit mal (epilepsy), 243–45, 289–90
Petroleum products and distillates, poisoning by, 156, 161, 162
   protection, 156, 161, 162
   symptoms, 156
Phosphorous poisoning, 160
Pimples, 86–87
Plant poisoning, 44
   See also Poisonous plants
Poison Control Centers, 46–47, 150–51
Poison ivy, 44, 214–24
   identification, 218–19
   prevention, 222–23
   protection, 44, 221–22
   toxic agent (urushiol), 217, 221
Poison oak, 44, 214, 217, 219–24
   identification (two types), 219–21
   prevention, 222–23
   protection, 44, 221–22
   toxic agent (urushiol), 217, 221
Poison sumac, 44, 217, 221–23, 226
   identification, 221
   prevention, 222–23
   protection, 44, 221–22
   toxic agent (urushiol), 217, 221
Poisoning, 64, 149–50, 279–80
   causes and modes of entry into the body, 149
   internal, 64
   prevention, 150
   See also Food poisoning; Gas poisoning; Poisoning, drugs and chemicals; Poisonous bites and stings; Poisonous plants; Poisons, corrosive; Poisons, noncorrosive
Poisoning, drugs and chemicals, 157–161
   alcohol poisoning, 157, 159
   arsenic, 160
   atropine, 158
   barbiturates, 157
   belladonna, 158
   boric acid and borates, 159

   camphor, 159
   carbon tetrachloride, 149, 162
   cardiovascular drugs, 158
   cyanide, 161
   depressant drugs, 157
   iodine, 159
   iron, 158
   lead, 160
   methyl alcohol (wood alcohol), 159
   narcotics, 157
   petroleum distillates, 162
     See also Petroleum products and distillates
   phosphorous, 160
   protection, 157
   same as for noncorrosive poisoning, 151–53
   sedatives, 157
   strychnine, 160
   See also Poisons, corrosive; Poisons, noncorrosive
Poisoning, gas. See Gas poisoning
Poisonous bites and stings, 44, 64, 196–211
   arachnids, 197, 208–11
     chiggers, 197, 210–11
     scorpions, 197, 209
     spiders, 197, 209–10
     ticks, 197, 210
   classification of venomous animals, 197, 208
     arachnids, 197, 208
     insects, 197
     mammals, 196, 197, 198
     reptiles, 197
   rabid animals, 196, 197, 198–200
   reptiles, 197, 200–208
     lizard (Gila monster), 197
     snakes. See Snakebites; Snakes, species and habitats in the U.S.
   stinging insects (Hymenoptera), 44, 64, 197, 211
     allergy problem, 197, 211
     prevention, 211
     protection, 44, 54, 211
Poisonous drugs and chemicals. See Poisoning, drugs and chemicals
Poisonous plants, 44, 214–33
   oral, 225–33, 234–35
     castor bean, 225
     common field, garden, and house plants, 231–32
     jewelry containing plant substances, 233
     mistletoe, 229–30
     mushrooms, 225, 227–29
     oleander, 230
   prevention, general, 233
   protection, general, 231
   skin irritation, 44, 214–24
     number of plants in the U.S., 214

Index

Poisonous plants (cont.)
   poison ivy. *See* Poison ivy
   poison oak. *See* Poison oak
   poison sumac. *See* Poison sumac
   prevention, 222–23
   protection, 44, 221, 222
   symptoms, 214
  summary list of, 234–35
Poisons, corrosive, 136, 137, 138, 153–56
  acids. *See* Acid poisoning
  alkalis. *See* Alkali poisoning
  eyes, emergency care, 137, 138, 156
  skin, emergency care, 137, 138, 156
  See also Poisons, noncorrosive
Poisons, noncorrosive, 151–53
  antidotes, 151–52
  protection, 151–52
    conscious victim, 151–52
      use of activated charcoal, 152
      use of epsom salts, 152
    convulsions, 153
    unconscious victim, 152–53
  See also Poisons, corrosive
Potthoff, Carl J., 84, 171, 238, 243
Pressure points for controlling arterial bleeding, 81–83
Protection, 32, 35–57
  concept of, 35–37
  defined, 32
Psychological first aid, 187–93
  principles, fundamental, 187–89
  reactions to emergencies, 189–92
    depressed reactions, 190–91
    individual panic, 190
    normal reactions, 189–90
    overactive responses, 191
    physical or bodily, 191–92
  suicidal tendencies, 192–93
Psychological shock, 95
Psychomotor (epilepsy), 243–45
Public accidental deaths, number of, 11, 284
  See also Public-recreational accidents
Public-recreational accidents, 11, 43–44, 284–91
  boating, 286–87, 288
  camping, 289
  causes, 291
  cold, excessive, 289
  deaths and disabling injuries, annually, 11, 43, 284–85
  drowning, 11, 285
  epilepsy, with relation to swimming, 289–90
  falls, 11, 285
  firearms, 11, 285
    deaths from, 285
  fire burns, 288
  first-aid principles, 43–44
  flying, 288
  heat, excessive, 289
  lightning, 289
  railroad, 11, 288
  safety training programs available, 291
  transport, 289
Puncture-type wounds, 74–75

Q fever, 210

Rabies, 196, 197, 198–200
  caused by, 198
  how transmitted, 197
  protections, 198–99, 200
  signs, 199
  statistics, 198
  vaccinations, 198–99
Rabies Immune Globulin, 199
Radiological monitors, 258
Records and accident-reporting, 44–45, 314
  school accidents, 314
  system of, 44–45
Recreational accidents. *See* Public-recreational accidents
Reptiles. *See* Poisonous bites and stings, reptiles; Snakebites; Snakes
Respiratory arrest, 106–107, 109–12
  artificial resuscitation, 106
  artificial ventilation, 109
  causes, 106, 108
  chances of recovery, 106
  problems, 110–12
    anaphylactic shock, 108
    carbon monoxide and other gases, 106, 110–11
    compression, 106, 112
    drowning, 106, 108
    drugs, 111–12
    electricity, 106, 108, 112
    hanging, 111
    strangulation, 108
    suffocation, 108
  situations resulting in, 107
  symptoms of, 107, 109–10
  See also Asphyxia
Respiratory resuscitation, 103–28
  See also Cardiopulmonary resuscitation; Artificial ventilation
Respiratory system. *See* Breathing system
Rocky Mountain spotted fever, 210
Rupture (hernia), 249–50

Safety, 22–23
  concept of, 23–25
    betterment of society, 24–25
    objectives, 25
    as a positive concept, 23–24

Index

risk acceptance, 24
defined, 32
emergency care, 25, 28
  defined, 25
  need for trained first-aiders, 25, 28
philosophy, 22–25
  See also Safety movement
Safety movement, organized, 28–31
  forces behind the movement, 28–29
  organization behind the movement, 29–31
Salicylate poisoning, 157–58
Salmonella, 164–65
School accidents, 15–16, 40, 41, 44–45, 306–314
  administrative and teacher's roles, 41
  college and university, 16, 308–309
  elementary and secondary schools, 16, 307–308
  first-aid principles, general, 40
  reporting, 44–45, 314
  student accident rates, boys and girls, 306–307, 311–12
  types of, elementary and secondary, 309–10, 313–14
Score sheet for community emergency medical care, 390
Scorpions, 197, 209
Sedative poisoning, 157
Shock, 90–100
  anaphylactic, 95–96
  electric. See Electric shock
  insulin, 98, 99–100
  psychological, 95
  traumatic, 90–94
Shulman, Dr. Alex, 131, 132
Skin infections, 86–87
Skin irritation by poisonous plants. See Poisonous plants, skin irritation
Snakebites, 196, 197, 201–208
  death of victims, statistics, 196, 197, 201–202
  methods, 206–208
  precautions against, 204, 205–206
  prevention, 204, 205
  protection, 64, 206, 207–208
  symptoms, 206
  See also Snakes
Snakes, species and habitats in the U.S., 202, 204
  See also Snakebites
Spiders, poisonous, 197, 209–10
Splinter and thorn wounds, 76, 78–79
Splinting, 326, 336, 338–52
  fixation, 338–49
    ankle, 343
    collarbone and shoulder, 340
    elbow joint, 342
    finger, 342–43
    kneecap (knee or patella), 344
    lower arm and wrist, 339
    lower leg (tibia and fibula), 343–44
    neck and back, 346–48
    pelvis or hip, 346
    rib injuries, 348–49
    upper arm (humerus), 340
    upper leg (femur), 344–45
  need for, in case of broken bones, dislocations, suspected fractures, 336–37
  traction, 349–52
    Thomas splint for arm and leg, 349–52
    triangular bandage for, 326
    wooden, improvised, for leg, 351–52
  See also Splinting material
Splinting material, 337–38
  improvised, 338
  purchased, 337
  self-made, 337–38
Sprains, 176–79
  defined, 176
  protection, 178–79
    at a distance from help, 179
    at school and at home, 178
  symptoms, 177
Stahnke, Herbert L., 206, 209
Staphylococci poisoning, 165
Stings, poisonous. See Poisonous bites and stings
Strain. See Muscle strain
Stroke. See Apoplexy
Strychnine poisoning, 160
Subclavian artery, 82–83
Suicidal tendencies, 192–93
Sunburn, 131
Sunstroke, 141–42
Symptomatic epilepsy, 244

Temperature, body, methods of taking, 145
Temperature problems. See Heat problems
Temporal artery, 82
Test of foreseeability, 52
Tetanus infection, 72, 74–75, 78–79, 87–88
  abrasions, 71–72
  fishhook wounds, 78
  puncture-type wounds, 74–75
  thorns and splinters, 76, 78–79
  prevention, 87–88
Thorn and splinter wounds, 76, 78–79
Ticks, 197, 210
  diseases spread by, 210
  protection, 210
Tort liability, 50–51
Tourniquet, 84–85, 326
  triangular bandage for, 326
  use of, 84–85

Index

Traction splinting. *See* Splinting
Traffic accidents. *See* Motor-vehicle accidents
Transporting the injured, 355–72
  by air, 371–72
  litters, 367–69
    army cot, 368
    army-type stretcher, 367
    blanket, 367
    jacket or hunting coat, 368
    platform, 369
    two-chair, 368
    two-sack, 368
  motor vehicle, 357, 371
  objectives for, 355
  one-man method, 357–59
    arm carry, 358–59
    blanket drag, 357
    fireman's carry, 358
    fireman's drag, 357–58
    piggyback, 359
    support and carry, 359
  two-man method, 359, 361
    chair carry, 361
    fore-and-aft carry, 361
    pack saddle (four hands), 361
    two-man support, 359
  three-man method, 363–65
    hammock carry, 363–65
    lift, one side, 363
  four-man method, 365–66
  six-man method, 367
  precautions and directions, 355–57
Trauma Program, 257–58
  Trauma Center, 257–58
  Emergency Medical Technician (EMT) course, 257–58
Traumatic shock, 90–94
Treatment, defined, 32
Triangular bandages. *See* Bandaging techniques, triangular bandages
Tularemia, 210

Unconsciousness, 95, 237–45, 247–49
  apoplexy, 239–41
    little strokes, 239
    protection, 240–41
    symptoms, 240
  causes, 237
  characteristics of causal factors, 238
    protection, 238
  concussion, 241–42
  convulsions, 242–43
  epilepsy, 243–45
  fainting, 95, 247–48
  intoxication, 248–49
Urticaria (hives), 250
Urushiol (toxic agent in plants), 217, 221

Venous bleeding, 80
Ventricular fibrillation, defined, 107

Warning signals, disaster, 260
Watt, Charles, 196, 207, 208
Wood alcohol (methyl alcohol) poisoning, 159
Work accidents. *See* Industrial accidents
Wounds, 44, 71–79
  avulsions, 75
  closed (contusions or bruises), 75–76
  minor, treatment of, 44
  open, 71–75
    abrasions, 71–72
    incisions, 72–74
    lacerations, 74
    punctures, 74–75
  special, 76–79
    eye, 76–77
    finger, 78
    fishhook, 78
    gunshot, 77–78
    nosebleed, 76
    thorns and splinters, 76, 78–79